AF775856

MANAGING PANDEMICS IN EARLY MODERN GERMANY

SPEKTRUM: Publications of the German Studies Association

Series editor: Birgit Tautz, Department of German, Bowdoin College

Published under the auspices of the German Studies Association, *Spektrum* offers current perspectives on culture, society, and political life in the German-speaking lands of central Europe—Austria, Switzerland, and the Federal Republic—from the late Middle Ages to the present day. Its titles and themes reflect the composition of the GSA and the work of its members within and across the disciplines to which they belong—literary criticism, history, cultural studies, political science, and anthropology.

Recent volumes:

Volume 34
Managing Pandemics in Early Modern Germany
Edited by Peter Hess

Volume 33
Agency and Author: German Literature Beyond the Bestseller List
Rachel J. Halverson and Benjamin D. Schaper

Volume 32
This Horrible Uncertainty: A German Woman Writes War, 1939–1948
Erika Quinn

Volume 31
Faith in War: Religion and the Military in Germany, c.1500–1650
Nikolas M. Funke

Volume 30
Religious Plurality at Princely Courts: Dynasty, Politics, and Confession in Central Europe, ca. 1555–1860
Edited by Benjamin Marschke, Daniel Riches, Alexander Schunka, and Sara Smart

Volume 29
Healing and Harm: Essays in Honor of Mary Lindemann
Edited by Erica Heinsen-Roach, Stephen Lazer, Benjamin Marschke, Jared Poley, and Daniel Riches

Volume 28
Former Neighbors, Future Allies?: German Studies and Ethnography in Dialogue
Edited by A. Dana Weber

Volume 27
The Origins of German Self-Cultivation: Bildung *and the Future of the Humanities*
Edited by Jennifer Ham, Ulrich Kinzel, and David Tse-Chien Pan

Volume 26
Invested Narratives: German Responses to Economic Crisis
Edited by Jill E. Twark

Volume 25
Football Nation: The Playing Fields of German Culture, History, and Society
Edited by Rebeccah Dawson, Baston Heinsohn, Oliver Knabe, and Alan McDougall

Volume 24
What Remains: Responses to the Legacy of Christa Wolf
Edited by Gerald A. Fetz and Patricia Herminghouse

For a full volume listing, please see the series page on our website: http://berghahnbooks.com/series/spektrum

Managing Pandemics in Early Modern Germany

Edited by

PETER HESS

berghahn
NEW YORK • OXFORD
www.berghahnbooks.com

First published in 2026 by
Berghahn Books
www.berghahnbooks.com

© 2026 Peter Hess

All rights reserved. Except for the quotation of short passages for the purposes of criticism and review, no part of this book may be reproduced in any form or by any means, electronic or mechanical, including photocopying, recording, or any information storage and retrieval system now known or to be invented, without written permission of the publisher.

Library of Congress Cataloging-in-Publication Data

A C.I.P. cataloging record is available from the Library of Congress
Library of Congress Cataloging in Publication Control Number: 2025045257

British Library Cataloguing in Publication Data

A catalogue record for this book is available from the British Library

EU GPSR Authorized Representative

LOGOS EUROPE, 9 rue Nicolas Poussin, 17000, LA ROCHELLE, France
Email: Contact@logoseurope.eu

ISBN 978-1-83695-425-5 hardback
ISBN 978-1-83695-426-2 epub
ISBN 978-1-83695-427-9 web pdf

https://doi.org/10.3167/9781836954255

∾ CONTENTS ∾

Part III. Broader Academic and Social Responses to Plague

~: ILLUSTRATIONS :~

Figures

Maps

Tables

Introduction

HANNAH MURPHY

Early modern German people were intimately involved with plague, which occurred with what seemed like divinely ordained frequency in cities and territories across Europe. In sixteenth-century Nuremberg alone, plague was officially recorded almost every eleven years.[1] Once a micro-generation, plague decimated the population—decimated in its original meaning, killing one in ten. That meant that with the exception of children who died young from other ailments or accidents, or those who were only temporarily resident in the city, every Nuremberger was a survivor of plague: in some cases they avoided contracting plague, in others they recovered from it. All those who survived knew someone who had died—collaborators and partners, neighbors and friends, kin and extended family, brothers, sisters, parents, husbands, wives, children. The relationships spared by one epidemic would be threatened again in the next. When it raged, plague disrupted all aspects of daily life, but when it was dormant it was equally and always latent in the fabric of the early modern everyday. In household provisions and storehouse cupboards, in carefully kept recipe books, and professional libraries, in daily practices and familial memory, in curated practices of hygiene, perfuming, and grooming, in talismans and devotional objects, in civic chronicles and built memorials, the materials of the household, the body, the city, and the land spoke to anxiety about the prevention of plague and the management of its outbreak.[2]

The scale of such death, loss, and destruction might seem almost unthinkable, but in fact it was rendered with acute numerical clarity. Starting in 1533, the city marked plague with new forms of recordkeeping. Nuremberg civic scribes began to keep tables which tallied the weekly deaths with forensic granularity. As the century progressed the city compared these numbers to previous epidemics and began to study their quantitative patterns.[3] Plague tables were not the only mechanisms of control deployed by the city. Plague pamphlets were another paper tool in the fight against plague. Written for the most part (though not exclusively) by municipal physicians, plague pamphlets were some of the most frequently published texts in the early modern period, particularly in the category of vernacular medicine. At their height, Carolin Porzelt estimates that up to six thousand copies of Nuremberg's plague ordinances and plague remedies circulated within the city.[4] As well as circulating advice and information, the Nuremberg council banned multiple products thought to potentially carry the plague, including used clothes and feather mattresses. They closed bathhouses and brothels. They issued decrees about burial times, and who could be exposed to dead bodies.[5] They safeguarded civic order by appointing experts and councilors to temporary positions of oversight, and safeguarded governance (i.e. themselves) mostly by fleeing to safer pastures.[6] They opened and closed plague hospitals and formed and dissolved temporary structures of oversight.[7] The relationship of these various strategies to the numbers of dead recorded in the plague tables was a matter of concern for sixteenth-century policy-makers, as well as historians today.

The contemporary preoccupation with counting as a coping strategy marks a moment where the intersection of recordkeeping, representational strategy, and the experience of pandemic intersected to critical affect. Much like the COVID-19 infographics, which occupied prime place on the front pages of newspapers until the deaths tapered off (but never ended) and their recordkeeping became a matter of rebuke and not management, Nuremberg's plague tables remind us of the aspirational and fictive nature of recordkeeping itself. Such representational strategies for management rehearsed entire disciplines of public health.[8] They carried with them the potential for new ways of thinking, but they also rendered invisible the individual experiences which undergirded them. Deaths in such numbers obscure the tragedies of individual loss: they allowed the city to go on and ultimately to forget. These recordkeeping practices and their relationship to the city's strategies pose important questions about the ways in which pandemics were recorded as narrative events with a beginning and an end. They remind us that the crafting of narrative about pandemics is itself central to public health, and that the supposedly liminal temporality of "the pandemic" is a core component of narrative strategy. Challenging and critiquing those narratives as historically situated and historically constructed allows us to see the continuing dynamics by which we are comforted, silenced, and "managed" today.

What is pandemic management? What does it mean for a pandemic to be "over"? Does the ending of a pandemic mean it has been managed? The essays in this volume address the management of pandemics in early modern Germany in broad strokes, as strategies enacted in times of crisis, policies of prevention, and diverse practices of governance which cohered around a particular claim: that the social experience of disease could (and should) be dependent on governance, or, to put it another way, that governance could (and should) trump nature. Unpacking the development of this thinking is no small thing. The essays gathered here cover a chronology spanning roughly the end of the fifteenth century through to the middle of the eighteenth century, showcasing important changes in these strategies, but also highlighting long continuities. The ubiquity of outbreaks of infectious disease, their intersections with large-scale historical processes and phenomena, the familiarities and discontinuities with modern public health, plus their occurrence in the midst of new forensic methods of recordkeeping serve to make early modern pandemic management a subject of compelling relevance.[9] The essays here offer lessons in the agency of societies and individuals in times of crisis, as well as insight into changing medical and moral understandings of disease, contagion, and bodily integrity. But before addressing their contents more directly, and reflecting on the lessons they offer, a few essential terms and concepts used in this volume deserve consideration, not least the term "pandemic" itself.

The *Dictionary of Epidemiology* defines an epidemic as "the occurrence in a community or region of cases of an illness, specific, health-related behavior, or other health-related events clearly in excess of normal expectancy," and pandemic as an especially widespread epidemic.[10] As a relatively new medical science, applying a definition derived from epidemiology to the early modern period is anachronistic. Neither disease, nor contagion, nor "health-related behavior" were understood or experienced in the same way in the early modern period. The German term used was *Seuche* or *Pest*, both of which could sometimes be conflated with plague, and like plague were also affixed to instances of pox, smallpox, leprosy, typhoid, flux, as well as their symptoms such as fever, buboes, diarrhea, etc.[11] For this reason, in her still-unsurpassed survey of early modern medicine, Mary Lindemann uses the term "pestilence" as the best descriptor for this encompassing phenomenon in the early modern era.[12] Recent collaborations between historians and geneticists have seen greater specificity brought to bear on the epidemiology of the early modern period, as well as a broader kind of evidentiary record available to historians, and there is much still be learned from this pursuit.[13] As a medical term, pestilence was remarkably capacious and pliant. It linked concepts of corruption and putrefaction, miasma and infection, allowing writers to layer seemingly discrete and sometimes incompatible medical ideas on top of each other.[14] It also transcended the medical. Pestilence, as scholarship on plague also notes, had both medical and moral connotations; it was understood not just as a disease, but as problem of social and moral order.[15] Plague management thus brought together the social, the religious, and the medical in profoundly exigent ways.

It is therefore important that the essays in this volume span a chronology in which important changes were taking place in each of these spheres. The well-known complexities of the Holy Roman Empire, with its proliferate territories, divergent structures of governance, and contested areas of jurisdiction and degrees of autonomy, created a unique situation for the structuring of responses to plague.[16] The essays in this volume take place in different political settings, from imperial free cities to absolutist principalities, and at very different moments in the early modern history of the empire. Considering what might appear at first glance as a set of temporal or political "tensions" is key, allowing us to disaggregate strategies of management across geography, chronology, and political context. This has particular implications for our understanding of the movement and appropriation of policies from place to place. Despite an emphasis on local authority during times of plague, edicts issued in one territory or principality were often circulated to and adopted by others.[17] Plague ordinances throw up the dynamics both by which local states, territories, and cities exercised and thought about their own independence and by which they made decisions in practice, often drawing on "best practice" and the innovations of their neighbors or rivals. As Nükhet Varlik's approach to plague in the Ottoman Empire observes, "a conceptualisation of disease along a set of relations in time and space can also expose social, political, and economic structures and inequalities."[18]

Such structures and inequalities, as well as the spatial management of plague, were shaped and framed by the confessional disputes which divided the lands of the Holy Roman Empire across new axes in the sixteenth century. Few areas of the printed landscape escaped these debates entirely, including medicine. Erik Heinrichs has shown both in this volume and in his monograph, the degree to which these plague pamphlets were mobilized as vehicles for confessionalization.[19] Luther's famous pamphlet on whether one could or should flee the deadly plague was just one example of the way in which religious authorities debated the appropriate responses to plague. But the ways in which Catholic and Protestant territories organized and thought about plague and pandemic management were also informed by confessional attitudes to charity and welfare, good works and penance, and the role of religious rituals.[20] Obvious examples are the role of pilgrimage and other devotional works which remained a resource for Catholics and were reconfigured in Protestant areas. Prayer was an intrinsic part of prevention, as were piety and good order. Sermons and the tools of liturgy and ritual were all mobilized to help manage the emotional vicissitudes of plague.[21] And in the confessional disputes, these forms and genres were equally vehicles for propaganda. In this sense plague and its management formed a strand of the religious repertoires of the later sixteenth century, to borrow a term coined by Kat Hill, and could be themselves a useful barometer of the relationship between confessional division and pragmatic political association.[22]

As the political and religious landscape of the Holy Roman Empire was in flux, so too was the landscape for medical practice. This was particularly evident in sixteenth-century civic spaces, as university-trained practicing physicians carved out protected roles for their authority.[23] Plague exposed the reach but also the limit of this "new order" of medicine.

Not only did it complicate the role of physicians, who were in theory required to attend plague victims, but who in practice often fled the city; it also created opportunities for other practitioners. Surgeons and barber-surgeons wrote plague texts and advertised their prowess as successful practitioners, but they simultaneously used plague to think through and theorize other aspects of their medical practice.[24] Midwives and nurses received extra pay and sometimes the opportunity to prescribe medical remedies. New positions were established during times of plague, including hospital personnel and cooks, but also ministers, grave-diggers, and porters who carried the dead from their place of death to the graveyards.[25] The question was how the measures and management of crises spilled over into the maintenance and dispersal of power and authority in times of good health. The links between pandemics and the creation of public health regimes have long been asserted.[26] More recently, some historians have argued that one outcome of the plague was the (slow) medicalization of disease management more broadly. As Paul Slack has observed, from 1665 there were fewer religious treatises on plague than there were medical treatises.[27] Andrew Wear demonstrated that even within such medical texts a lessening of religious sentiment can be clearly discerned.[28] While the overall framing of this shift as a secularizing phenomenon has received pushback, the link between the management of plague and a more assertive medical authority is generally accepted.[29] The essays here re-entangle medical, political, and religious forms of authority, showing how each discourse could serve the needs of local elites; but they equally do much to complicate any portrayal of a linear, or straightforward development of authority. This volume shows that pandemic management was crucial to the emergence of public health, but not as a faceless, people-less governmental force, nor still as a secularized body of medical theories, but, rather, as a highly contested, interpersonal set of debates between local and competing experts, played out in temporally specific and changing ways.

To be clear: this is not an origin story. As the robust literature on the Black Death in Europe and beyond comprehensively demonstrates, very few management strategies adopted in the early modern period were truly novel.[30] Plague texts, temporary quarantine, practices of fumigation, and the establishment of hospitals were all elements of management strategy which dated back to 1347, and in some cases even earlier.[31] No responsible early modernist, however tempted, can assert the sixteenth century as something dramatically new. At the same time, while resisting an overly positivist teleology, it is equally important to avoid a kind of ahistorical assertion of continuity or "ever-presentism" in pandemic management. The dynamics of continuity are frequently invoked in the study of epidemics.[32] But I do not feel that the justification for addressing pandemic management in early modern Germany lies in significant continuities between its experience and our present moment. Indeed, I suggest that it is precisely this veneer of continuity which demands critical attention and engagement. The recent (or ongoing) COVID-19 pandemic has offered us this challenge with renewed urgency, not least because it evidenced a collective desire to make sense of strangeness by assimilating it to past experience, particularly in the popular media landscape, which featured endless thinkpieces on the similarities between policies of isolation and early modern quarantine. These temporal collapses and contrivances mark another way of looking at the important dictum that "the distinctiveness of the plague is that it ultimately destroys all forms of distinctiveness."[33] But such a tendency runs the risk of naturalizing plague, of excusing deaths, of explaining away as inevitable what were highly preventable deaths occasioned and caused by public health policies, by equating commercial interests and corruption with limitations of the state and government, by accepting global inequities as unfortunate medical causalities.[34] As historians, but also as historically literate global citizens, we must resist this temptation. It is a historical imperative to consider temporality and disjuncture carefully, to denaturalize and think critically about causation, culpability, and agency, and to scrutinize the way in which narrative—historical narrative—has served to further or bolster the power of the state and the inequities of pandemic management. The essays in this volume elucidate highly idiosyncratic and complex case studies, all of which do work to disaggregate and think critically about the structures by which meanings around plague were made.

Contents

The first group of essays take plague texts as their primary provocation. Strategies for managing plague required first the successful recruitment or engagement of a general public. In Chapter 1 Christopher Hutchinson offers an illuminating example of how early plague writers sought to engage non-literate communities in literate texts. Focusing on three pamphlets in particular, by Hans Folz and Hieronymus Brunschwig, the chapter draws our attention to the dissonances within the texts which claimed to address the common man but provided costly recipes. Hutchinson provides a deep analysis of the oral and aural dimensions of text, with a focus on instruction for reading left by the writer themselves. Complicating a simple assumption that vernacular texts were intended for the "common man," Folz's verse format engaged a more aural dimension which explicitly addressed a non-learned audience, while his prose text was directed to more literate individual readers. Hieronymus Brunschwig, offered a tripartite set of remedies, including (as Hutchinson delightfully renders it) "some fancy ones for the lords, some middling ones for the townspeople, and some for the common people in the countryside who can't reach an apothecary." In considering the multilayered work that texts do to reflect (and create) inequality, Hutchinson offers insight into what medical historians have termed the "plurality" of medical practice, and a mode of interpretation applicable to source material that will recur throughout the volume.

Hans Folz appears again in the second chapter of the volume, by Peter Hess, which focuses on pandemic management as an ambivalent ethical challenge bracketed by the writings of this early author and the better-known Hans Sachs in 1563. The locus of Hess's focus is Nuremberg, a city which, as we have already seen, attempted numerous measures to combat pandemics. Nuremberg was famous for the unusual degree of control its patrician city council exercised, and its strategies during times of plague have often been interpreted (including by me) as evidence of this. However, through a careful reading of dozens of plague texts, including both consilia and ordinances, Hess unpicks any straightforward depiction of control. He reveals instead a deeply conflicted patrician council, caught between a desire to exercise authority, a moral obligation to provide care and discharge their duty, and a strong sense of self-preservation. Luther's well-known 1527 pamphlet on whether one can flee the deadly plague has meant that fleeing has taken on specific valences of confessional conformity in historiography, but this too was less straightforward than we might expect. In Nuremberg, local preachers Veit Dietrich, Wenzelaus Link, and Andreas Osiander all debated the issue carefully. Not only did patrician flight reinforce the entrenchment of inequalities between those who could afford to leave and those who had no recourse but to remain, it also acted as a spur to enshrine new forms of social control to replace the council's physical presence. The deep and extensive deliberation that went into these decisions is significant; they were not the knee-jerk reactions of self-preservation, but carefully and extensively justified. The moral framework created by these debates materialized in practical strategies, which in turn enshrined inequalities. Political control, rather than presence, duty, or obligation, thus became the moral answer to plague. As we shall see in later chapters, this would play out through the following centuries.

Chapter 3 by Erik Heinrichs addresses plague pamphlets in ducal Bavaria. Heinrichs has been a leading scholar in the study of this literature, demonstrating its decisive role in the Reformation as a material by which preachers, particularly Protestant writers, could think about embodiment, sin and salvation, and devotional practice. Here Heinrichs picks up the question of Catholicism and illustrates with great subtlety the ways in which mobilization of piety as a defense against plague could allow authors, writers, and even princes to push highly specific religious agendas. In sixteenth-century Bavaria, mainly Catholic but with significant tendencies amongst nobles to Protestant reform, the confessional nature of the pamphlets turned primarily on saints and their role in broader devotion. The authors Heinrichs traces were unusual, with attitudes shaped by theological beliefs but also by institutions and by (extremely) local altercations and rivalries. They were also reactionary—shaping their writing by dint of anxiety about the waning role of long-standing traditional practices.

Heinrichs' treatment of plague writing offers lessons in how to read ordinances and pamphlets more generally, demonstrating that pamphlets rarely reflected in an uncomplicated way the dominant attitudes or behaviors of the audiences for which they were intended. His concentration on Bavaria allows for disaggregation of the experiences of epidemics over the course of a century and shows how strategies even between epidemics only ten years apart could differ in ways that individuals found terrifyingly exigent, not just for their personal health but for religion, salvation, and the future of their communities as well.

The second group of essays turn to political strategies for managing pandemics. In Chapter 4 Mona O'Brien offers us an example of two city councils and their approach to French Pox in the earliest years of the disease, 1495–1510. Unlike plague, pox was recognized as a new disease, and in their responses, civic councils provide a good example of the way in which older measures could be rethought for new contexts. O'Brien's chapter is useful for contextualizing many of the other essays in this volume, since the timeline of her comparison takes place before confessionalization occurs. What is particularly compelling is that there were still clear differences between cities and their disease-management strategies, which cannot be explained away by religious differences. Here the critical importance of recordkeeping and the structures of the archive are once more to the fore. As O'Brien's reminds us, the written sources present the council operating with one voice, when in fact, the results could be arrived at after significant debate.

A very different political context is considered in Chapter 5 by Thomas Wozniak, whose intimate portrayal of civic devastation focuses on an extraordinary set of sources in late sixteenth-century Quedlinburg Abbey and its surrounding towns: tax registers on which scribes have noted the numbers of the dead. Unlike the purpose-drawn plague tables kept by Nuremberg, these were longer-standing forms of recordkeeping, amended in highly idiosyncratic ways. Crosses or annotations transformed one kind of record into another, a good analogy for the way in which plague politics more generally could overlay otherwise familiar-looking political decisions. As Wozniak observes, the records allow for a graphic (rather than simply numerical) representation of the dead, and close attention to the neighborhood, gender, age, and sometimes occupation of the dead allows for a detailed study of how waves of pandemics reshaped communities in profound ways. In the wake of population devastation, Quedlinburg turned to recuperative measures, creating new citizens, appointing guardians for bereaved children, and seeking to restore the health of society. As Wozniak argues, this was not just reactive, but evidence-based decision making, and the role of quantitative recordkeeping in producing political decisions should be seen a sign of the way in which futurity and strategy was itself codified within reaction to pandemics.

If plague was generally a crisis, what happened when it occurred in a time of catastrophe? In Chapter 6 Sigrun Haude offers a comparative study of plague in Munich and Nuremberg during the Thirty Years' War, when broader emergency drastically changed the parameters of pandemic experience. Haude's chapter assesses the cities' strategies for control, but also their limits in application, traced through records of violations. While governments threatened severe punishment for violations, not only did many citizens simply ignore the ordinances, in practice city councils often made exceptions for individuals or were more lenient in prosecuting violations of ordinances than the legislation might suggest. This was especially true for cases arising in the countryside. In Munich, Brigitta Millerin, for example, who lost her father to plague in 1634, sold some of his clothes and was duly reprimanded, but was not punished. Haude offers us ad hoc adaptability and decision making as a site of resilience, warning at the same time that ad hoc should not be confused with carelessness or indifference. These practices demonstrate a level of self-reflection and reflexiveness with which plague policy continually grappled.

Ulf Wendler, in Chapter 7, drills down on one of the most foundational practices to characterize pandemics across times and spaces, the practice of quarantine in the political entity most characteristic of the eighteenth century, the "absolutist" principality of Electoral Hanover, where quarantine served to delineate and articulate with granular precision the elector's political agenda. In forty-seven edicts issued over only seven years, the targets became, in gradual stages, the itinerant poor ("vagrants"), Jews (specifically "poor Jews," "Betteljuden," as opposed to the more limited category of "protected Jews," "vergeleitete Juden" or "Schutzjuden"), "dissolute craftsmen," and Roma. Broader eighteenth-century debates about quarantine are usually interpreted through the lens of trade and developing concepts of the free market, but here an alternative emphasis on control and moral order is revealed as an animating throughline from the patrician to the absolutist prince. The time-consuming and costly effort put into this—border checks every fifteen to twenty kilometers, manned by numerous bureaucrats as well as soldiers—shows how resources and emergency measures could be transformed into a mobilization of the power of the state. This was a level of political control which was not simply pragmatic or reactive, but, like the strategies studied by Peter Hess in Nuremberg almost two centuries earlier, was carefully crafted as a moral good in its own right. By revealing very different foci to inequality, Wendler shows how overt similitude of practices can sublimate the broader question of control, who wields it, and who falls victim to it.

Having explored the ad hoc, messy world of practice, and the critical throughline of control in which it resulted, the third section of this collection pivots again, addressing questions of theory in the broader context of scholarship, the nonhuman animal, and public health. In Chapter 8 Benjamin Wallura explores the variety of approaches to plague evident in the University of Helmstedt between academics from medicine, natural philosophy, and law, all of whom contributed dissertations and plague texts. Focusing on the period immediately following the Thirty Years' War, Wallura shows how "discourses of possibilities" were debated by local academics. Wallura's chapter reframes pragmatic decisions, flight, burial practices, personal health, and hygiene, not as well-established, still less inevitable strategies of plague management, but as profound intellectual quandaries to which a generation of local academics saw themselves offering meaningful contribution. His chapter therefore establishes a circular dialogue or dialectic with the political, practical decisions explored by the previous section. The continued vitality of these debates is important, not least because the end of the seventeenth century is more often interpreted as an era where the prevalence of plague began to wane.

Ansgar Schanbacher, Philip Knäble, and Malte de Vries remind us in Chapter 9 that epidemics were not experienced only by humans but also by animals, and that experiences of disease was an interspecies question. Animal epidemics or epizootics occurred on a roughly similar timeline to human epidemics: eleven outbreaks of Rinderpest, cattle-plague, foot and mouth disease, anthrax, rabies, or other highly contagious epizootics were recorded in the sixteenth century, and thirteen in the seventeenth century. Medical attention to these diseases became more formalized as the centuries progressed, while social authorities reacted with a variety of attempted solutions, many of which were similar to those deployed in "human" plague. The changes to the way in which animal plague was managed tracked developments on agriculture and husbandry more generally. This involved an emphasis on quarantine and "enclosure," with cattle in particular the subject of increasing "interior" dwellings in barns. While partly informed by confession, responses to the disease were also increasingly framed as a danger to the economy. While the shapes of this study echo other chapters here, the focus on the nonhuman animal reminds us that while we need to think critically about social and medical policy, we also need to be critical of the centrality and moral imperative of human agency within it. Even when the desire was to cure or treat nonhuman animals, their pain and suffering was too often a result.

The degree to which measures formulated around the crisis points of epidemics went on to structure the development of broader notions of public health remains one of the most formative questions in the history of pandemics. Martin Christ focuses in Chapter 10 on plague cemeteries as a site of pandemic management, and on the pandemic as a factor in the development of cultures of burial more generally. Using the case studies of Nuremberg and Munich in comparative context, he demonstrates that the ability of specific places to manage their epidemics also depended on contingent external factors. Nuremberg, for example, was able to speedily establish plague cemeteries, despite opposition from town clergy, because its well-known strong council held sway, while other cities saw a different balance of power. What were enacted as contingency measures created enduring change, since strong efforts to disassociate burial spaces from plague and dishonor gradually meant that what were once sites of "dishonorable" burial became the main sites of civic interment. Despite the relative absence of archaeological and archival records for smaller-scale cemeteries, there is evidence to suggest that small towns and villages also opened plague cemeteries, but that upon the passing of pandemics, these sometimes fell into disuse, or in rare cases were used to inter other liminal or marginal members of society: unbaptized infants, travelers, or Jewish people, for example. Fittingly, at the end of this collection, the temporalities of pestilence come once more into view. Debates about cemeteries and burial speak to the futurity of plague planning: to the expectations of magistrates and clerics alike for the future. The way in which these burial spaces dragged the plague into the literal foundations of the cities' dead is a good metaphor for how plague management as a historical phenomenon functions. We still carry it with us.

Conclusion

As Sigrun Haude reminds us, there are lessons to be learned here. For early modernists, these essays show clearly the centrality of pandemic management to normal social function—as Martin Christ puts it, "how important responses to outbreaks of disease are to understanding early modern society at large." Likewise, for historians of medicine and science asking broader questions about pandemics and the history of disease management, it should be clear that the early modern period offers valuable and specific insights into the way in which social authorities, medical practitioners, and individuals constructed narratives about morality and order, necessity and culpability, which allowed for the exercise of state control in increasingly restrictive ways.

Together, these essays make clear the duty of care ascribed to social authority during times of plague. They show the way in which plague and pandemics functioned as a testing ground for civic authority—they were a "demonstration of the councils' growing control over municipal healthcare systems and, indeed, their cities." But they also reveal the contingency at the heart of what is often regarded as a relentless paternalistic direction in the governances of German cities. Changes in regimes of order make a case for the temporal and cultural specificity of plague, which, like "carnival" saw a temporally limited suspension of the mechanisms of social life. Perhaps less like the world turned upside down, here the world was turned inside out, with minute degrees of stratification around new and contingent social professions. If control and order during times of plague subverted or restricted social freedoms, control and order after times of plague resulted in enduring inequalities. These challenge any self-satisfied notions of modernity. Plague regimes speak to the way in which reckoning with pandemic's own temporality—when it will pass and what wreckage and residue it will leave in its wake—is part of the challenge of managing it. What is it, then, to "manage" a pandemic? Is it to survive it? To protect those infected, or those not yet infected? Is it to ensure a quality of life for those who come after it? While attention to the way in which these pandemic managements produced social regimes of control is critical, it is equally important to remember to take seriously the gravity with which these questions were debated, and the deeply contingent circumstances through which they were enacted. In what civic governments and early modern people managed to effect and in what they failed to achieve—what they wrought, and what they won from these changes—we see the gauntlet of the early modern period laid down for us.

Hannah Murphy is Senior Lecturer in Early Modern History and Director of the Centre for Early Modern Studies at King's College London. Her first book, *A New Order of Medicine: The Rise of Physicians in Reformation Nuremberg*, was published in 2019 by the University of Pittsburgh Press and was the winner of the Society for Renaissance Studies 2020 Biennial Book Prize. In 2021 she was the recipient of a £1.4 million UK Research and Innovation Future Leaders' Fellowship for her current project, which examines the role of medical practitioners in the transatlantic slave trade.

Notes

1. Porzelt, *Die Pest in Nürnberg*.
2. For a recent account of these challenges in an Italian context see Henderson, *Florence under Siege*.
1. StadtArchiv Nürnberg, B/19, 480. See Murphy, *A New Order of Medicine*.
2. Porzelt, *Die Pest in Nürnberg*, 56–57.
3. Newhouse, "Outside the Walls."
4. Beer, *Eltern und Kinder*.
5. Mummenhof, *Die öffentliche Gesundheits- und Krankenpflege*.
6. This is better studied in the English context. See Slauter, "Write Up Your Dead"; McCormick, *Human Empire*.
7. The literature on plague is too great to adequately summarize, but for formative works on early modern Germany see Swan, *Negotiating the French Pox*; Feuerstein-Herz, *Gotts verhengnis*; Eckert, *The Structure of Plagues*; Ulbricht, *Die leidige Seuche*.

8. Byrne ed., *Encyclopedia of Pestilence*, vol. 1, 197–200. For historical reflections on definitions see Vögele et al., "Epidemics and Pandemics."
9. Arrizabalga et al., *The Great Pox*; Brenner, *Leprosy and Charity*; Demaitre, *Leprosy in Premodern Medicine*; Herlihy, *The Black Death*; Berco, *From Body to Community*; Stein, *Negotiating the French Pox*.
10. Lindemann, *Medicine and Society*, 51.
11. Monica Green lays out the importance of historical engagement with these developments. See M. Green, "The Four Black Deaths"; M. Green, "Plague (Yersinia pestis)."
12. Kinzelbach, "Infection, Contagion, and Public Health"; Dross, "Vergesellschaftung unter Ansteckenden," 198.
13. Burschel, *Die Erfindung der Reinheit*; also Douglas, *Purity and Danger*.
14. For consideration of this specificity see Wendler, *Pest, Fleckfieber, Ruhr und Typhus*. On the constitution of the Holy Roman Empire see Brady, *German Histories*; Wilson, *The Holy Roman Empire*; Stollberg-Rillinger, *The Holy Roman Empire*; Hardy, *Associative Political Culture*.
15. Christenson, "Politics and the Plague," 374.
16. Varlik, *Plague and Empire*, 9.
17. Heinrichs, *Plague, Print, and the Reformation*.
18. Cunningham and Grell, eds, *Four Horsemen of the Apocalypse*.
19. Rittgers, *The Reformation of Suffering*.
20. Hill, "Introduction."
21. Murphy, *A New Order of Medicine*. See also Mendelsohn et al., *Civic Medicine*.
22. Murphy, "Skin and Disease," 191–201.
23. Newhouse, "Outside the Walls."
24. Mummenhof, *Die öffentliche Gesundheits- und Krankenpflege*.
25. Slack, *The Impact of Plague*, 228–47.
26. Wear, *Knowledge and Practice*, 291.
27. Relevant, though an older framing on the contest between "state-control" and religion see Palmer, "The Control of Plague."
28. Cohn, *Cultures of Plague*; Cohn, *The Black Death Transformed*.
29. Wray, *Communities and Crisis*.
30. See Cohn, *Epidemics*; Vögele et al., *Epidemics and Pandemics*.
31. Girard, "The Plague in Literature and Myth," 834.
32. T. Green, *The Covid Consensus*.

Bibliography

Arrizabalga, Jon, John Henderson, and Roger French. *The Great Pox: The French Disease in Renaissance Europe*. New Haven: Yale University Press, 1997.

Beer, Matthias. *Eltern und Kinder des späten Mittelalters in ihren Briefen*. Nuremberg: Korn & Berg, 1996.

Berco, Christian. *From Body to Community: Venereal Disease and Society in Baroque Spain*. Toronto: University of Toronto Press, 2016.

Brady, Thomas A., Jr. *German Histories in the Age of Reformations, 1400–1650*. Cambridge: Cambridge University Press, 2012.

Brenner, Elma. *Leprosy and Charity in Medieval Rouen*. Woodbridge, Suffolk: The Boydell Press, 2015.

Burschel, Peter. *Die Erfindung der Reinheit, Eine andere Geschichte der Frühen Neuzeit*. Göttingen: Wallstein, 2014.

Byrne, Joseph P., ed. *Encyclopedia of Pestilence, Pandemics and Plagues*. 2 volumes. London: Bloomsbury, 2008.

Christenson, Daniel Eric. "Politics and the Plague: Efforts to Combat Health Epidemics in Seventeenth-Century Braunschweig-Wolfenbüttel, Germany." PhD dissertation. University of California, Riverside, 2004.

Cohn, Samuel K., Jr. *The Black Death Transformed: Disease and Culture in Early Renaissance Europe*. London: Arnold and Oxford University Press, 2002.

Cohn, Samuel K., Jr. *Cultures of Plague: Medical Thinking at the End of the Renaissance*. Oxford: Oxford University Press, 2009.

Cohn, Samuel K., Jr. *Epidemics: Hate and Compassion from the Plague of Athens to AIDS*. Oxford: Oxford University Press, 2018.

Cunningham, Andrew, and Ole Peter Grell, eds. *Four Horsemen of the Apocalypse: Religion, War, Famine, and Death in Reformation Europe*. Cambridge: Cambridge University Press, 2008.

Demaitre, Luke. *Leprosy in Premodern Medicine: A Malady of the Whole Body*. Baltimore: Johns Hopkins University Press, 2007.

Douglas, Mary. *Purity and Danger: An Analysis of Concepts of Pollution and Taboo*. London: Routledge, 2002.

Dross, Fritz. "Vergesellschaftung unter Ansteckenden—für eine Körpergeschichte der Seuche." *NTM—Zeitschrift für Geschichte der Wissenschaften, Technik und Medizin* 28, no. 2 (2020): 195–202.

Eckert, Edward A. *The Structure of Plagues and Pestilences in Early Modern Europe: Central Europe, 1560–1640*. Basel: Karger, 1996.

Feuerstein-Herz, Petra. *Gotts verhengnis und seine straffe. Zur Geschichte der Seuchen in der Frühen Neuzeit*. Wiesbaden: Harrassowitz, 2005.

Girard, Rene. "The Plague in Literature and Myth." *Texas Studies in Literature and Language* 15, no. 5 (1974): 833–50.

Green, Monica H. "The Four Black Deaths." *American Historical Review* 125 (2020): 1600–31.

Green, Monica H. "Plague (Yersinia pestis)." *Encyclopedia of the History of Science* (May 2024), accessed 20 April 2025. https://doi.org/10.34758/dy11–5697.

Green, Toby. *The Covid Consensus: The New Politics of Global Inequality*. London: Hurst, 2021.

Hardy, Duncan. *Associative Political Culture in the Holy Roman Empire: Upper Germany, 1346–1521*. Oxford: Oxford University Press, 2018.

Heinrichs, Erik A. *Plague, Print, and the Reformation: The German Reform of Healing, 1473–1573*. Abingdon: Routledge, 2018.

Henderson, John. *Florence under Siege: Surviving Plague in an Early Modern City*. New Haven: Yale University Press, 2019.

Herlihy, David. *The Black Death and the Transformation of the West*. Edited by Samuel K. Cohn, Jr. Cambridge, MA: Harvard University Press, 1997.

Hill, Kat. "Introduction: Making Lutherans." *Past & Present* 234, Supplement 12 (2017), *Cultures of Lutheranism: Reformation Repertoires in Early Modern Germany*, edited by Kat Hill, 9–32.

Kinzelbach, Annemarie. "Infection, Contagion, and Public Health in Late Medieval and Early Modern German Imperial Towns." *Journal of the History of Medicine and Allied Sciences* 61 (2006): 369–89.

Lindemann, Mary. *Medicine and Society in Early Modern Europe*. Cambridge: Cambridge University Press, 2010.

McCormick, Ted. *Human Empire: Mobility and Demographic Thought in the British Atlantic World, 1500–1800*. Cambridge: Cambridge University Press, 2022.

Mendelsohn, J. Andrew, Annemarie Kinzelbach, and Ruth Schilling, eds. *Civic Medicine: Physician, Polity, and Pen in Early Modern Europe*. Abingdon: Routledge, 2020.

Mummenhoff, Ernst. *Die öffentliche Gesundheits- und Krankenpflege im alten Nürnberg. Festschrift zur Eröffnung des Neuen Krankenhauses der Stadt Nürnberg*. Nuremberg: self-published, 1898.

Murphy, Hannah. *A New Order of Medicine: The Rise of Physicians in Reformation Germany*. Pittsburgh: University of Pittsburgh Press, 2019.

Murphy, Hannah. "Skin and Disease in Early Modern Medicine: Jan Jessen's *De cute, et cutaneis affectibus* (1601)." *Bulletin of the History of Medicine*, 94, no. 2 (2020): 179–214.

Newhouse, Amy. "Outside the Walls: Civic Belonging and Contagious Disease in Sixteenth-Century Nuremberg." PhD dissertation. University of Arizona, 2015.

Palmer, Richard. "The Control of Plague in Venice and Northern Italy, 1348–1600." PhD dissertation. University of Kent, 1978.

Porzelt, Carolin. *Die Pest in Nürnberg: Leben und Herrschen in Pestzeiten (1562–1763)*. St Ottilien: EOS Verlag, 2000.

Rittgers, Ronald K. *The Reformation of Suffering: Pastoral Theology and Lay Piety in Late Medieval and Early Modern Germany*. Oxford: Oxford University Press, 2012.

Slack, Paul. *The Impact of Plague in Tudor and Stuart England*. Oxford: Clarendon Press, 1984.

Slauter, Will. "Write Up Your Dead. The Bills of Mortality and the London Plague of 1665." *Media History* 17 (2011): 1–15.

Stein, Claudia. *Negotiating the French Pox in Early Modern Germany. The History of Medicine in Context*. Farnham: Ashgate, 2009.

Stollberg-Rillinger, Barbara. *The Holy Roman Empire: A Short History*, translated by Yair Mintzker. Princeton: Princeton University Press, 2021.

Swan, Claudia. *Negotiating the French Pox in Early Modern Germany*. Aldershot: Ashgate, 2009.

Ulbricht, Otto, ed. *Die leidige Seuche: Pest-Fälle in der Frühen Neuzeit*. Cologne: Böhlau Verlag, 2004.

Varlik, Nükhet. *Plague and Empire in the Early Modern Mediterranean World: The Ottoman Experience, 1347–1600*. Cambridge: Cambridge University Press, 2015.

Vögele, Jörg, Luisa Rittershaus, and Katherina Schuler. "Epidemics and Pandemics—the Historical Perspective. Introduction." *Historical Social Research / Historische Sozialforschung* 33. Supplement: *Epidemics and Pandemics—the Historical Perspective* (2021): 7–33.

Wear, Andrew. *Knowledge and Practice in English Medicine, 1550–1680*. Cambridge, Cambridge University Press, 2000.

Wendler, Ulf. *Pest, Fleckfieber, Ruhr und Typhus: Epidemien auf dem Land und Ihre Deutung im Fürstentum Lüneburg, 1565–1666*. Göttingen: Wallstein Verlag, 2024.

Wilson, Peter. *The Holy Roman Empire: A Thousand Years of Europe's History*. London: Penguin, 2016.

Wray, Shona Kelly. *Communities and Crisis: Bologna during the Black Death*. Leiden: Brill, 2009.

PART I

Textual Strategies: Plague and Print

CHAPTER 1

Plague for a Popular Audience

Suspicions of Print in Late Fifteenth-Century Germany

CHRISTOPHER HUTCHINSON

Introduction

At the end of his 1482 plague treatise, the Nuremberg barber-surgeon and poet Hans Folz (ca. 1440–1513) outlines his reasons for composing the treatise in verse. He explains that he chose to write this work in verse, rather than prose, so that the treatise's audience could more easily commit the text to memory. The work has been:

> Composed in verse,
> So that it will be more easily recalled,
> And equally so that the things may be grasped in such a manner
> That everyone remembers a little piece of information,
> In order for one person to support another.[1]

The work (to which I refer henceforth as Folz's verse treatise) should be remembered piecemeal by those who read or hear it, and the information should then be reconstructed from memory in a group by its audience.[2] Folz thus appears to advocate a form of community medical practice that is not dependent on an individual's consultation of his printed text. Instead, his audience should collaborate to reconstruct from memory the information that his text had provided. Folz does not intend his text to be received by an individual reader, but to be received by a group, committed to memory, then pieced back together orally by the group. Folz's explanation of his work's intended function is unusual—fifteenth-century plague treatises do not typically provide instructions on how the audience should consume the work. This passage raises a number of questions about what the group reception of texts in the first decades of print actually looked like. How did print change the reception of medical knowledge in less literate communities? Who made up these groups of consumers and how large were they? Folz suggests his readers divide the labor of memorizing his plague treatise so each person takes responsibility for one section of the work. How organized, then, were these groups of readers? Would an entire group reassemble to recite the whole work or would certain consumers be consulted on a particular aspect of plague treatment as and when the need arose? How many less literate listeners would this work have reached?

Although there has been a great deal of scholarly work on the oral reception of early printed texts, we cannot definitively know the answers to these questions about how texts like Folz's would have been consumed in a group environment.[3] Yet this text, and other texts that explicitly reference modes of communal, presumably oral reception, form a fruitful area of study to help us inquire into the way fifteenth-century Germans grappled with the proliferation of printed texts that aimed to target less literate, or less wealthy, audiences. This work, one of a small number of fifteenth-century plague treatises in verse, demonstrates one approach to a contradiction of early vernacular print: many incunabula—especially broadsides and pamphlets—lay some claim to be of use to a less literate readership in a time when as little as 3 percent of the population of the Holy Roman Empire may have been fully literate in the vernacular.[4] Yet almost all printed works rely principally on text to communicate the information they contain. Writers and printers employ strategies like verse, woodcuts, or indexes, to make their works more accessible to a less literate audience, but the underlying hurdle of illiteracy remains. The development of print made texts commodities that could be produced at scale and sold and distributed more widely than manuscripts had previously allowed. This sudden expansion of the potential audience of books forced those involved in book production to consider what information should be made available to various segments of the population of fifteenth-century Germany; how this information should be presented; and what roles less literate and less Latinate consumers of knowledge could play in transforming the information they consumed in texts into real-world practice.

This chapter investigates these concerns about audience and print in fifteenth-century vernacular German plague treatises. Plague is an especially pertinent disease to investigate here, as its devastating effects were regularly felt by rich and poor alike. It is difficult to overstate the prominent position that plague would have occupied in the consciousness of fifteenth-century Germans. Outbreaks were frequent: over the course of the fifteenth century, plague struck German cities approximately once a decade. This made plague a regular feature of existence in all but the most isolated—and fortunate—settlements.[5] Although the mortality and morbidity rates of the disease had declined over the first hundred years since the Black Death (1347–51), this trend reversed starting in the middle of the fifteenth century. In the century's second half, plague's recurrence accelerated and its mortality rate grew. Medical thinkers and practitioners therefore had to newly reckon with the fact that plague was a recurring feature of contemporary experience.[6] The disease's rapid spread and devastating impact on all segments of society meant that all Germans—rich and poor, urban and rural, illiterate and literate—needed useful medical advice on the disease. Many vernacular plague treatises were designed to fill this need.

The running assumption in much scholarship is that print expanded the audience of vernacular medical treatises, making medical knowledge available to audiences that manuscripts rarely reached.[7] This is hard to dispute—the scale of vernacular medical printing suggests audiences grew substantially in the last half of the fifteenth century. However, this commodification of print and the expansion of the audience for medical texts also encountered ambivalence toward print's growing audience. While most vernacular treatises billed themselves as suitable for a broad audience, not all authors took this claim equally seriously. Writers on plague take different approaches to the expanding audience which the new technology allowed them to target. Sometimes they develop strategies that are conceivably useful; other times, their attempts to provide useful information for a less literate audience ring a little hollow. Some express significant concerns that the expansion of print may even cause harm to its growing audience.

This chapter compares three plague treatises—two 1482 treatises by the Nuremberg barber-surgeon Hans Folz and a 1500 treatise by the Strasbourg barber-surgeon Hieronymus Brunschwig (ca. 1450–1512/13)—and reveals these writers' anxieties and ambivalence toward print's popularization of medical knowledge. Folz and Brunschwig take different approaches to the question of how best to address a wide audience comprising more and less literate readers. While Folz produces two separate treatises—one in verse, the other in prose—that primarily target separate audiences, Brunschwig seeks to create a common audience for his plague treatise, deploying strategies of information organization for more and less literate readers and including medical information useful to wealthier and poorer, urban and rural readers alike. By examining the two authors' different approaches to the expanding audience of printed plague treatises, we see how writers on plague innovated both in the informational strategies their books deployed and in the kinds of medical information they chose to include. Examining these differences in Folz's and Brunschwig's approaches to audience sheds light on the strategies writers and printers employed to reach different categories of vernacular consumers—from the rural, illiterate poor to wealthier, urban elites and learned physicians—and complicates our understanding of the democratization of medical writing through print.

Plague Treatises for a Mass Market

The rapid expansion of print over the course of the second half of the fifteenth century allowed texts on plague—as well as on other medical topics—to reach more people than manuscripts had previously allowed. This expansion contributed to changes in the functions that plague served in fifteenth-century literature. Plague became a commodity of sorts as writers on the disease grappled with the mass-market potential of information on the disease. There were no printers' guilds in Germany until the 1490s, and printing was largely unregulated.[8] Consequently, the body of incunabula printed was largely determined by market demand, although it was also influenced by the preferences of individual patrons, cities, or printers themselves. Rolf Engelsing has demonstrated that approximately 5 percent of German-language books printed before 1520 have medical subject matter.[9] Of these, plague treatises counted among some of the most widely read German-language printed works, as judged by the number of editions they went through and the signs of use in the surviving copies.[10] Many successful treatises were reprinted several times every few years. In all, sixty-nine individual editions of secular plague incunabula printed in Germany are recorded, of which twenty-five were printed in Latin and the rest in German.[11] These texts have many features in common: they typically outline general principles concerning the maintenance of health, the origins and symptoms of plague, and a handful of recipes for substances that can prevent plague infection or reduce the chance of death in those infected.

Despite these similarities in content, plague treatises often differ in length, in form (most of these works are in prose, but a handful, like Folz's treatise, are in verse), and in the social status of their author: many were adapted from older manuscripts by learned doctors, some were written by barber-surgeons or other less elite practitioners, and many are anonymous. This large and varied corpus also attests to the social breadth of the audience many writers and printers sought to target with their works on plague. Early printed vernacular plague treatises have received little scholarly attention, although Erik Heinrichs' recent monograph is a notable exception.[12] Yet these texts form a rich and compelling corpus of texts that can shed light on fifteenth-century Germans' responses to epidemic disease and on the role new forms of media played in supporting, or undermining, their efforts to fight disease.

The second half of the fifteenth century is a fruitful time period for examining these questions about print and audience, as it saw an expansion not just of printed books, but of commodities and consumption more broadly. Lisa Jardine has shown how the fifteenth and sixteenth centuries formed a period characterized by the ownership of things; by "a celebration of the urge to own, the curiosity to possess the treasures of other cultures, and pride in a new craftsmanship which can make the most humdrum commodities desirable."[13] The expansion of global trade networks, the development of urban middle classes in many parts of Europe, and innovations in diverse fields such as mining, bookkeeping, and navigation all contributed to this growing culture of commodities and consumption in Europe.[14] The development of print media in the mid-fifteenth century also made knowledge a mass commodity for the first time. Information could be printed, reproduced, and distributed quickly and cheaply, allowing it to circulate to a wide audience. The growing culture of consumption in fifteenth-century Germany is also reflected in print media as books, pamphlets, and broadsides were sold, passed on, and traded like other commodities. Therefore, writers, printers, and booksellers had to consider the economic viability of their works and reflect on how best to market a particular product for specific consumers.[15]

In a practice indicative of the growing audience for books, vernacular printed books on a variety of subjects began to cite their audiences explicitly as the "gemeine man" (common man), a segment of the population that was not in a position of social or political control. Scholars have generally sought to define this social group according to certain professions or the ability to read and write.[16] However, the frequency with which writers on all manner of topics invoke the "common man" suggests its meaning is more mutable. This term rarely connotes a predefined social and cultural group. It is a term that, as Lyndal Roper suggests, "derives its meaning in its use."[17] There are frequent variations across texts as far as what social and cultural functions the common man can be expected to perform—whether the common man is urban or rural, literate or illiterate, rich or poor. The term represents an at times banal idea of an audience that stands in for society at large. It is everyone and no one, an authorial or publishing shorthand for precisely the audience that a writer or printer should be seen to address in order for their work to be seen as contributing to the healthy functioning of society. Vernacular writers' frequent appeals to the common man illustrate the expanding audience of printed books, as writers and printers navigated shifting expectations of audience and reception.

Fifteenth-century plague treatises that explicitly target the common man support this understanding of the term as a stand-in for society at large; they seek to appeal to social groups that are at once urban and rural, literate and illiterate, rich and poor. The strategies the writers and printers of these treatises employ to make the works more accessible to a wider readership speak to the changing media landscape. They employ a variety of formal strategies, such as rhyming verse, indexes, and woodcuts, to cater to readers or listeners less familiar with knowledge in written form. Many include recipes derived from everyday herbs readily available to a poor, rural audience alongside more complex, costly medicines. These texts show a clear interest in their usability; that is, in the reader's ability to translate the information they contain into practices that could mitigate the spread of plague.

The innovations of printed plague treatises in their treatment of audience stand within a broader context of shifting emphases of medicine in fifteenth-century Europe. Vivian Nutton has argued that the fifteenth century saw significant changes in medical writing that testify to a shift from theoretical orthodoxy to an emphasis on medical practice itself.[18] While medical humanists of the early sixteenth century would return to theoretical and etymological discussions of canonical texts, the previous century was marked by a concentration on empiricism and pragmatism that contributed to, and was reflective of, vibrant and adaptable medical thought. More specifically, Danielle Jacquart has highlighted the fifteenth century as the time when medical writers began to incorporate alternative, non-canonical ideas into their works. Although these writers never jettisoned Greek and Arabic models, those older works were increasingly becoming "dead texts," as their inability to inhibit the spread and mortality of diseases like plague became more and more evident.[19] Fifteenth-century writers began to integrate alternative sources of medical knowledge into their writings.

By the mid-fifteenth century, we have a medical discourse in which, while the ultimate authority of canonical texts was never explicitly challenged, the body of texts on learned medicine came to be reflective of the plurality of types of medical practice; where alchemical, magical, and empirical medicine were more frequently acknowledged in texts, even if they were not always accepted. It was also a time when medical practice was not limited to professionals but was regularly practiced within households as part of people's everyday lives, as Elaine Leong has shown.[20] In other words, there was considerable overlap between learned medical texts and the lived experience of people. Ann Carmichael has highlighted how print stimulated this already existing emphasis on experience as a significant foundation of medical thought and practice, providing writers with "ready reference to the experience of people elsewhere."[21] Print also allowed this process to work the other way, disseminating writers' ideas broadly. The printed medical text began to address an audience of practitioners composed, frequently, of medical professionals and laypeople alike. This manifest concern that printed texts be of use to the public, rather than primarily to medical professionals, also revealed obstacles to print's ability to expand the reach of medical knowledge. How could the printed word communicate useful information widely when only a very small segment of the proposed readership was literate and, in many cases, lacked the means to undergo the cures and acquire the medicines that canonical medicine proposed? Two plague treatises by Hans Folz, the Nuremberg barber-surgeon, printer, and poet, engage with this question.

Two Forms for Two Audiences: Hans Folz's Plague Treatises in Verse and Prose

Hans Folz is the only fifteenth-century German printer known to regularly have printed works that he himself composed. There are forty-one known works that have been attributed to his press, mostly small pamphlets covering a variety of genres, from medical works and other instructional manuals to poems in rhymed couplets and Shrovetide plays. The limited number of surviving texts printed by Folz suggests printing was at most a subsidiary pursuit for him, and not a primary source of income.[22] Although his printing operation was limited in scope, Folz's unusual status as both writer and printer of his works, as well as a medical practitioner, makes him a central figure for an investigation of the relationship between medical authority, audience, and the circulation of useful information.

In 1482, Folz wrote and printed two texts on how best to avoid and treat the plague that was afflicting Nuremberg. The first is a 474-line verse adaptation of a prose plague treatise written by the Ulm physician, Heinrich Steinhöwel (1410/11–79), in 1473. Like most of Folz's printed works, the verse treatise is a *Reimpaarspruch*; a non-strophic series of rhymed couplets in iambic tetrameter. The second plague treatise (to which I refer as Folz's prose treatise) is a sixteen-page commissioned work in prose, one of only two prose works authored and printed by Folz. These two texts differ substantially in how they conceive of the audience they address: the verse treatise is designed to target a non- or partially literate audience, as it can be memorized and circulated, whereas the prose treatise appears to be designed for individual reading. The differences in audience between the two texts also inform the tone of the works, as well as the medical information they contain. Folz's careful attention to audience in his two plague treatises shows the social and political concerns that informed his publication of these works. It also reflects Folz's own concern with printed works' appeals to a broad audience—a concern through which Folz implies that other printed texts, whose writers and printers may be less attentive to audience than Folz himself, spread information unsuitable for less literate, lay consumers.

In his introduction to the prose work, Folz claims the work is largely the same as the verse treatise, only "not rhymed, like the previous one." Indeed, there are many similarities between the verse and prose treatise. Both contain some information about the origins of plague, practical tips for preventing infection, and general advice about the importance of prayer, the validity of earthly medicine, and the wisdom of fleeing a plague-afflicted city. The pamphlets are similar in size, so the cost to purchase them would probably have been comparable. Both also contain medical recipes: some partly in Latin, others fully in German; some explicitly for a wealthier audience, others explicitly for a poorer audience.

Both texts, for instance, include a regimen derived from an unidentified citizen of Pavia who successfully avoided plague by eating a handful of dried dock leaves each morning.[23] To a certain extent, then, both verse and prose treatise have something to offer elite and non-elite readers alike.

But there are a number of key differences as well: in the rhetorical strategies Folz employs to reach each work's audience; in the relative weight Folz gives to the information he includes in each work; and in the warnings these pamphlets contain about quack practitioners. Folz may claim the content of verse and prose treatise is similar, but the differences reveal his attention to tailoring each work for a particular audience: the prose treatise for a wealthier and more literate audience; the verse treatise for the common man. One central difference is the form itself of each work, which is suggestive of two different models of reception.

We have already seen how Folz includes instructions in his verse treatise that the work's audience should memorize the text piecemeal, then reconstruct its contents in a group. Folz suggests a different model of reception for his prose treatise. The work opens with a dedication to the Nuremberg patrician Antonius Haller, who had asked Folz to write a prose text on the plague: "but not, like the previous one, set in verse, for the benefit of the many people who are better accustomed to prose."[24] The assertion that the prose work's audience is "better accustomed" to prose is probably a euphemism for this audience's literacy and suggests this treatise would more likely have been consulted by an individual reader. In other works, Folz explicitly suggests verse is the ideal form for the less educated and less literate: in his pamphlet on confession, Folz explains he composed the work in verse "because one finds many young, unlearned people who can learn such rhyme or verse by heart more easily than otherwise, so [verse] can then be of use to them and other unlearned or simple people."[25] Folz identifies two separate groups here: those who can learn the text by heart and "other" simple people. The implication is that those partially literate readers who learn the text by heart can further circulate the work's contents, presumably orally, to those who cannot read at all or to those who do not own a copy of the pamphlet. Given Folz's association of verse with memorization by a less learned audience, and a wider, public reception, his characterization of the prose plague treatise's audience as one "accustomed to prose" thus implies that readership is more educated and more literate than that of his verse treatise. It also suggests this audience would not have learned the text by heart but might instead have kept a physical copy for private consultation.[26] Moreover, given that the work's dedicatee, Haller—a member of the Nuremberg elite—commissioned Folz's prose plague treatise, it is likely Folz had a wealthier, more urban audience in mind when composing its text.

The dedication of Folz's verse treatise also offers clues about that work's intended audience. Whereas the prose text was commissioned by Haller, the verse text includes a dedication "in honor of the city of Nuremberg."[27] This line could suggest that the city had commissioned the work or that Folz had composed it opportunistically, in the hope of financial reward from the council.[28] Whichever of these motivations is more accurate, this does suggest that Folz is not only writing for the common man, but also for the council. The Nuremberg city council, alongside private philanthropists, was obliged to take a particularly high interest in the care of its poorer residents. This was partly because guilds, which took some responsibility for public welfare in other cities, had been banned in Nuremberg since the mid-fourteenth century.[29] Furthermore, unlike many other polities in the German lands, the Nuremberg council maintained strict controls on the distribution and performance of literary works. A 1502 law required all printers in the city to obtain permission from the council for each individual work that they intended to print, and there is evidence the council had been censoring works by the gunsmith and dramatist Hans Rosenplüt as early as 1459.[30] A good relationship with the council would have been important for writers and printers, and demonstrating a commitment to the medical care of the city's population would have gone some way towards achieving this. This dedication, then, would seem to reinforce the fact that Folz is aiming his treatise at the less literate and, most likely, poorer residents of Nuremberg and its environs. The difference in how Folz conceives of his texts' reception speaks to the political and social benefits writers and printers stood to gain by producing plague texts for specific audiences.

Curating Information for Different Audiences

Folz's consideration of audience not only determined the form of the two plague treatises; it also informed how these works presented information concerning the disease, its prevention, and its treatment. I now turn to three specific differences between the verse and prose treatises. First, the verse text displays a greater focus on the sufferers' lived experience of the disease, whereas the prose text discusses the disease's symptoms in a more perfunctory manner. Second, the prose treatise contains a number of discursive passages, in which Folz comments on trends in contemporary medicine, while the verse treatise consists primarily of pithy instructions. The third difference concerns Folz's frequent warnings in the prose treatise about quack medicine and the dangers of consulting irregular practitioners or the recipes contained in the printed works they produced, warnings which are absent in the verse treatise. While both texts have many recipes in common, Folz omits certain recipes from each treatise and uses his prose treatise to explicitly highlight the social dangers of printing recipes in German for the unlearned reader. These differences between the two treatises are deliberate, and they show how Folz considers the suitability of various categories of information for an elite and a non-elite audience, respectively. Folz's sensitivity to the particular needs and priorities of the different audiences of his two plague texts reflects his wider concern with the dangers inherent in distributing medical information in print for a broad readership.

While his account of the disease's symptoms in the verse treatise is tense, emotive, and detailed, the equivalent passage in the prose treatise is strikingly perfunctory. In his verse treatise, Folz dedicates a forty-two-line section to outlining the symptoms of plague. He begins by describing the early symptoms (fever, foul breath, weak pulse), then recounts the progression of the disease: the sufferer's tongue will turn black, they will develop a dry cough, they will become delirious, and boils will start to appear on their body. There is a poignant quality to Folz's discussion of plague's symptoms in the verse treatise. By setting the symptoms in narrative—moving from the first signs of the disease to the patient's likely death—this passage creates tension and seems designed to have an emotional impact on the reader. Folz concludes this section of the treatise by outlining the signs that death is near:

> Hope for his salvation when black appears,
> Because black in stool and urine mean,
> It is true, that death is near.
> The more these signs appear,
> The closer they are to death.
> But God, who knows of life and death,
> Has everything in his hand.[31]

Folz heightens the emotional impact of the symptoms in this passage. His euphemistic reference to death as salvation and his abstraction of the black color of the patient's excreta to black itself in the first line—a color with a powerful symbolic meaning in the late medieval imaginary—lend his description of plague's symptoms a vividness that mimics the despair a patient or their loved ones might feel when they reach this stage in the disease's progress. The final two lines, in which Folz reassures the audience that God alone knows who will live and die, take on a cathartic quality, concluding the narrative progression of symptoms and offering solace to the despairing patient.

The emotive character of Folz's language is not solely attributable to the literary quality of verse itself and the emotional impact of its rhyme and rhythm. Compare the above to the hurried, sober list of symptoms the prose treatise contains: "And also the signs of death are ... sudden hunger, disappearance of the boils, unquenchable thirst, unsteady pulse, black urine, then grace in God."[32] These are largely the same symptoms Folz outlines in the verse treatise, yet he presents them as a simple list with no editorializing—one cannot say that this list is designed to have the same emotional impact on the audience as the lines in the verse treatise. The final "grace in God" conveys some of the pathos of the last lines of the passage from the verse treatise, but in a far more perfunctory form. Indeed, Folz may even have included the list of symptoms in his prose treatise as an afterthought. They appear on the final page, occupy around half a page of text, and do not follow logically from the previous section of the work, which concerns printing errors in plague treatises. His account of the symptoms of plague is more prominent in the verse treatise: occupying two sides of text (around one tenth of the work) toward the middle of the treatise.

This difference in prominence, details, and tone suggests that Folz viewed a detailed knowledge of the symptoms and lived experience of the disease as more relevant for the less literate audience of his verse treatise. It also implies that he viewed the emotive nature of literary language as more suitable for this less literate audience. Fritz Langensiepen has claimed the *Reimpaarspruch* in the late fifteenth century was "the optimal form for instructing the popular masses and the laity," as it was easily memorable.[33] The emotive quality of the verse treatise's list of symptoms could also support the audience's ability to memorize the text, employing imagery that would stick in their minds and stimulating an emotional response to the text. Moreover, the prominence of symptoms in the verse treatise speaks to the work's focus on practical usefulness. It aims principally to help its audience deal as best they can with the spread of plague among their communities, giving them simple, memorable strategies for recognizing infection and realistic expectations of the disease's prognosis. While the prose treatise also contains several points of practical advice, its slapdash inclusion of a perfunctory list of plague's symptoms suggests that dealing with the material reality of plague infection may not have been a primary concern for its intended readership. Rather than being instructional and focused on practical solutions, Folz's prose treatise is more focused on theoretical questions surrounding the disease. In it, he expounds on ethical, religious, and social topics related to the plague as well, such as the ethics of fleeing an approaching plague, the religious validity of earthly medicine, and explanations for his instructions concerning certain medicines, dietary prescriptions, and healthy habits. In the verse treatise, by contrast, Folz limits himself largely to matters of direct practical use to the consumer, with only sporadic and brief discussion of some of these more theoretical concerns.

Folz's directions on bloodletting are another instructive example of the difference in tone between verse and plague treatise. The bloodletting instructions in his verse treatise succinctly direct the audience to let certain veins to drain the poison infecting specific parts of the body:

> Should a person feel pain in the head,
> Then empty out the cephalic vein.
> If he notices a boil on his ear,

He should let the same vein.
If he feels something around the breast,
He should let the median vein.[34]

These instructions are to the point, and seem designed to be translated into specific treatment practices—letting certain veins—if a sufferer should feel symptoms in their head, ear, or breast, respectively. The prose treatise gives essentially the same instructions as the verse treatise, although the phrasing Folz employs is less imperative: "And so, generally speaking, an infected brain lets out by the ears and in that area. Its poison is to be extracted through the head vein [i.e. the cephalic vein] on the thumb. Also, the heart lets out by the armpits and can be extracted through the median or basilic vein."[35] The reference to actual medical practice in this passage is less direct than the equivalent in the verse treatise. He speaks "gemeinclich" (generally) about the relation of areas of the body to the veins of the arm and even introduces an additional level of theoretical knowledge that the verse treatise does not include: where the body part in question lets out into the associated vein (as distinct from the place where the vein itself should be cut). Rather than directly instruct the reader to let certain veins in response to specific symptoms, Folz here presents this information in the form of established principles of medical learning. This information does not instruct in the actual practice of letting certain veins but constitutes fundamental theoretical knowledge underlying the practice. The expository tone of this passage differs from the direct, uncomplicated instructions of the verse treatise. These differences suggest the intended audiences of the two treatises had different priorities: while Folz assumed the consumers of the verse treatise required explicit, practical instructions, he thought the readers of the prose text were more interested in the principles that underlie various facets of plague treatment.

As Heinrichs has shown, vernacular plague treatises typically include both theoretical principles (for a more learned and perhaps wealthier audience) and practical instructions for the less learned.[36] In his two plague treatises, however, Folz distills these two components out into separate concerns for separate audiences, emphasizing principles in his prose treatise and practical solutions in his verse treatise. There may be significant overlap in much of the content of the two works, but Folz attends to the nuances of audience in a way that is uncommon among writers of fifteenth-century vernacular plague treatises.

Literacy and Quackery

One of the reasons for Folz's sensitivity to audience is the potential danger he associates with the spread of certain forms of misinformation; a risk he attributes to the spread of vernacular print. Publishing books for a broad audience requires careful attention to the information presented, so that the book will not mislead the reader. More and less learned consumers require different kinds of information, and different strategies for presenting it. By emphasizing simple, practical solutions in his verse treatise and expounding on broader aspects of plague treatment in his prose treatise, Folz shelters the unlearned and less literate reader from more complicated theoretical questions they may not fully understand. It is, counterintuitively, the more literate reader of the prose treatise who has the greatest risk of being duped by false information, as they are more likely to read other books. Folz's concern for the potential harm of certain types of information for his different audiences takes on tellingly different implications in his reflections on quack medicine.

Folz writes at considerable length about quackery in his prose treatise, but does not mention the subject at all in his verse treatise, suggesting that this information is more relevant for the more literate audience of the prose treatise. In this work, Folz associates an incomplete understanding of medical principles with quacks, who prescribe medicines to any customer without the faintest idea of the patient's complexion or the condition that ails them. The implication of Folz's diatribe against quacks is that treatment should be left in the hands of the professionals:

> These [lay] doctors think all purgatives only exist to push out shit and don't pay attention to driving the harmful material from all parts of the body or how they might introduce other sicknesses. At the same they would drive out of the body of someone with a damp temperament those things they think there are too little of and keep those things they think there are too much of because they do not know the difference, either between diseases or the complexions of patients. And so a blind man leads another blind man and both fall into the ditch. I myself have seen one [practitioner] who quickly caused his own death with a purgative he had been handing around.[37]

According to Folz, unlearned practitioners present various dangers. These quacks have an overly simplistic understanding of the human body and view treatment as a simple, mechanical process: by taking a laxative, the patient will excrete the poisonous material at the root of their ailment. However, they do not understand the various other factors that should inform the choice and dosage of purgative: the patient's humoral complexion, the condition they suffer from, and the qualities of the drug itself. The consequences of their ignorance, Folz suggests, are often fatal. However, the solution to the problem of irregular practitioners is certainly not to broaden medical education so these quacks gain a deeper understanding of the nuances of diagnosis and treatment. Folz morbidly remarks that these practitioners belong in "their own hospital or churchyard."[38] Instead, the reader should avoid unauthorized practitioners altogether and only seek medical advice from "those who know and have long experience."[39] It is telling that Folz centers his excursus on quackery on the prescription of purgatives, because these drugs were paradigmatic of simplistic and popular views of medicine. They are a particularly important topic in discussions of quack medicine and appear in many Nuremberg *Fastnachtspiele*, including ones by Folz himself. Plots centering on constipation and laxatives offer a healthy dose of toilet humor but they also reflect the central role of excreta in the popular image of medicine in late medieval Europe: diagnosis was conducted by examining urine and the archetypal treatment was the laxative.

Folz's diatribe about quackery covers three sides of text—about five times as long as his brief list of the symptoms of plague. He appears to view quackery as a central topic for the audience of his prose treatise. We can read this interest in quackery as Folz's attempt to distance himself from irregular practitioners in the minds of the Nuremberg elite. Folz himself was no university-educated physician. A barber-surgeon, he occupied a median position in the hierarchy of Nuremberg medical practitioners, below apothecaries and academically trained doctors but above midwives and hospital masters.[40] Despite his lack of formal education, Folz seems to have been a respected figure in the Nuremberg medical community. He knew the physician Hartmann Schedel (1440–1514), compiler and editor of the Nuremberg chronicle, and there is evidence he and Schedel treated each other for various ailments.[41] Moreover, as already mentioned, Schedel kept a copy of Folz's verse treatise on plague in his library, and Haller, the commissioner of Folz's prose treatise, was Schedel's father-in-law. By including this jeremiad on quack doctors in his prose treatise, the non-university-educated but generally respected Folz could further distance himself from the city's uneducated, irregular practitioners and cast himself as one of the responsible, knowledgeable few. He was also probably motivated, in part, by professional rivalry. Even social elites routinely consulted empirics, alchemists, and other practitioners not licensed by city authorities.[42] These healers were competitors of barber-surgeons like Folz, or indeed of physicians like Schedel. Here, Folz also uses his work to slander his professional rivals.

As Heinrichs has pointed out, authors like Folz "sought to use their vernacular plague texts to establish clear lines between legitimate and illegitimate healers."[43] However, why does Folz not also seek to draw this distinction between respectable practitioners and quacks in his verse treatise? After all, a less learned, less wealthy, and less literate audience would have less recourse to learned doctors and might be more susceptible to seeking treatment from irregular healers. Indeed, this concern with the prevalence of quackery among non-elite consumers motivates a number of sixteenth-century writers to pen vernacular treatises for the common man dedicated to combating medical malpractice.[44]

The key difference is that whereas Folz assumes the reader of his prose treatise has the means to seek help from a medical practitioner, he intends his verse treatise to actually assume the role of doctor, providing the audience with all the practical information they need. In the prose treatise, Folz advises the reader to seek the advice of a doctor at various points, and it is notable that, while both treatises contain various recipes in Latin and German, the prose treatise is the only one containing a recipe in apothecaries' weights and measures, suggesting Folz intended the reader of his prose treatise to consult an apothecary to obtain this particular concoction. In his verse treatise, by contrast, Folz does not presume his audience will have access to a medical practitioner. In the introduction to a 1530 reprint of the verse treatise, the title page explains the work is intended for "the common man whom the doctor and apothecary cannot reach."[45] While Folz's prose treatise can supplement consultation of a medical professional, then, his verse treatise should replace it, offering helpful advice for those who either cannot afford to consult a doctor or who live far from the nearest town. This function of the verse treatise as a stand-in for a doctor is supported by the woodcut that introduces Folz's edition of the verse treatise (Figure 1.1), which depicts a doctor lancing a plague sufferer's boil. Although this procedure is performed on an external part of the body—typically the domain of barber-surgeons—the doctor's beret and long-sleeved gown suggest he is a learned physician.[46] The verse treatise also includes two woodcuts at the end of the work: portraits of Hippocrates and Galen. Caroline Huey has argued that the high frequency of text–image combinations in Folz's printed works relative to the works of other contemporary printers suggests that he viewed printed documents as versions of theatrical performance.[47] By bookending his text with three images of learned doctors, Folz clarifies its function. The work itself stands in for the learned doctor. Folz does not need to warn the audience of his verse treatise about the lies and deceptions of quacks because they, unlike the readers of the prose treatise, are not likely to consult any medical practitioners in the first place.

It is the audience of the prose treatise—more urban, more literate, and possibly wealthier—that is more at risk of being duped by quacks. In some ways, Folz suggests, it is their literacy that makes them more vulnerable to deception. Toward the end of his prose treatise, he discusses his reasons for leaving a particular recipe out of the treatise and reflects on the mistakes found in printed vernacular medical texts:

> And the second regimen on strengthening the heart and cooling the mind I leave to the doctors and apothecaries so that they are not misunderstood by the unlearned. I have seen wrong names in many German recipes: horseradish (mirretich) instead of myrrh (mirra); snake blood (sangwis draconis) instead

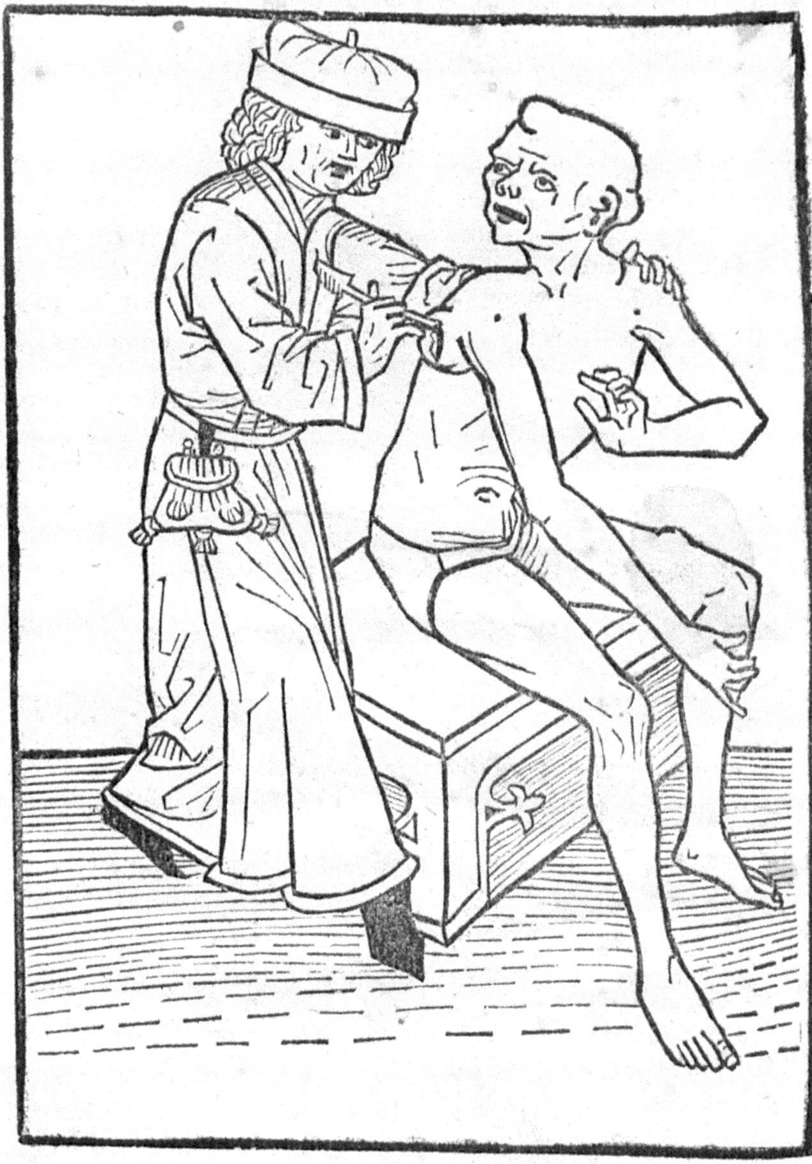

Figure 1.1. Woodcut of a doctor lancing a patient's boil. Folz, *Verse Treatise*, 1v. Bayerische Staatsbibliothek, Munich. BSB-Ink. F-184. CC0 1.0 Universal.

> of sandarac (sandaracam); pimpenella (bibneln) instead of bdellium; terpentine instead of serpentinite; cinnamon bark (ciment rinten) instead of cumin (ciminum); orache (scheiß molten) instead of goat's whey (geiß molken). There are enough of these mistakes in a German printed book called Ortolffus.[48]

The literate person's ability to read printed vernacular medical texts creates two problems: first, it introduces the risk that they may misunderstand the information these texts contain. Although they may be able to understand the text on a surface level, it is very possible that they lack the background medical knowledge necessary to fully grasp the broader context of a particular piece of information. Second, the text itself may be inaccurate, and the reader has no way of discerning accurate from false information. Giving examples of errata in a popular printed medical work originally written by the thirteenth-century Bavarian physician Ortolf and printed in five separate editions before 1482, Folz suggests mistakes are not limited to Ortolf's text but are pervasive in vernacular printed treatises.

The consequences of these mistakes are serious: including the wrong substance could make a medicine ineffectual, or even harmful. In the context of preventing plague, which decimated German cities roughly once a decade in the fifteenth century, the stakes were particularly high. Printing errors and misunderstandings could exacerbate the spread of plague and increase the risk of death for those infected. Folz, then, is recognizing the danger not only of quacks but of print itself, at least if improperly produced: print could either help combat a disease or facilitate its spread. By drawing the reader's attention to the inadequacies of vernacular medical works, and the risks of reading them, Folz offers valuable medical information. Print could facilitate the spread of disease, but it could also combat it.

By outlining the medical risks of printed vernacular texts, Folz anticipates a more substantial medical discourse in the sixteenth century that warns readers about the misinformation contained within vernacular herbals. In a 1534 vernacular treatise on the medicine theriac, the Marburg physician Euricius Cordus (1486–1535) complains about German-language herbals that "cause considerable damage among the ignorant people, who, having read these books, think they're doctors and become murderers many times over."[49] Printed herbals, Cordus claims, enable uneducated and unqualified readers to practice medicine, with fatal consequences for those they treat. The "ignorant people" Cordus discusses does not connote illiteracy. On the contrary, Cordus links these murderers with the ability to read the vernacular. We are dealing with a social group that is literate, though not Latinate, and wealthy enough to be able to afford books. This audience resembles the intended readership of Folz's prose treatise: they read books in the vernacular, have the resources to consult medical professionals, and their interest in medicine extends beyond survival strategies into more theoretical, disciplinary questions. Folz does not mention the risks of vernacular books in his verse treatise at all, perhaps because the "common man" he addresses in this work—poor, rural, and less literate—would have less access to the books in question than the audience of his prose treatise. If they cannot visit an apothecary, they are unlikely to visit a bookseller. Printed texts present less of a danger to this audience than to more literate, urban, wealthier consumers.

Folz's attention to audience in these two plague treatises reveals the precarious position vernacular print occupied for fifteenth-century medical writers. This new technology allowed information on plague to reach a wider audience than manuscripts had allowed, and writers like Folz employ strategies like verse and woodcuts to take advantage of the broad reach of print. At the same time, the democratization of information that print promised presented significant risk. Especially in a medical context, printing errors or the literate but insufficiently learned reader's misuse of information could cost lives. By attending carefully to the different needs of the audiences of his two plague treatises, Folz demonstrates how a responsible medical writer and printer might mitigate the risk that vernacular print presents while profiting from its expanding audience. For the less literate audience of his verse treatise, he concentrates on simple, practical solutions and is not concerned that this audience will have been misled by competing voices. His prose treatise, though—aimed at a more literate, wealthier, and more ambitious readership—must directly address the risks of consulting quacks or certain vernacular texts. In these two treatises, Folz demonstrates how different the vernacular audiences of medical texts could be, as the spread of print presented different benefits and risks for different groups of consumers. The choices Folz makes concerning what information to include in his two treatises and how best to present information for different audiences show one approach to the popularization of medical information in the second half of the fifteenth century.

Brunschwig's Plague Treatise: The Book as Ersatz Doctor

Folz's treatises are a particularly germane case study of the stumbling blocks writers and publishers faced in combating plague with the printed word. The tension between, on the one hand, a programmatic desire to expand the audience of plague texts beyond the wealthy and educated and, on the other, the need to tailor different works to the needs of different audiences is to some extent reflected in the genre of the printed plague treatise as a whole. Similar issues come to the fore in a 1500 plague treatise by the Strasbourg surgeon Hieronymus Brunschwig. Unlike Folz, who distills his information into separate treatises for separate (but overlapping) audiences, Brunschwig presents his work as a catch-all book for learned and less learned, urban and rural, wealthier and poorer audiences. There is a financial calculus here—the more potential consumers a book has, the more copies can be sold—but this is also a medical decision. Plague threatens all social classes, so any effort to combat it must account for the differences in literacy and in financial resources that potential victims of the disease may face.

Brunschwig's books were tremendously successful and most of them explicitly target a broad audience. Born in Strasbourg around 1450, Brunschwig spent a large period of his life as a military doctor in Alsace, Swabia, and Bavaria, before settling back in Strasbourg, where he obtained the post of city surgeon.[50] He authored a series of medical textbooks at the turn of the sixteenth century, including his *Buch der Cirurgia*, a manual for apprentice surgeons, and his *Liber de arte distillandi*, a work on pharmacological distillation. In all of these works, all written in German, Brunschwig seems interested in making medical knowledge available to as wide an audience as possible. Brunschwig's *Liber pestilentialis* is a forty-leaf volume in folio format that provides primarily prophylactic information on the plague. Like Folz's verse treatise, and most other vernacular plague treatises, Brunschwig cites the "common man" as the intended audience of the work. He also, however, targets the book at learned doctors and apprentice barber-surgeons. Indeed, the book should be suitable for "anyone" who "desires to learn … how to recognize an approaching epidemic or general principles of how to lead one's life."[51] Brunschwig's intended audience spans the entire social spectrum and includes more and less literate, urban and rural consumers alike. It should also be of use both to other medical practitioners and to the lay reader.

We have seen how we might read Folz's verse treatise as a stand-in for a medical practitioner. Brunschwig is more explicit about the fact that his book should play the role of doctor and replace the barber-surgeon himself, and there is a reason for this. In times of plague, Brunschwig writes, healers should avoid physically treating patients and instead just give advice, as the risk of infection is simply too great for doctors and their households.[52] At the end of the treatise, Brunschwig explains that he is about to leave Strasbourg and has left this book, "so as to not harm those who asked me to write it."[53] He thus envisions his book as a replacement for the practitioner: a book which, in the absence of Brunschwig himself, can perform all the professional responsibilities of the city surgeon, including providing advice and treatment for the citizens of Strasbourg, as well as instructing apprentices and less experienced practitioners. Brunschwig shows how printed books could function as ersatz medical professionals.

His treatise also shows a problem with this, however: books cannot perform the dual roles of the doctor at the same time—to teach students or apprentices, and to treat patients—as these roles require different ways of arranging, presenting, and disseminating information. Similarly, different audiences require different kinds of information on plague—an expensive remedy is of no use to a reader who cannot afford it. To support his aim of providing useful information for a broad audience, Brunschwig targets various remedies at various social groups. He divides the remedies that he prescribes into three categories: "Some fancy ones for the lords, some middling ones for the townspeople, and some for the common people in the countryside who can't reach an apothecary."[54] He provides recipes for the elites, for the urban citizenry, and for peasants. For instance, when discussing substances to burn in order to purify the air in times of plague, Brunschwig includes three recipes: the first is a recipe in Latin that includes Armenian bole and *terra sigillata* and is aimed at the wealthy. This is followed by a second recipe in Latin with less expensive ingredients such as turpentine and cloves. The reader is encouraged to copy out this recipe (in apothecary notation) and send it to the apothecary, suggesting a literate, urban target audience. The third recipe is in German and includes juniper and laurel roots and the sap of a plum tree. Brunschwig explains that this recipe is "for those in the countryside who do not have an apothecary or cannot reach one."[55] At one point, he even graciously offers to give a prophylactic powder to any poor Strasbourg residents who cannot afford to purchase it themselves (although one wonders how Brunschwig actually intended to fulfil this offer, given he planned to leave the city).[56] Brunschwig explicitly attempts to provide medical knowledge that is applicable and relevant to different social strata, as well as to poorer residents of both city and countryside. However, including information intended for a less literate, poorer, or more rural audience is one thing; presenting it in a way that is readily accessible to that audience is another question entirely.

Brunschwig's works have generally been viewed as examples of new vernacular, artisanal texts intended to communicate practical competences to a non-Latinate readership.[57] However, as I have argued elsewhere in reference to Brunschwig's 1500 *Small Book of Distillation*, sometimes the form of Brunschwig's book itself stands in the way of its practical usefulness to this audience.[58] The same is true of Brunschwig's plague treatise. The form of the book—the plague treatise is rather lengthy and is written in dense prose—suggests this less literate audience would have had great difficulty reading it. Brunschwig acknowledges this problem in the summary of the work. Reflecting on his intended audience, he admits the book so far has failed to meet his goal of producing a work on plague accessible to a wide audience of less literate and less wealthy consumers:

> If someone were to say that these teachings or lessons were in no way comprehensible for the common man in the countryside, or were scarcely comprehensible to him, truly they would not be wrong. … Because I said at the start of this

> book that I was writing for the common man and for the appreciation of my dear lords and citizens, I have extended my teachings and made them incomprehensible for the unknowing and unlearned. So, I want to make them available to their hands and minds in an intelligible manner in this summary. I hope that everyone, however little they can read and write, can be instructed in this way in what they desire to know.[59]

Brunschwig juxtaposes two target groups of his work in this passage: the "common man in the countryside"—a subsection of society he suggests is not fully literate and lives in more rural areas—and the citizens and social elites of Strasbourg, his "dear lords and citizens," who are presumably urban, relatively wealthy, and literate in German. Even if this first audience is an important target, Brunschwig admits to not having produced a work that is accessible to them because of the way he has "extended" these teachings for the more elite audience. By attempting to make his book a thorough teacher of medicine, Brunschwig admits, he has made the work less able to function as an effective doctor for a more rural and less literate public. To address the inaccessibility of his work to this less literate audience, Brunschwig introduces an abridged summary of the work, which spans two leaves and reiterates the key points of his treatise. He relates the importance of prayer and lists a few important measures, such as dispelling foul air by burning incense, where and when to let blood, and a small number of basic pills that a sufferer might take.

Nevertheless, even this summary falls short of its announced goal of accessibility. While this information would no doubt have had some medical use for its recipients, there is very little in this section of specific use to those without easy access to apothecaries or medical practitioners. All of Brunschwig's suggestions that specifically target a poor or rural audience, such as his juniper and laurel recipe, are buried within his dense prose. Moreover, Brunschwig's work itself would presumably have been fairly expensive. As the price of books in the fifteenth century was largely determined by the number of leaves and the size of the book, Brunschwig's text—printed in folio format, measuring 285 x 205 mm, and consisting of forty leaves—would have been significantly more expensive than more incidental publications on plague, such as broadsides or smaller pamphlets like Folz's. The high cost of Brunschwig's book contradicts his stated intention that it should be of use to the "common man in the countryside." At the very least, the "common man" would have been unlikely to buy the book outright.

Tillmann Taape has recently argued that Brunschwig's "common man" —the audience his books repeatedly claim to target—represents an "increasingly confident middling sort" that is literate, but not learned.[60] In his plague treatise, however, Brunschwig's common man occupies a lower social rank than this, perhaps representing differences in audience between works on epidemic disease and works on specific medical practices, like surgery and distillation.

At stake in the plague treatise is an audience whom vernacular books on less urgent and less life-threatening topics rarely address: the illiterate and rural poor. It is telling that Brunschwig should explicitly cite this audience in his plague treatise, even though the book's usefulness to less literate, less wealthy consumers is questionable. The discrepancies between his claims that the book should have a broad readership and the formal obstacles to the book's actual use by this readership show the difficulties authors and printers faced in producing treatises on plague that could be practically useful for both audiences and the more "common" audience to whom they hoped to expand their ideas.

There is a tension in a number of Brunschwig's works. They are invested in the common man's material engagement with the practices the books describe, yet the formal elements of the book—dense prose or unclear woodcuts—hinder this project. In the case of the plague book, Brunschwig aims to empower the less learned reader to transfer the book's contents into actions and techniques that should ward off, or cure, the plague. Many of his works contain woodcuts of a striped figure representing the layman—a recurring figure whose stripes, in Taape's analysis, stand for the common man's status as half-learned—performing various medical or surgical practices.[61] In the plague treatise, woodcuts depict the striped layman making an electuary, letting blood, and even martyring St. Sebastian, the saint often invoked by plague sufferers (Figure 1.2). While this last example raises interesting questions about how the reader should engage with plague saints, generally speaking the woodcuts in this work depict practical tasks that the reader should be able to perform and may prompt the reader to imagine themselves in the roles depicted.

However, a number of these woodcuts do not make logical sense with the text that surrounds them. In fact, some of them might confuse certain practices for the less literate reader Brunschwig cites as a target audience. In the section on bloodletting, for example, Brunschwig, or his printer, Johannes Grüninger (1455–1531), includes a woodcut that depicts the striped layman letting a man's blood (Figure 1.3). The woodcut includes a short poem on a banderole: "You should have the blood of a sanguine man of thirty years old, so long as he chooses it." In the surrounding text, Brunschwig outlines a general procedure for letting blood, and explains which veins should be cut to address pain in certain areas, much in the same way as Folz does in his treatises. Brunschwig does not mention specific ages in this section of text, aside from stressing that "all people should have their blood let, unless they are under eleven or twelve."[62] It is curious, then, that the woodcut should discuss letting the blood of a thirty-year-old. Moreover, the use of the verb "hon" (to have) to describe the practitioner's actions rather than the more typical "lassen" (to let) suggests the woodcut is not actually depicting bloodletting. Combined with the reference to the patient's consent ("so long as he chooses it"), it suggests the

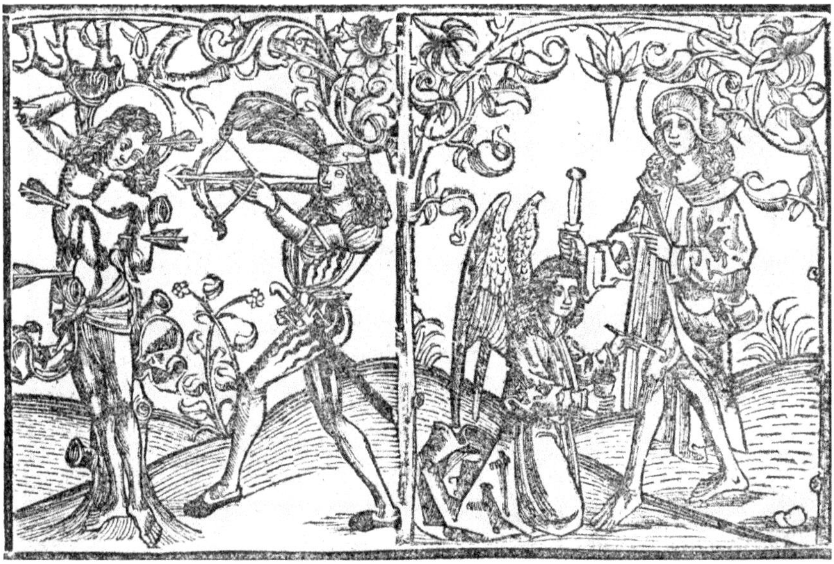

Figure 1.2. Woodcut of a striped figure shooting St. Sebastian alongside an image of St. Roch. Brunschwig, *Liber pestilentialis*, B5r. Countway Library of Medicine, Harvard University, HOLLIS ID 990093699060203941.

woodcut actually depicts blood harvesting for the benefit of the practitioner, rather than the patient.

The same woodcut also appears in Brunschwig's 1500 treatise on distillation, the *Liber de arte distillandi de simplicibus*. There, it appears in a catalogue of substances that can be distilled, alongside plants and animal by-products, in a section in which Brunschwig describes how to distill human blood and feces and the medical uses of the distillates derived from these substances. This woodcut fits more logically in the context of the distillation treatise: the text in its banderole can be plausibly interpreted as describing whose blood would make the most suitable distillate and stressing that the donor must consent to the procedure. In the plague treatise, this woodcut muddies the waters, conflating the prophylactic practice of bloodletting with the pharmacological practice of distilling blood.

We cannot know whether readers were actually misled by this woodcut—given how ubiquitous bloodletting was in early modern dietetics, it is unlikely a reader would look at this woodcut and assume only thirty-year-old men with a sanguine constitution should have their blood let. However, the awkward juxtaposition of the woodcut with the surrounding text shows the multivalence of Brunschwig's and Grüninger's approaches toward the uses

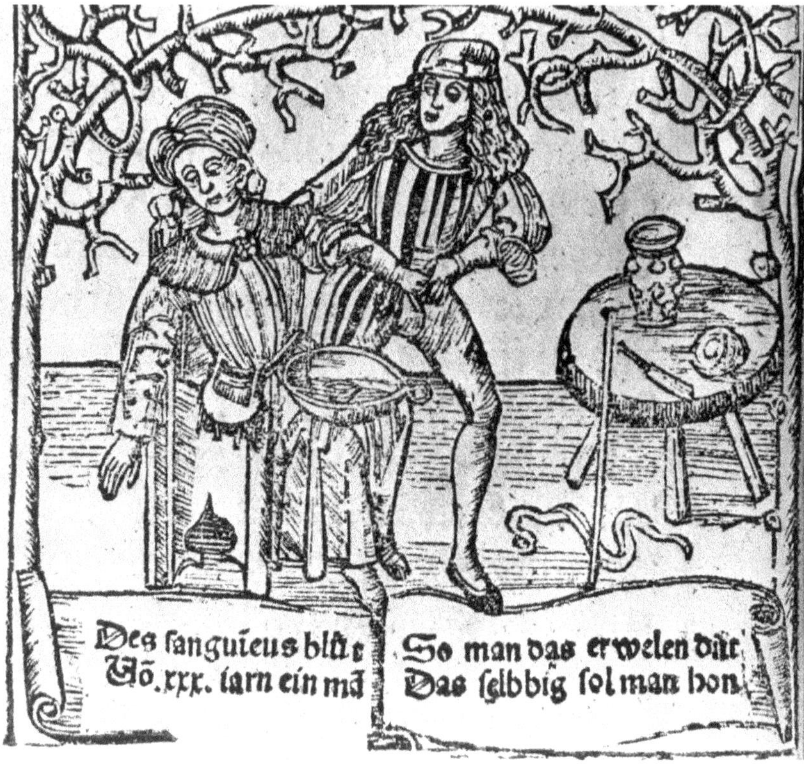
Des sanguieus blůte
Vō.xxx. iarn ein mā
So man das erwelen dût
Das selbbig sol man hon

Figure 1.3. Woodcut of a striped figure drawing blood from a patient. Brunschwig, *Liber pestilentialis*, F1v. NLM ID 2211022R, National Library of Medicine, Bethesda, public domain.

and effects of printed pictures in communicating actionable information on medical treatment to a wide audience.[63] It was common practice for printers to reuse woodcuts in various contexts, and they frequently sold and traded woodblocks with other printers. Johannes Grüninger, the printer of most of Brunschwig's treatises, is no exception, and he frequently reused woodcuts from various sources.[64] Nevertheless, the decisions printers (and, perhaps, writers) made to include particular woodcuts in certain contexts are meaningful editorial choices. Woodcuts can decorate certain passages or elucidate particular phenomena. Sometimes they confuse and obscure certain pieces of information. While we might read Brunschwig's and Grüninger's use of woodcuts, which sometimes include short poems in rhyme, as evidence for their concern with making their plague treatise more accessible to a less literate audience, a reader who focuses primarily on the information contained within this treatise's woodcuts could derive little usable information on preventing and treating plague.

There is a disconnect in Brunschwig's treatise between his expressed desire to provide useful medical information for the "common man in the countryside" and the formal constraints of the printed prose treatise itself. Brunschwig intends his text both to allow its audience—literate and illiterate, rich and poor, urban and rural—to assume a level of responsibility for their own medical treatment, and simultaneously to function as a teaching manual for apprentice practitioners. In other words, he intends, as we have seen, for the printed book to function as an ersatz doctor, fulfilling both the therapeutic and pedagogical duties of the city doctor. His plague treatise, Brunschwig claims, can replace the doctor as a teaching aid. The work is a rich and thorough compendium of all facets of medical knowledge concerning the plague—it is perhaps the most encyclopedic of German-language plague incunabula. However, the ability of the book to replace the doctor as healer hinges on its ability to communicate practical solutions effectively to a general audience; that is, in its ability to overcome the hurdle of illiteracy. It also depends therefore on the appropriate selection of information, which is hard to reconcile with this work's encyclopedic qualities. While he does summarize several important pieces of advice in his concluding summary of the work, he buries a number of practical, simple recipes within the dense main body of prose. Perhaps he intends this information to be mediated by more literate readers, but he does not outline any model through which this would happen.

The different approaches Folz and Brunschwig take to the question of how best to present useful information on plague to a poorer and less literate audience demonstrate the ambivalent relationship medical writers had with new forms of print media. Print allowed text to be reproduced cheaply and distributed widely, enabling publications on important topics like plague to circulate in rural and less literate communities. Folz and Brunschwig recognize the public health benefits of this expanding network of knowledge distribution—printed works on plague can, at least in theory, reach a wider audience than manuscripts had previously allowed. They both employ formal strategies—verse, woodcuts, summaries—and specific types of information to enable their treatises to better reach this audience. However, each of these works attests to problems with and doubts about the ability of print to spread useful information on plague to this broad audience, although they highlight different problems. In Folz's case, print brings with it errata and misinformation that can cause medical harm. Producing medical treatises thus requires particular care to a work's audience to ensure it does not mislead particular groups of consumers. Brunschwig's treatise illustrates a particular tension between the book's stated aim to provide useful information for a less literate audience and the formal constraints of the book itself: the book's size, its dense prose, and some of its woodcuts stand in the way of the work's usability by this audience and cast doubt on print's ability to spread information widely in the first place.

Conclusion

In a master song from the 1480s, known as the "Song of Gutenberg," named after the Mainz goldsmith who introduced print to Europe, Folz reflects on the impact of print on the dissemination of information. The song consists of fourteen strophes that outline the effect print has had on the spread of religious learning: "It is clear what usefulness and worry has come from this craft."[65] Its effect has been both positive and negative. On the one hand, print has allowed all monasteries to own a copy of the Bible and has spread the word of the gospel far and wide. On the other hand, it has led to the proliferation of vernacular scripture, which "lead the world astray" by corrupting the authentic word of God. Weighing the benefit and harm brought by print, Folz concludes that this new media technology—despite the risks it presents—is a divine blessing bestowed on Germans: "The strength of God gave print to the German people." In the "Song of Gutenberg," Folz reflects more explicitly on the ambiguous impact of print than in his plague treatises. However, all of these works contain analogous concerns: the spread of print promotes the circulation of valuable information—religious teachings or medical advice—and so serves a common good. At the same time, the fast, uncontrolled spread of printed texts, especially those in the vernacular, increases the likelihood that mistakes and misinformation may also be circulating. When the stakes are so high—the reader's survival or their salvation—the consequence of these errors is grave.

Many plague writers tried to produce treatises that had something to offer to the whole spectrum of possible consumers for a vernacular text—from the rural poor to urban elites and medical professionals—as we saw in Brunschwig's treatise. Hans Folz's publication of two different treatises for different audiences is unique in the corpus of plague incunabula. His careful attention to the distinct needs and priorities of the consumers of these texts speaks to his unique perspective on the new technology of print. A printer, a writer, and a medical practitioner, Folz held an ambiguous opinion of the usefulness of vernacular print in spreading medical information. His equivocation anticipates later suspicions of new media in the field of medicine, from anonymous pamphlets on the 1529 epidemic of the English sweating sickness to social media posts advocating bogus cures for COVID-19. Not all medical writers saw the proliferation of print as a positive development. Folz's and Brunschwig's plague treatises highlight the ambivalent view some medical professionals held of new forms of media and the democratization of medicine they promised.

Christopher Hutchinson is Assistant Professor of German at the University of Mississippi. He received his PhD from Stanford University in 2019. His research interests include book history, the history of disease, and the popularization of scientific discourses in literature. He has published articles in *The German Quarterly* and in *Seminar*, and his book on print and epidemic disease in German medical writing and literary texts at the turn of the sixteenth century is forthcoming with the University of Delaware Press.

Notes

A version of this chapter also appears in Christopher Hutchinson, *Medical Misinformation in Early Modern Germany* (forthcoming with University of Delaware Press).

1. Folz, *Verse Treatise*, 11v. [*Reimpaarsprüche*, 427–28]. All translations my own unless otherwise stated.
2. The dismembering of texts and decontextualization of words and sentences by the popular reader also finds expression in the figure of Ginzburg's miller, Menocchio. See Ginzburg, *The Cheese and the Worms*, 33–41. Readerly fragmentation and decontextualization of textual passages was also key to elite reading practices. See Chartier, *Forms and Meanings*, 94–95.
3. There has been significant work on the oral reception of early printed texts. See, in particular, Chartier, *Cultural Uses of Print*; Chartier, "Orality Lost."
4. Engelsing, *Analphabetentum und Lektüre*, 20.
5. The disease struck most cities on average once a decade. Naphy and Spicer, *The Black Death*, 57.
6. Cohn, *Cultures of Plague*, 13.
7. See, for instance, Heinrichs, *Plague, Print and the Reformation*, 8.
8. Knape and Till, "Deutschland," 252.
9. Engelsing, *Analphabetentum und Lektüre*, 16. Heinrich Dormeier has claimed that vernacular plague treatises counted among the most widely read German-language printed works of the fifteenth century, as judged by the number of editions they went through and the signs of heavy use on the surviving copies. Dormeier, "St. Rochus," 33.
10. Dormeier, "St. Rochus," 33.
11. My calculations are drawn from Klebs's catalogue of plague incunabula. See Arnold C. Klebs, " Geschichtliche und bibliographische Untersuchungen."
12. Heinrichs, *Plague, Print, and the Reformation*. See also Esser, *Pest, Heilsangst und Frömmigkeit*.
13. Jardine, *Worldly Goods*, 34.
14. On the link between globalization and early modern commodity culture, see, in particular, Brook, *Vermeer's Hat*; Johnson, *German Discovery*.
15. See Giesecke, *Buchdruck*, 419.
16. Schenda, "Der 'gemeine' Mann," 20; Lutz, "Wer war der gemeine Mann?"
17. Roper, "Common Man," 18.
18. See Nutton, "Medicine in Medieval Western Europe," 200. Katharine Park has traced this empirical flourishing into the sixteenth century with particular reference to Italian literature on healing springs. See Park, "Natural Particulars," esp. 360–61.

19. Jacquart, "Three Fifteenth-Century Physicians," 160.
20. Leong, *Recipes.*
21. Carmichael, "The Last Past Plague," 133.
22. Ursula Rautenberg has calculated that Folz spent no more than twenty-two days per year printing. Rautenberg, "Das Werk als Ware," 27–31. Rautenberg bases this calculation on the time she estimates it would have taken Folz to print the forty-one texts attributed to his workshop. However, thirty-six of these forty-one works survive in only one copy, and Rautenberg estimates an average print run for a work by Folz would have consisted of between 150 and 500 copies. This suggests Folz may have printed many more works that have since been lost, and it is almost impossible to estimate the total number of works that Folz printed.
23. Folz, *Verse Treatise,* 6v [*Reimpaarsprüche,* 419]. Folz, *Prose Treatise,* 21r [*Reimpaarsprüche,* 435].
24. Folz, *Prose Treatise,* 1v–2r. [*Reimpaarsprüche,* 429].
25. Folz, *Beichtspiegel,* 2r. [*Reimpaarsprüche,* 188]. Fritz Langensiepen has argued the *Reimpaarspruch* is "the optimal form for instructing the popular masses and the laity." Langensiepen, *Tradition und Vermittlung,* 38.
26. Brian Murdoch reaches a similar conclusion in his study of Folz's two versions of the Adam legend: like the plague treatises, one is in prose, the other is in rhymed couplets. He has argued that Folz conceived of the prose version of the legend as a text for private consumption and the verse version as a text for public consumption. Murdoch, *Hans Folz and the Adam Legends,* 33.
27. Folz, *Verse Treatise,* 11v. [*Reimpaarsprüche,* 427].
28. Langensiepen, *Tradition und Vermittlung,* 37; Krohn, "Hans Folz," 119. The Nuremberg *Stadtrat* was known to give out modest sums to literary works dedicated to it, although very infrequently. In the seventeenth century, the *Stadtrat* even threatened poet Wilhelm Weber with punishment if he did not stop dedicating poems to the council in the hope of financial reward. See Reichel, *Der Spruchdichter,* 157.
29. Reichel, *Der Spruchdichter,* 108.
30. Reichel, *Der Spruchdichter,* 159–60.
31. Folz, *Verse Treatise,* 8r [*Reimpaarsprüche,* 422].
32. Folz, *Prose Treatise,* 16r [*Reimpaarsprüche,* 437].
33. Langensiepen, *Tradition und Vermittlung,* 38.
34. Folz, *Verse Treatise,* 9v [*Reimpaarsprüche,* 424].
35. Folz, *Prose Treatise,* 7r [*Reimpaarsprüche,* 432].
36. Heinrichs, *Plague, Print, and the Reformation,* 24.
37. Folz, *Prose Treatise,* 9r–v [*Reimpaarsprüche,* 433].
38. Folz, *Prose Treatise,* 9v [*Reimpaarsprüche,* 433].
39. Folz, *Prose Treatise,* 10r [*Reimpaarsprüche,* 433].
40. Rautenberg, "Das Werk als Ware," 33.
41. Fuchs, "Hartmann Schedel als Arzt," 77.
42. Nummedal, *Alchemy and Authority,* 9; Moran, *The Alchemical World*; Stolberg, "Learning"; Rankin, *Panaceia's Daughters*; Nummedal, *Anna Zieglerin.*
43. Heinrichs, *Plague, Print, and the Reformation,* 40.
44. See, for instance, Cordus, *Von der vielfaltigen Tugend*; Cordus, *Von der kunst.*
45. Folz, *Regiment vnd Ertzney,* A1r.

46. Jurina, *Quacksalber*, 167.
47. Huey, *Hans Folz*, ch. 2.
48. Folz, *Prose Treatise*, 15v–16r [*Reimpaarsprüche*, 437].
49. Cordus, *Von der vielfaltigen Tugend*, A3r.
50. Sigerist, "Hieronymus Brunschwig and his Work," V.
51. Brunschwig, *Liber pestilentialis*, G5r.
52. Brunschwig, *Liber pestilentialis*, A2v.
53. Brunschwig, *Liber pestilentialis*, G6r.
54. Brunschwig, *Liber pestilentialis*, D2v.
55. Brunschwig, *Liber pestilentialis*, D2v.
56. Brunschwig, *Liber pestilentialis*, F1r.
57. Taape, "Common Medicine," 2; Rankin, "Golden Vein," 121.
58. Hutchinson, "Printing Things," 210.
59. Brunschwig, *Liber Pestilentialis*, G5r.
60. Taape, "Common Medicine," 2.
61. Taape, "Common Medicine," 23.
62. Brunschwig, *Liber Pestilentialis*, XXVIr.
63. See Hutchinson, "Printing Things."
64. Zimmermann-Homeyer, *Illustrierte Frühdrucke*.
65. Folz, "Gutenberglied." See also Flood, "Hans Folz," 14–18.

Bibliography

Primary Sources

Brunschwig, Hieronymus. *Liber Pestilentialis*. Strasbourg: Johann Grüninger, 1500. GW 05596.

Cordus, Euricius. *Von der vielfaltigen tugent vnnd waren bereitung / Deß rechten edlen Theriacs*. Marburg, 1532. VD16 C 5108.

Cordus, Euricius. *Von der kunst auch missbrauch vnd trug des harnsehens*. Magdeburg, 1536. VD16 C 5105.

Folz, Hans. *Die Reimpaarsprüche*, edited by Heinz Fischer. Munich: Beck, 1961.

Folz, Hans. "Gutenberglied," translated by Christopher Hutchinson, Stanford Global Medieval Sourcebook. Retrieved 28 May 2021 from https://sourcebook.stanford.edu/text/folz-gutenberg.

Folz, Hans. *Item ein fast köstlicher spruch von der pestilencz* (=Verse Treatise). Nuremberg: Hans Folz, 1482. GW 10146.

Folz, Hans. *Item von der pestilencz ein hübsch nüczlich vnd kurcz begriffes tractetlin* (=Prose Treatise). Nuremberg: Hans Folz, 1482. GW 10111.

Folz, Hans. *Ain seer gut nützlich vnd cöstlich Regiment vnd Ertzney / wider die Pestilentz / vnd andere Pestilentzische Fieber*. Vienna: Johann Singriener the Elder, 1530. VD16 F 1779.

Folz, Hans. *Von der beichte* (=Beichtspiegel). Nuremberg: Hans Folz, 1479. GW 10116.

Ortolff von Baierland. *Artzneybuch*. Augsburg: Anton Sorg, 1479. GW M28456.

Steinhöwel, Heinrich. *Büchlein der Ordnung der Pestilentz*. Ulm: Johann Zainer, 1473. GW M43865.

Secondary Sources

Brook, Timothy, *Vermeer's Hat: The Seventeenth Century and the Dawn of the Global World.* New York: Bloomsbury, 2008.

Carmichael, Ann. "The Last Past Plague: The Uses of Memory in Renaissance Epidemics." *Journal of the History of Medicine and Allied Sciences* 53, no. 2 (May 1998): 132–60.

Chartier, Roger. *The Author's Hand and the Printer's Mind*, translated by Lydia Cochrane. Princeton: Princeton University Press, 2014.

Chartier, Roger. *The Cultural Uses of Print in Early Modern France*, translated by Lydia Cochrane. Princeton: Princeton University Press, 1987.

Chartier, Roger. *Forms and Meanings: Texts, Performances and Audiences from Codex to Computer*. Philadelphia: University of Pennsylvania Press, 1995.

Chartier, Roger. "Orality Lost: Text and Voice in the Sixteenth and Seventeenth Centuries." In *Across Boundaries: The Book in Culture and Commerce*, edited by Jonquil Bevan et al., 1–28. Winchester, UK: St. Paul's Bibliographies, 2000.

Cohn, Samuel K., Jr. *Cultures of Plague: Medical Thinking at the End of the Renaissance.* Oxford: Oxford University Press, 2009.

Dormeier, Heinrich. "St. Rochus, die Pest und die Imhoffs in Nürnberg vor und während der Reformation. Ein spätgotischer Altar in seinem religiös-liturgischen, wirtschaftlich-rechtlichen und sozialen Umfeld." *Anzeiger des germanischen Nationalmuseums* (1985): 7–72.

Engelsing, Rolf. *Analphabetentum und Lektüre. Zur Sozialgeschichte des Lesens in Deutschland zwischen feudaler und industrieller Gesellschaft.* Stuttgart: J. B. Metzler, 1973.

Esser, Thilo. *Pest, Heilsangst und Frömmigkeit. Studien zur religiösen Bewältigung der Pest am Ausgang des Mittelalters.* Altenberge: Oros, 1999.

Flood, John L. "Hans Folz zwischen Handschriftenkultur und Buchdruckerkunst." In *Texttyp und Textproduktion in der deutschen Literatur des Mittelalters*, edited by Elizabeth Andersen, Manfred Eikelmann, and Anne Simon, 1–27. Berlin: De Gruyter, 2005.

Fuchs, Franz. "Hartmann Schedel als Arzt in Nördlingen, Amberg und Nürnberg." In *Welten des Wissens. Die Bibliothek und die Weltchronik des Nürnberger Arztes Hartmann Schedel (1440–1514)*, edited by the Bavarian State Library, 74–77. Munich: Allitera, 2014.

Giesecke, Michael. *Der Buchdruck in der frühen Neuzeit.* Frankfurt am Main: Suhrkamp, 1991.

Ginzburg, Carlo. *The Cheese and the Worms: The Cosmos of a Sixteenth-Century Miller*, translated by John and Anne Tedeschi. Baltimore: Johns Hopkins University Press, 1980.

Heinrichs, Erik A. *Plague, Print and the Reformation: The German Reform of Healing, 1473–1573.* London: Routledge, 2017.

Huey, Caroline. *Hans Folz and Print Culture in Late Medieval Germany. The Creation of Popular Discourse.* Farnham: Ashgate, 2012.

Hutchinson, Christopher. "Printing Things: Materiality and Immateriality in Hieronymus Brunschwig's *Liber de arte distillandi de simplicibus.*" In *Things and Thingness in European Literature and Visual Art, 700–1600*, edited by Jutta Eming and Kathryn Starkey, 193–210. Berlin: De Gruyter, 2022.

Jacquart, Danielle. "Theory, Everyday Practice, and Three Fifteenth-Century Physicians." *Osiris* 6 (1990): 140–60.

Jardine, Lisa. *Worldly Goods: A New History of the Renaissance.* New York: Doubleday, 1996.

Johnson, Christine. *The German Discovery of the World: Renaissance Encounters with the Strange and Marvelous.* Charlottesville: University of Virginia Press, 2008.

Jurina, Kitti. *Vom Quacksalber zum Doctor Medicinae. Die Heilkunde in der deutschen Graphik des 16. Jahrhunderts.* Cologne/Vienna: Böhlau, 1985.
Klebs, Arnold C. "Geschichtliche und bibliographische Untersuchungen." In *Die ersten gedruckten Pestschriften,* edited by Arnold C. Klebs and Karl Sudhoff, 1–167. Munich: Verlag der Münchner Drucke, 1926.
Knape, Joachim, and Dietmar Till. "Deutschland." In *Geschichte der Buchkultur,* vol. 6, *Renaissance,* edited by Alfred Noe, 231–304. Graz: Akademische Druck- und Verlagsanstalt, 2008.
Krohn, Rüdiger. "Hans Folz." In *Deutsche Dichter der frühen Neuzeit (1450–1600): ihr Leben und Werk,* edited by Stephan Füssel, 111–24. Berlin: Erich Schmidt, 1993.
Langensiepen, Fritz. *Tradition und Vermittlung. Literaturgeschichtliche und didaktische Untersuchungen zu Hans Folz.* Berlin: Schmidt, 1980.
Leong, Elaine. *Recipes and Everyday Knowledge: Medicine, Science, and the Household in Early Modern England.* Chicago: University of Chicago Press, 2018.
Lutz, Robert H. *Wer war der gemeine Mann? Der dritte Stand in der Krise des Spätmittelalters.* Munich: Oldenburg, 1979.
Moran, Bruce T. *The Alchemical World of the German Court: Occult Philosophy and Chemical Medicine in the Circle of Moritz of Hessen (1572–1632).* Stuttgart: Steiner, 1991.
Murdoch, Brian. *Hans Folz and the Adam Legends: Texts and Studies.* Amsterdam: Rodopi, 1977.
Naphy, William G., and Andrew Spicer. *The Black Death and the History of Plagues 1345–1730.* Stroud: Tempus Publishing Ltd, 2000.
Nummedal, Tara. *Alchemy and Authority in the Holy Roman Empire.* Chicago: The University of Chicago Press, 2007.
Nummedal, Tara. *Anna Zieglerin and the Lion's Blood: Alchemy and the End Times in Reformation Germany.* Philadelphia: University of Pennsylvania Press, 2019.
Nutton, Vivian. "Medicine in Medieval Western Europe, 1000–1500." In *The Western Medical Tradition. 800 BC to AD 1800,* by Lawrence I. Conrad et al., 139–205. Cambridge: Cambridge University Press, 1995.
Park, Katharine. "Natural Particulars: Medical Epistemology, Practice, and the Literature of Healing Springs." In *Natural Particulars: Nature and the Disciplines in Renaissance Europe,* edited by Anthony Grafton and Nancy Siraisi, 347–67. Cambridge, MA: MIT Press, 1999.
Rankin, Alisha. *Panaceia's Daughters: Noblewomen as Healers in Early Modern Germany.* Chicago: The University of Chicago Press, 2013.
Rankin, Alisha. "How to Cure the Golden Vein: Medical Remedies as Wissenschaft in Early Modern Germany." In *Ways of Making and Knowing: The Material Culture of Empirical Knowledge,* edited by Pamela H. Smith, Amy R. W. Meyers, and Harold J. Cook, 113–37. New York: Bard Graduate Center, 2014.
Rautenberg, Ursula. "Das Werk als Ware. Der Nürnberger Kleindrucker Hans Folz." *Internationales Archiv für Sozialgeschichte der deutschen Literatur* 24, no. 1 (1999): 1–40.
Reichel, Jörn. *Der Spruchdichter Hans Rosenplüt. Literatur und Leben im spätmittelalterlichen Nürnberg.* Stuttgart: Franz Steiner, 1985.
Roper, Lyndal. "'The Common Man', 'The Common Good', 'Common Women': Gender and Meaning in the German Reformation Commune." *Social History* 12, no. 1 (1987), 1–21.
Schenda, Rudolf. "Der 'gemeine Mann' und sein medikales Verhalten im 16. und 17. Jahrhundert." In *Pharmazie und der gemeine Mann. Hausarznei und Apotheke in der frühen Neuzeit,* edited by Joachim Telle, 9–20. Braunschweig: Waisenhaus, 1982.

Sigerist, Henry E. "Hieronymus Brunschwig and his Work." In *The Book of Cirurgia by Hieronymus Brunschwig*, edited by Henry E. Sigerist, I–XVI. Milan: R. Lier, 1923.

Stolberg, Michael. "Learning from the Common Folks. Academic Physicians and Medical Lay Culture in the Sixteenth Century." *Social History of Medicine* 27, no. 4 (2014): 649–67.

Taape, Tillman. "Common Medicine for the Common Man: Picturing the 'Striped Layman' in Early Vernacular Print." *Renaissance Quarterly* 74, no. 1 (2021): 1–58.

Zimmermann-Homeyer, Catarina. *Illustrierte Frühdrucke lateinischer Klassiker um 1500: Innovative Illustrationskonzepte aus der Straßburger Offizin Johannes Grüningers und ihre Wirkung*. Wiesbaden: Harrassowitz, 2018.

CHAPTER 2

The Ethics of Surviving Plague

Political, Social, and Moral Considerations in Sixteenth-Century German Plague Texts

PETER HESS

Introduction: Plague and Print

Living with plague was a common reality in Germany from 1348 until the early eighteenth century. In Nuremberg and elsewhere in Germany, plague commonly occurred approximately every ten to twelve years.[1] Some outbreaks were massive, others mild; some affected large regions, others spread only locally. Patterns of plague outbreaks changed after 1500 as a sharper bias became apparent. Plague became more regional, appearing and disappearing at different times in different regions. Cities tended to be hardest hit, and here the poor were more likely to be infected and die than the rich. During the plague of 1437–39, for instance around thirteen thousand persons died in Nuremberg and surroundings.[2] Plague mortalities decreased after 1500, but there are notable exceptions to this trend.[3] The city of Nuremberg, one of the largest in Germany with perhaps as many as forty thousand residents in the sixteenth century, was hit repeatedly after 1500.[4] Notable were the outbreaks of 1533 with over 8,000 deaths,[5] of 1562–63 with 9,034 recorded deaths,[6] and of 1574–75 that claimed over 6,500 lives.[7]

Managing plague to prevent or survive outbreaks and to increase general resilience therefore became an existential concern. Early moderns had no clear understanding of bacteriology and epidemiology, yet their pragmatic observations allowed for two generalizations. First, there was some form of contagion in play that made possible both interhuman transmission and indirect transmission through cloth and other objects. Second, there was a keen sense that plague was associated with place and that outbreaks could be highly localized, based on the observation that not all locations were afflicted with plague equally, which furthered the idea that plague was transmitted by miasma or other contamination of the environment.[8]

Italian city-states established fairly detailed plague ordinances in the sixteenth century, but the standardized Italian models were not copied consistently in Germany until the middle of the seventeenth century.[9] This chapter will show how Nuremberg, a major German city, struggled with establishing consistent rules, although a trend toward standardized rules is evident. While measures against plague were haphazard around 1500, we see the gradual formation of a canon of preventative measures and of public policies designed to manage outbreaks of the disease in the sixteenth century.

With the advent of book printing, published plague texts, many of them just brief pamphlets, became an increasingly important tool to respond to this perennial threat. Plague benefited the spread of the printing press, which in turn helped create awareness of plague and disseminate information on how to prevent or fight the disease. While plague statutes and ordinances inform us about specific actions taken by governing bodies, plague texts give us more comprehensive insights into thinking about plague in the early modern period.

German physicians started to publish vernacular literature to advise local people on preventing and curing the plague.[10] The growing demand for such pamphlets allowed both physicians and printers to profit from outbreaks of plague. Inversely, the rapid expansion of vernacular print had notable effects on medicine,[11] allowing physicians to peddle their own remedies to generate additional income. The physician Caspar Kegler (ca. 1461–1537) promoted his own medicines that, in his own words, "are the most reliable amongst all medicines since I experienced their effectiveness, whenever I experimented with them."[12]

Plague texts fall into three broad categories. (1) Devotional and religious texts offered consolation and spiritual support in adverse times but also focused on the divine hand guiding outbreaks of the plague. (2) Medical texts focused on how infection could be avoided by protecting house and body against invading toxic vapors and miasmas, and on how the disease could be diagnosed and treated, although there was no unified medical understanding of plague in the early modern period.[13] (3) Texts focusing on public policy dealt with the role of urban and territorial governments to prepare for and manage pandemics, but they also provided behavioral advice for individuals, a distinction that holds for the other two areas as well. The focus of these texts could vary, alternatively dealing with institutional issues, cleanliness of private dwellings and public spaces, avoidance of large assemblies of people, isolation of infected people, and extramural treatment and burials.[14]

Few texts focused on one area only; if so, they were mostly religious texts, which are not the main focus here. Texts in the other two categories were mostly written by university-trained physicians, yet typically referred to religious and spiritual dimensions of plague in introductions or dedications. While this chapter is mainly interested in the third area, that of public policy, we have to consider that the three broad themes blended into each other, just as there was no clear demarcation between natural aspects of epidemics and those related to chastisement by God.[15] While the faithful may have been summoned to church to pray for forgiveness and the end of plague, churches were also fumigated before and after service to prevent the spread of plague.[16] Furthermore, not just clergy but also secular authorities castigated perceived lapses in morality, and "governmental regulations continued to take seriously the religious response to plague as part of a broader civic concern."[17] The introduction to the semi-official Nuremberg plague pamphlet *Ein kurtz Regiment für den gepresten der pestilentz* (A brief primer for the disease of pestilence) from 1520 admonishes citizens to "reconcile with God your creator, as the righteous, veritable physician of souls and bodies."[18]

Erik Heinrichs identified 392 vernacular German plague books and pamphlets that were printed between 1473 and 1573, and an additional 551 texts printed by 1682. German plague texts became widespread during the Reformation in the 1520s, peaked in the 1560s, remained prolific until the 1620s,[19] but declined later in the century, along with plague outbreaks. In Nuremberg alone, dozens of such texts were published, with a peak during the plague outbreak of 1562.[20]

While many of these texts are derivative and appeared in similar form in different cities, they tended to consider local circumstances and address local audiences, which is why this chapter focuses on about fifty texts with a Nuremberg connection. I am interested in how plague narratives evolved, how a clear set of public policy tools emerged in this period, and how ethical concerns and moral dilemmas were addressed. This chapter will be framed in a temporary sense by contributions from two literary writers: Hans Folz in 1482 and Hans Sachs in 1563.

The Origin of Plague: Divine Punishment versus Natural Causes

The idea that plague was God's punishment for an immoral and godless life and for the loss of faith is one of the staples of all plague texts in the early modern period. While many texts only generically addressed this in their introductions, some writers enumerated specific sinful moral failings. The influential Nuremberg council member Lazarus Spengler (1479–1534) held those responsible who were seduced by "worldly enchantment and prosperity" to indulge in "pride, physical lust, and many other evils" and who "entirely forget about God their lord, creator, and sustainer, abuse His gifts, and despise

His word, will, and commands."[21] Like many writers in the early years of the sixteenth century, Caspar Kegler berated the growing influence of foreign fashions, manners, and even speech patterns that displaced a more wholesome, modest, and virtuous German way of life. Moreover, Kegler placed plague into a Reformation context by denouncing confessional divisions and the rise of the Lutheran faith as the work of the devil.[22]

It was generally agreed that plague did not target individuals but, rather, entire communities, and that plague indiscriminately struck the good as much as the evil, the young and the old, the rich and the poor. God's punishment was directed at humanity, not at individuals. This becomes evident in letters of consolation where the death of an individual had to be accepted as a mystery. The Nuremberg patrician Sebastian Imhoff (1511–72), for instance, commented on a friend's passing from plague in a 1562 letter: "Because it is the will of God, one must commend the situation to him. Whatever God allows here on earth is most fitting."[23]

Martin Luther's influential 1527 pamphlet, *Whether One May Flee from a Deadly Plague*, stressed the dual function of plague; it was God's punishment for sin, but also a test for the faithful. The idea that God's punishment afflicted all humans, good Christian people as well as godless and evil ones, was promoted both by followers of Luther and of the Roman Church. The Lutheran pastor Johannes Ulenbeck (fl. 1556) raised the same question, why the righteous died of plague just as the wicked did. He followed Luther's argument that plague also served as a test of faith:

> While death and pestilence appear to be horrible and cruel, they judge everybody's righteousness and explore the hearts of humankind, whether the healthy wanted to serve the sick, whether friends exercised neighborly love, whether masters had mercy on their sick servants, whether physicians abandoned their pleading patients. … For the Christians and followers of God, death serves to prepare their souls, through the contempt of death, for crown and glory.[24]

The physician Alexander Seitz (ca. 1473–ca. 1545) insisted, rather unconventionally, that the quick death brought on by plague should be seen as an act of mercy, since God let inflation, shorthand for famine and destitution, follow a course of the plague, which brought true horror and devastation: "In inflation there is crying and screaming toward God and all His Saints for grace and mercy. … O how blessed is this death, as Boethius says at the beginning of his book. Inflation thus makes humans eager and enraptured to die."[25]

Luther interpreted plague as an adversity in the world, like hunger and inclement weather, and admonished his contemporaries to vigorously fight it,[26] also with the use of medicines. To Luther, the strong divine hand behind the disease did not absolve individuals from the ethical obligation of rendering aid to those afflicted by the disease, particularly since sick people bore no individual responsibility for their infection. For Luther, taking care of the sick therefore was an act of neighborly love and amounted to a test of faith.[27] Even followers of the Roman Church, like the Tyrolean pastor Balthasar Conradinus (fl. 1562–94), agreed with this principle: "A human should help the other and definitely not abandon him like a badly bitten dog in dire need, even though this is a punishment from God."[28]

Nuremberg council member Lazarus Spengler, an early Luther supporter, urged Christians to endure all hardship and adversity with patience and constancy, knowing that they were part of God's will and judgment and imposed on humans as a healing medicine. He urged Christians to trust the divine promise "that all adversity, toil, labor, worries, and fear, and whatever God inflicts on them in this life, is not a damnation but rather a medicine, not a poison but a healing theriac."[29] However, this medicine, God's grace, was available only to believers: "While suffering, afflictions, and hardship are common to the pious and evil ones, only the godly ones who trust in God are preserved by it and delivered from it."[30] This view was shared by the Nuremberg preacher Veit Dietrich (1506–49). While God clearly used plague as a form of punishment—so his 1544 sermon on the 91st Psalm—God was gracious and benevolent towards those who accepted him. Where God's grace was in play, "neither the devil nor pestilence" could inflict harm.[31]

Spengler's text spoke to the desire of Nuremberg authorities to embed plague outbreaks in teachings about sin, repentance, and divine punishment in an attempt to promote social stability. Similarly, the preface of the semi-official but anonymous 1520 Nuremberg plague primer urged citizens to accept plague as part of a divine verdict:

> He who places his trust in God with a properly ordered faith will be able to accept joy and sorrow, happiness and difficulty, health and sickness, death and life exactly the same, and everything that happens to him in this life will be entirely joyous and agreeable. Fear of death does not scare him at all. Therefore, he is able to speak to God with a steadfast heart and spirit: for you I live, for you I die, yours I am, dead and alive.[32]

God also was a healer, yet his medicine was of a spiritual nature: "First seek the medicine of salvation from this doctor."[33] This was the foundation on which secular rules were pitched and indeed could be effective. Likewise, the Nuremberg preacher Wenzeslaus Link (1483–1547), an early promoter of the Lutheran doctrine, stated: "This is why God sends all kinds of plagues into the world, so that the godless will perish, and the faithful ones will be tested and saved through it. Amen."[34]

The Nuremberg theologian Andreas Osiander (1498–1552) argued in 1533 that both good and evil people died of plague, but that God took the evil ones prematurely as punishment and the pious ones at their right time as a reward. Death by plague therefore was just, which in Osiander's view not only removed the need to fight plague but made it a violation of God's commands: "Therefore such untimely fear and flight are truly against God's commands and nothing other than an indication of a great and severe disbelief, namely that one does not believe nor trust God that he can and wants to save."[35] Osiander created a dichotomy between scientific knowledge and divine knowledge, divine wisdom clearly being superior.[36] Thus he stood in clear opposition to medical and other secular authorities. His viewpoint was not reflected in plague texts of the time, which indicates that its influence was limited to the theological community. However, preachers like Osiander were at the source of conflict with secular authorities who wanted to limit attendance at church services and in funeral processions to curb infections.

Theological explanations rose in the immediate aftermath of the Lutheran Reform, which was introduced in Nuremberg in 1525. For most post-Reformation physicians, integrating theological and medical etiologies of plague became an increasingly difficult task. Their entire professional ethos was designed to use scientific insight to heal patients. Therefore, integrating the theological premise of disease as God's punishment required some delicate argumentation. If plague was God's punishment for an immoral and godless life and for the loss of faith, how should humans modify their behavior, and how could humans protect themselves against plague without defying God's will?

Even though plague could be seen as part of the providential order, the Christian view also created space for action, be it the search for scapegoats, the condemnation of poor and disreputable diseased persons, or attempts to address conditions that threatened moral and physical health.[37] For this reason, the relationship between divine will and natural vectors of disease was explored in many plague tracts to illuminate the questions what the punishment was for exactly, how humans could recognize God's will, and how God possibly could be pacified to avert an outbreak of plague. While plague commonly was seen as an expression of divine will, simultaneously a range of natural causes were identified to explain outbreaks of plague, such as toxic and putrid air or unfavorable planetary constellations.

The medical text by the physician Achilles Pirmin Gasser (1505–77), published in Nuremberg in 1544, can serve as an illustrative example for many others:

> For sure, according to Holy Scripture, diseases are punishments for sins on earth. Aside from that, death originates from natural causes, such as the influence of stars, toxic air, harmful vapors and exhalation of the earth, impure and putrid water, and the like. This is probed by physicians and is reported and described here. Yet, there is no doubt that the most prominent and topmost cause of this common plague and pestilence is our unchristian, wicked life.[38]

These natural causes were generally framed as the natural outlet through which God's will manifested itself. While natural vectors of disease were real, they mostly served as divine tools for punishment: "Like with all punishments, therefore, our sins and not the natural effects are the most important cause, even though God utilizes natural means," as the physician Hieronymus Oder (fl. 1536–50) argued in 1550.[39] The Ingolstadt physician Michael Fenk (fl. 1533) conceded that God mandated the plague in principle, yet asserted that it fell on humanity to fight or escape it through their efforts: "As learned people confirm, pestilence is caused by poisoning or putrefaction of the air that, as it stains a body, may poison many humans, which may occur in accidental fashion, but never without the consent of the almighty."[40]

The pastor Haimeran Schweller (fl. 1547–50), a follower of the old faith, in his 1550 theological tract claimed that "God our Lord effects good and evil through nature that He created."[41] Schweller argued that plague could arise in the environment as well within the human body. Infection from the environment was transmitted through toxic air due to a disruption of seasonal weather patterns, due to smelly and foul air produced by putrid standing water or poorly buried bodies, or due to celestial constellations and events. Plague could arise within a human body when the humidity within began to putrefy. Once humans were contaminated by any method, they could pass it on to others.[42] Authorities could contain plague by combating contaminated air by keeping streets and houses clean of reeking waste and by limiting contact with infected people by shunning inns, bathhouses, shops, dance halls, markets, houses of sick people, and cemeteries where victims of the plague were buried.[43]

God could send warning signs through nature before releasing a pestilence wave, as the physician Jacobus Theodorus (1522–90) asserted in his 1564 tract. Invoking Avicenna as authority, Theodorus elaborated that such punishment was first anticipated through lunar and solar eclipses, comets with tails, other extraordinary celestial phenomena, and certain planetary constellations. This led to toxic air that sickened humans and cattle and that gave fruit and grains a toxic quality, which all marked the beginning of the pandemic.[44] Likewise, Theodorus viewed unusual climate patterns as ominous signs for a deadly outbreak of the plague.[45]

Luther's views on plague as a form of divine punishment made reference to it as a required part of any plague text. While some texts addressed theological points in some detail, the majority only paid lip service. By the middle of the sixteenth century, a dominant consensus had emerged that God used natural means to unleash plague onto humanity as part of his punishment. Given that plague was transmitted through natural means, the opportunity and indeed obligation for human intervention arose. Prevention strategies were developed to help individuals protect themselves and their homes, and communities to create institutions and policies in anticipation of outbreaks. Medical interventions could be prepared to protect individuals during outbreaks of plague and to treat them in case of infection, to be discussed in the next section.

Consequently, authorities had the obligation to mandate measures that would prevent or contain outbreaks of plague, to be discussed in more detail in the final section. The 1562 Nuremberg plague ordinance is a good example of this. Its preamble stated that God used plague, war, and inflation as his rod to punish human sins and infractions. The honorable council acted out of a "fatherly benevolent disposition" to remind citizens to return to a god-pleasing life.[46] The second part of the preamble established that plague had natural causes, and therefore measures to counter its progress had to be taken: "Thus the honorable council thought of useful and necessary measures and had them enshrined in the following ordinance."[47] The nine articles of the ordinance, therefore, did not mention the idea of divine punishment and instead addressed individual citizens directly and prescribed certain actions. Theological references were relegated to the preamble and were completely absent from the ordinance.

Medicine versus Theology: The Ethics of Fighting Disease

As plague was universally seen as a form of God's punishment, plague pamphlets were compelled to raise the difficult ethical question whether humans had the right to fight a disease and if they would defy divine will by doing so. This section examines whether medical intervention against plague was seen as legitimate, justified, and even required.

The earliest printed plague text strongly favored medical responses. The Nuremberg barber-surgeon Hans Folz (ca. 1437–1513) in his 1482 tract denied that plague was a scourge sent by God but asserted that it rather was caused by the poisoning of the body that resulted in infection and inflammation.[48] He mocked pretend-clerics who maintained that humans did not have the right to fight plague or to flee house, city, or region because God's punishment was not to be resisted.[49] In his view, all those were wrong who claimed "that this is a special affliction that nobody is able to withstand, and that no such poisoned person has to be shunned and to be fled from, nor the house, city, or the region where such disturbance takes place."[50] In his counterargument, Folz stressed the central role of medicine: "if nobody was allowed to withstand then God would have created medicine for nothing and physicians would not be needed, and Solomon would have said in vain, honor the physician to benefit your own cure."[51]

His support for medical interventions led him to urge city councils to set up plague hospitals and to support medical professionals, such as himself, to increase preparedness for pandemics. Folz's 1482 texts fell into a time of renewed interest in surgery, which created an opportunity to prioritize "diseases, empirically based observation, and clinical diagnosis." Medical practitioners, like Folz, started to rely on practical expertise and to introduce pragmatic approaches to addressing health issues.[52] Folz's practical and pragmatic approach created a prototype of medical plague texts that dealt only with a single disease and that sought to emancipate themselves from theological considerations.

The physician Joachim Vadianus (1484–1551) in his 1519 tract presented the idea of a helping God. He insisted that not actively fighting plague would lead to a foolish death. Rather than relying on saintly intercessors,[53] his biblical rhetoric encouraged individuals to fight for their own well-being, "for there is a common saying, if humans help and take care of themselves God will help them as well."[54] Vadianus added that avoiding harm to oneself and one's family also was in the interest of the common good.

Likewise, the physician Alexander Seitz affirmed the requirement to use God's medicine, since God wanted humans to live; humans had to seek to prolong life as a way of honoring God. Not fighting plague would be like hanging oneself, which would lead to sanctions from the Church. To Seitz, physicians and medicines were God's tools: "Revere the physician for God created him out of need, the Supreme created medicine out of the earth. A reasonable person would not shy away from it, etc. From this we can clearly judge that God the Almighty created a comforting treasure, namely medicine, which helps humans eke out a life."[55]

The physician Caspar Kegler picked up on the dual nature of God as punisher and healer. As human life invariably was heading toward death, so wrote Kegler in his introduction, "we don't have to seek someone other than God, our Lord, who is our helper and just punisher even though the illness under discussion here, pestilence, at times is born and caused from natural causes and influence of the cosmos."[56] He stressed that "in Holy Scripture, in several places, God the Lord punished the disobedience of his people commonly with war and pestilence." Therefore, he admonished his readers to maintain faith and a pure conscience and "to prefer spiritual to physical medicine," as medication only has the desired effect in the faithful.[57]

Likewise, Achilles Pirmin Gasser admonished humans to return to faith and lead a God-pleasing life so that the natural remedies given by the creator himself could do their work. Based on Luther's teachings on this matter, medicines were a gift from God and thus could and indeed had to be used to fight disease, even plague that was sent by God as punishment.[58] Faith was the key for medicines to be able to fight the toxins in the human body. Having established this in his introduction, Gasser proceeded with his medical advice on how to prevent plague and how to recover from it.[59]

To Kegler, God's helping hand served as justification for human intervention. Helping plague sufferers thus did not thwart God's plan, rather it was pleasing to a compassionate, helping God. By defining God as a paternal figure, developing remedies against plague—Kegler's professional enterprise—and accepting them as a gift from God could become a God-pleasing activity.[60] By developing and promoting his own secret recipes, Kegler contributed one of the few truly original treatises on the plague.[61]

The herbalist and physician Tarquinus Schnellenberg (d. 1561) in 1546 published *Experimenta*, a guide on how to use twenty German herbs and roots to fight a plague infection. As the book's title indicates, Schnellenberg confidently prioritized his own observations and experiences over the authority of classical authors.[62] In his poetic address to the reader, he praised God's goodness and grace that made simple herbs grow on German soil to treat plague and other illnesses.[63] Schnellenberg stressed his strong preference for simple herbs grown in German soil: "As we have so many good and precious simple remedies in the German nation, they are more compatible with and closer to our nature than those called trans-oceanic or alien."[64]

Schnellenberg was part of a movement of German herbalists in the first half of the sixteenth century who promoted native herbs and medicines to provide cures for Germans. Locally grown herbs and roots were more attuned to the humoral composition of the German body. Imported herbs and spices from India and Arabia, on the other hand, inflicted harm on German bodies because of their hot nature. In these herbalists' view, God provided ample food and medicine in the native environment to sustain and to provide cures for German bodies.[65]

The pastor and early reformer Jakob Strauß (1480–1533) elaborated that God provided for his creation: "God feeds the birds in the air and the fish in the water and dresses the flowers in the meadows."[66] God exposed sinners to hunger as a form of punishment but provided for the faithful: "Each pious Christian shall adhere to Christ's affirmative words without doubt, then he shall not lack nourishment."[67] Hunger and lacking or ineffective medicine therefore were signs of deficient faith.[68]

This is in line with the Lutheran idea of a God who sustained believers. Luther reminded his followers in his 1527 plague tract that "God has created medicines and provided us with intelligence to guard and take good care of the body so that we can live in good health."[69] Luther read this as a mandate to keep one's own body healthy, to use medicines provided by God, and to take measures to fend off disease through prevention and medication. Humans therefore had the ethical responsibility to keep their bodies in good health and to protect themselves against plague.

Following Luther's directive, instructions on how to protect one's body and preserve life became a standard part discussed in all plague books in some detail. A standard list of protective personal behaviors and body techniques was promoted by most of these texts.[70] People should get a good night's rest, eat regular but modest meals, and drink only moderately.

Some writers, like Adam Lonitzer (1528–86), stressed the harmful effect of strong affects and emotions and of excessive physical activity.[71] Both excessive mental strain and physical activity were draining energy that was needed to fend off the plague. The physician Theobald Fettich (fl. 1527–50) recommended that "one should pursue moderate joys in such time. Particularly suitable are all music and lovely song, the play of strings, as well as friendly and entertaining conversation."[72]

Protecting oneself to prevent infection with plague also had behavioral and social implications. Seeking social distancing and social isolation was a commonly promoted method to protect oneself against infection. The physician Johann Copp (1487–1558) advised his readers in 1521 to avoid the company of others, to avoid mass gatherings at churches or public bathhouses, and to seek social isolation at home instead: "Not that I want to forbid you to go to church. However, I believe that by staying at home in these circumstances a person easily can achieve something that is as pleasing to God as going to church."[73] Taking care of one's health and preserving one's life were God-pleasing acts, even if that meant staying away from worship in church.

Infected persons, in particular, should self-isolate, as the Nuremberg physician Johann Magenbuch (1500–46) wrote in his short plague tract from 1530: "Furthermore, one should avoid taverns and common bathhouses. Also, one should forbid people who had the disease to meet other people for three or four days, particularly if they were not healed yet."[74] Magenbuch's text was reprinted and disseminated by the city of Nuremberg to raise awareness during the plague outbreak of 1532.[75]

The anonymous pamphlet *Ein kurtz Regiment/ wie sich zu zeiten der Pestilentz zu halten sey* (A brief primer how to conduct oneself during a time of pestilence) from 1543, published on behalf of the Nuremberg council, recommended staying away from places like churches and bathhouses where large numbers of people congregated and infections easily could be passed on: "In these times gatherings and congregations of humans are to be fled, for who can tell the infected ones from the healthy ones?"[76] The Nuremberg council thus fully endorsed both social isolation and medical intervention to prevent the spread of plague. Restrictive theological views, like those of Osiander, increasingly became marginal positions that failed to influence public discourse and public policy.

The Ethics of Fleeing Plague: Self-Protection versus Social Responsibility

Giovanni Boccaccio's *The Decameron* framed the discussion of whether it was morally acceptable to flee a city afflicted by plague, as his native Florence was in 1348. Plague survivors "took one utterly cruel precaution, namely, to avoid the sick and their belongings, fleeing far away from them, for in doing so they all thought they could preserve their own health."[77] This theme played out in the subsequent discussion in Germany as well.

The physician and intellectual Alexander Seitz insisted on the right to flee plague because "God gave us our own will … and lets us run according to our will, which allows us to accrue merit or debt."[78] Fleeing locations inflicted by plague generally was accepted as a reasonable response, unless more pressing ethical concerns stood in the way. If the miasma theory was correct, meaning that transmission was caused by bad and toxic air or vapors, then removing oneself from the source of bad air represented a viable strategy.

In his enumeration of how to protect oneself against plague, Hans Folz listed flight second only to repentance and service to God: "Before fear takes root, one should flee soon, flee far, and return late so that the later times won't be worse than the earlier."[79] A possible source for Folz might have been the Nuremberg physician Hermann Schedel (1410–85), who was appointed Nuremberg city physician around 1467.[80] In his *Tractatus de Peste* that he prepared in manuscript form in 1453 he used the adverbs "cito, longe, tarde," indicating that one should flee quickly and far and return slowly.[81] This formulation was copied frequently in plague literature in subsequent decades,[82] for instance by the physician Anton Brelochs (ca. 1488–1559) in his plague book printed in Nuremberg in 1529: "Move quickly and far out of the lands where pestilence takes hold. Return slowly once it has dissipated, so you may live as it seems to me."[83]

The right to flee was invariably linked to an individual's responsibilities for family and community. Martin Luther insisted that certain individuals—preachers, physicians, public officials, and anyone who had a caretaker role—had to fulfill the ethical obligations of their estate, even if the personal risk was considerable. At the same time, a good Christian had to flee to safety if this could be done without neglecting obligations to others, just like one would run out of a burning house. To Luther, a Christian could not gain favor from God solely by staying behind in times of plague.[84] Therefore neither fleeing nor remaining was right or wrong per se.[85]

While those afflicted by plague had to be isolated to protect the community, they were not stigmatized and deserved to be fed and nursed, particularly as plague was not seen as God's punishment for the sins of individuals.[86] In Martin Luther's view, the command to love one's neighbor extended to those afflicted by plague: "If you wish to serve Christ and to wait on him, very well, you have your sick neighbor close at hand. Go to him and serve him, and you will surely find Christ in him, not outwardly but in his word."[87] When Elector John of Saxony on 10 August 1527 ordered the evacuation of Wittenberg University because of plague, Luther and Johannes Bugenhagen refused to leave, so as to minister to the sick and dying.[88]

Despite Luther's intervention, some writers continued to downplay the ethical implications of fleeing plague, like Johannes Castner (fl. 1540–56) in his didactic verses published in Nuremberg in 1542. Castner stressed that nobody could escape death, but that one certainly could avoid toxic air. Fleeing therefore was a normal act of self-preservation:

> Flee soon and far from the country,
> where the plague takes over.
> Don't heed calls to return home,
> unless the disease is well past.
> Meantime have joy and good spirit,
> for brooding and mourning don't do good.
> What help are property and wealth to you,
> when you depart from this world.
> Destitute is better than dead,
> God will help you against ruin,
> in whom you put your trust,
> that He will make up for all your sorrows.
> You must not resist His will,
> thus you can live here and there.[89]

Yet, even Castner recognized that some public officials who performed critical services had to remain in the city.[90]

Heinrich Stromer's (1482–1542) highly influential plague tract, first published in Leipzig in 1516 and reprinted many times, including in Nuremberg in the plague year of 1533, offers the most comprehensive discussion of the topic. It is noteworthy that post-Reformation editions of the text remained unchanged. Stromer defended the practice of fleeing plague against detractors: "While many quarrelsome people despise the flight because they believe that pestilence is not harmful to anyone since such deaths are intended and carried out by God, such presumption results in the premature death of many."[91] Stromer responded to a segment in the population that seemed to downplay the threat of plague, at least for believers, like the preacher Andreas Osiander, discussed below.

Stromer confirmed that fleeing very early in the plague cycle was the best way to protect oneself, provided that the destination had been plague free for at least nine months. If individuals hesitated too long, they could get infected and die during their flight or spread the disease to cities that took them in. Accepting plague refugees therefore posed great health risks for prospective host cities: "From this follows that it is very dangerous to admit and shelter those who had remained in dangerous air for a long time. For it often happens and is experienced that cities and villages, where those who had fled lands of death were taking refuge, were poisoned with great savage pestilence. For this reason, such people have to be avoided with great diligence."[92] Travelers who arrived from cities afflicted with plague, be it refugees, messengers, or merchants, had to be kept downwind at a safe distance, and talking to them or socializing with them was ill-advised.[93] Stromer thus addressed the issue from both perspectives: while it was legitimate to flee plague, host cities had to be wary of accepting plague refugees.

From his refuge in Wrocław, the Nuremberg patrician Michael Behaim (1510–69) wrote in a letter in October 1533 "that there is a great dying in Nuremberg and more than a third of the entire city fled and that therefore, as far as honorable citizens are concerned, nobody is in Nuremberg, other than the seven old councilors."[94] Behaim added that more artisans had deserted the city than ever before. The Behaim letter pointed to yet another problem caused by citizens fleeing plague: the threat to city governance and to critical services due to the absence of office holders. The Nuremberg city council made a first attempt to restrict travel for jurors at criminal courts and for council members during times of plague in a 1407 ordinance. The council wanted critical urban institutions to function by keeping key public officials from leaving the city.[95] Beginning in 1520, Nuremberg prevented a large number of critical city officials, such as council members, judges, physicians, customs officials, and others, from leaving the city during times of plague without special permission, in order to ensure the proper functioning of the city and to provide services needed during times of plague.[96]

Many writers acknowledged that the option to flee was open only to the privileged who had the financial resources to travel and to forego income during their absence. Johannes Castner in his 1542 tract, for instance, confirmed that many could not flee because of their poverty.[97] The 1621 *Neubauer Chronicle* confirmed that "the wealthy people all fled the city" during the deadly plague of 1562, leaving poor people behind.[98] Castner argued that the inability of poor people to flee the city created the ethical obligation for authorities to create good public policy to protect them, and in particular to keep the air clean, both indoors and outdoors. The practice of fleeing the city during plague outbreaks was politically fraught and ethically challenging as this option was open only to elites, causing tensions and even open conflict, like in Nuremberg in 1533.

The primer issued by the Nuremberg magistrates on 16 July 1533 generally promoted social distancing, such as staying away from churches, and preserved the option to flee the city.[99] However, this view was not universally accepted. Nine days after the Nuremberg primer was printed on 3 August 1533,[100] a sermon delivered by the Nuremberg theologian Andreas Osiander argued that both good and evil people died of plague but that God took the pious ones as a reward at their right time, as mentioned above. The decision of who lived and who died was up to God, and pious Christians therefore had nothing to fear from plague, as God invariably made the right decision for each Christian: "Therefore such untimely fear and flight truly are against God's commands. They are nothing other than an indication of a great and grave unbelief that one does not believe in God nor trusts that He can and will absolve."[101] To Osiander, fighting plague as well as fleeing from it out of fear were futile, godless, and selfish acts, as they invariably harmed the community: "Your love can easily see from all of this how unwise and un-Christian those act who leave their occupations and offices out of inappropriate fear of this plague, and who knowingly withdraw their love, help, and loyalty towards their next ones, which they were obligated to grant based on God's commands."[102] To Osiander, fleeing town was like fearing the wrath of God. The only path was to have faith and to trust the word of God, "for this is the only assured and redeeming flight in these dangerous times, by which one can escape this plague and can be saved."[103]

Osiander's position had few followers, and Luther's more moderate and pragmatic stance prevailed. However, Osiander's sermon displayed an open conflict with the 1533 version of Nuremberg's primer on plague that recommended social isolation, including staying away from church services, as well as fleeing the city altogether. As the option of fleeing town was open to the elites only, Osiander's interpretation offered consolation to the poor who did not enjoy this privilege. This may explain why Osiander's sermon was reprinted in 1543.[104]

The examination of the question of whether one may flee in times of plague in Nuremberg texts thus shows five trends: (1) Hans Folz's unconditional appeal to flee plague found few backers. (2) Luther's theological viewpoint that only those were allowed to flee who did not neglect obligations to others became a generally accepted norm. (3) We see a gradual shift toward stressing individual responsibility for the well-being of others as well as for the protection of the community. (4) Public policy took an increased role and, in some cases, created conflict with religious authorities. (5) While fleeing the city remained common practice, it disappeared as a discussion point in plague texts by the middle of the sixteenth century. The tract by the physician Johannes Rympffer (fl. 1538–52), published in Nuremberg in 1538 and 1552, did not address the topic. Furthermore, the 1562 city plague ordinance or its discussion by Hans Sachs in his poem dated 12 December 1563 did not mention it.

However, the fictitious dialogue between the poet and a friend that followed Sachs's poem addressed this issue. The poem ended by introducing the topic of the dialogue: "A good friend asked me whether I did not want to flee the dying to protect myself against this plague and move out of the city to a safe place for a while."[105] In the dialogue, the friend noted that the poet had no esteem for those who fled and added: "Don't you see how the wealthy and powerful flee the city on a daily basis in order to sustain their lives?" He added that they were leading happy lives elsewhere, while feasting, promenading, and seeking joy. The poet insisted that they would not escape death by fleeing: "Fear will haunt them daily and will torment them inside in their hearts with frequent sighing pain, and fear will grow the longer the more."[106] While the friend insisted on seeking a place of safety, the poet closed the dialogue by taking the moral high ground: "I said: friend, I tell you in loyalty, you will regret your escape from the bottom of your heart. I, on the other hand, want to stay in Nuremberg, committed to drafting poetry and writing, where God will bestow life to me and in addition will grant me grace and assistance so that I can write many lovely poems in these times of death."[107] What was framed as a political and ethical obligation in earlier texts, Sachs pitched as a personal choice, informed by a moral core, a commitment to the community, and psychological well-being.[108]

The Authorities' Growing Regulatory Role: The Case of Nuremberg

As argued before, a consensus gradually arose in the first half of the sixteenth century that plague was transmitted by natural means, the fact that it was a form of divine punishment notwithstanding. This gave rise to the opportunity, and indeed obligation, for human intervention. As stated in the introduction, intervention strategies were generally guided by the two basic insights: contagion occurred through interhuman transmission or indirectly through cloth and other objects, and outbreaks of plague were associated with place.[109] Prevention strategies were developed to help individuals protect themselves, their homes, and their communities. At the same time, there was growing pressure on authorities to mandate measures to prevent or contain outbreaks of plague and thus to protect the entire community.

Hans Folz was one of the earliest advocates for the intervention by urban authorities. With the rise of university-trained physicians, the reputation of barber-surgeons like Folz had started to slip. In 1482, Folz urged councils to establish a plague hospital and to support all members of the medical community, including barber-surgeons, while shunning ignorant laypeople and even unqualified physicians.[110] Folz quipped sarcastically that times of plague brought about a large number of quacks: "Just like one calls on a shoemaker to mend pants, one now looks for medicines with bakers, armorers, coppersmiths, goldsmiths, and old women, and with many other country swindlers who seek to authenticate their medicines with phony affidavits; even worse, one also looks for medicines with Jews."[111] It is worth noting here that antisemitic references in plague literature had become rare by the late fifteenth century and disappeared in the sixteenth century entirely. The increasingly questionable status of barber-surgeons became clear in the remarks by the physician Johannes Copp in 1521; he included barber-surgeons among the medical imposters. He warned plague patients against seeking help from "old women, barbers, and pharmacists," who, as unlearned charlatans, did more harm than good.[112]

The example of Nuremberg shows how cities in the late fifteenth and early sixteenth centuries gradually created public policy and institutions regarding plague and expanded their authority over matters that either had been the responsibility of the church or had been left up to individuals. The burial of those who died of plague became one of the first and most important issues the city council sought to gain control over. In a first timid attempt in 1474, Nuremberg passed an ordinance that outlawed the burial of non-residents in the city and limited the ringing of bells for the dead to Fridays. Early on, authorities took a great interest in concealing the real impact of plague by limiting bell ringing and minimizing the size of funeral processions to project a sense of normalcy,[113] yet could not enforce these provisions against the resistance of the Church.[114] The city council attempted to move the cemetery outside the city walls as early as 1483. It finally ordered in 1505 that no deceased person could be brought into the city for burial. In 1518, the city established the new extramural Saint Rochus Cemetery. A year later, the city council issued an ordinance regulating how people should be buried during times of plague.[115]

Nuremberg's council considered a plague ordinance in 1517, a year without plague, but the effort gained traction only after a new outbreak of plague in fall 1519, which prompted the plague ordinance of 9 November 1519.[116] Nuremberg's council passed its first comprehensive plague ordinance on 18 April 1520 and expanded it on 28 July 1520.[117] Perhaps in response to resistance in the population, this ordinance was printed in six thousand copies and distributed to all Nuremberg households[118] "so that no one can feign ignorance and escape punishment from the council."[119]

Measures to keep the air clean played a significant role in urban regulatory approaches, particularly to benefit those who had no opportunity to flee the city. Beginning in the early sixteenth century, there were recurring ordinances mandating to keep streets clean, particularly of animal manure and human waste, outlawing pigs in the city, regulating the processing of animal carcasses, draining standing water, and other measures to improve air quality.[120] In 1530, the Nuremberg physician Johann Magenbuch declared clean air a basic common good: "Plague is a disease that comes from toxic air, the air that is common to all human beings."[121] Guidance was also developed to keep private homes clean, fumigated, and well ventilated.[122] Many plague tracts provided recipes for herb combinations that could be used to clean the air of private dwellings.

Around 1500, the erection of plague hospitals outside city walls became increasingly common to contain plague by removing the source of contaminated air to a safe place outside the city. The city of Nuremberg in 1498 started to construct the *Sebastianspital*, a plague hospital, indicating a shift from reacting to present plague infections to anticipating health care needs arising during future waves of plague.[123] However, the hospital was completed only in 1528;

the number of construction interruptions points to a lack of commitment in years when plague was not present.[124]

Martin Luther was a strong promoter of the common good whose support depended both on actions by authorities and individual responsibility. His seminal 1527 plague tract, *Whether One May Flee from a Deadly Plague,* strongly pushed such an agenda. The command to love one's neighbor required both individuals and governments to assume responsibility for the sick. Cities and territorial states had to create more hospitals to ease the burden on families affected by plague: "It would be well, where there is such an efficient government in cities and states, to maintain municipal homes and hospitals staffed with people to take care of the sick so that patients from private homes can be sent there—as was the intent and purpose of our forefathers with so many pious bequests, hospices, hospitals, and infirmaries so that it should not be necessary for every citizen to maintain a hospital in his own home."[125] Where no such institutions existed, Christians had to "give hospital care and be nurses for one another in any extremity or risk the loss of salvation and the grace of God."[126]

This is the context in which printed plague texts around 1520 became much more prolific. The prototype for Nuremberg was the fourteen-page anonymous *Ein kurtz Regiment auß vil treffenlichen zůsamen geprachten tractaten verstendiger artzt gezogen/ wie sich zů zeiten der pestilentz zuhalten sey* (A brief primer, drawn and compiled from many relevant tracts by knowledgeable physicians, on how one should conduct oneself in times of pestilence), published in Nuremberg on 6 March 1520. This semi-official pamphlet became the model for future Nuremberg civic pamphlets, reissued by the city council throughout the sixteenth century, namely in 1533, 1543, 1562, 1574, 1575, 1582, and 1585.

Aside from the formulaic reference to divine intervention and the reminder to seek God's grace in the introduction, mentioned above, the text has a completely secular framework. It advised citizens to stay away from large groups of people and from infected neighbors. If possible, people should flee the city; if that was not possible, people should air out and fumigate their dwellings and consult with a pharmacist about certain preventive medications. The second part advised citizens how to deal with infections. The focus of the entire tract was on vague advice for individuals, while actions the government took or should have taken were excluded from discussion.

The next edition of this text, issued by the magistrates on 16 July 1533, had a more official look, as the coat of arms of the city of Nuremberg was added to its title page as well as to all subsequent editions. The plague advice given in the 1533 version, entitled *Ein kurtz Regiment wie sich zu zeiten der Pestilentz zu halten sey* (A brief primer on how one should conduct oneself in times of pestilence), differed only minimally. The only critical innovation was the entirely Lutheran religious framing of the introduction.[127] The only way to receive the divine gift of medicine and to make it "through these dangerous times" was "through a righteous, firm, constant faith in the gracious gospel of our Lord Jesus Christ."[128] Like other early Lutheran texts published in Nuremberg, the text urged common people, who had no means to flee or to protect themselves in other ways, to trust in God's goodness, knowing that God disciplined only those he loved.[129] Finally, the citizens should ask God to protect the Christian community "through his holy word, through his holy angels, through the pious and honest authorities, and through fruitful blessings and weather."[130]

The next version of the text, published on 16 October 1543, did not differ greatly from the 1533 version. Important is the indication of authorship, which was not present in earlier versions: "Augmented and improved by scholars and experienced doctors of medicine."[131] Readers now could trust that the text had the stamp of approval from the city's medical establishment. The main body of the text was still based on the 1520 version, as it followed the same structure and contained the same advice. The only difference was that some provisions were explained in more detail.

In 1562, the most severe outbreak in Nuremberg's history[132] forced the council to change their legal framework as well as their textual strategies. On 26 January 1562, Nuremberg's council passed the most comprehensive ordinance to date, which was printed and distributed to all households in the city in an effort to impose a sense of order. It was the duty of precinct captains to disseminate the ordinance to all households "so that nobody could use their ignorance as an excuse."[133] While the 1533 ordinance had given vague advice, like social distancing and maintaining the option of fleeing, the 1562 ordinance contained nine provisions defining specific measures, most of them addressing personal responsibility. As plague was still viewed as punishment from God, the "honorable council out of a good paternalistic spirit" reminded Nuremberg's citizens to turn away from sin and to return to God in prayer.[134] The ordinance was motivated by the desire to create order at a time when the social fabric of the city was stressed to the limit by the outbreak of plague.[135] Likewise, the physician Hieronymus Oder stressed the need to create order, as plagues in the past had led to insanity, mayhem, and war.[136]

Except for the maintenance of the Saint Sebastian plague hospital, all provisions related to obligations of individuals in the general public, such as not emptying human excrements onto streets, removing animal waste after two days, removing pigs from the city, no bloodletting, not selling clothes and bedding of infected and diseased people, and avoiding large congregations of people, particularly those infected or recovering. Heads of households had the obligation to isolate sick members of their household. Finally, pharmacists had to ensure that they stocked up.[137] The ordinance closed with the assurance that the city would continue to provide porters to carry the sick and the deceased out of the city and nurses to take care of diseased people and their households, all to provide for citizens and to maintain a "useful good order."[138] Indeed many, like the pastor Haimeran Schweller, reminded urban authorities that they had the obligation to take care of indigent plague victims in plague hospitals and fraternal houses.[139]

The 1562 ordinance was confirmed and reprinted in 1575, 1585, and 1600. Starting in 1585, a tenth provision, against dancing, was added, not on moral grounds but to enforce social distancing and to avoid the unnecessary heating of bodies, as enlarged sweat glands were believed to create an entry point for contaminated air.[140]

The 1562 version of the primer, entitled *Ein kurtz Regiment/ wie man sich in Zeit Regierender Pestilentz halten soll* (A brief primer on how one should conduct oneself in times of governing pestilence), made much stronger religious demands of individuals. The theological introduction stressed that plague was God's punishment for a sinful life and that humans first had to show humility toward God, confess, repent, and beg for forgiveness, coupled with the demand for increased future obedience: "There is no redress that is better and more useful than that we humiliate ourselves in front of his divine majesty, fall on our knees, confess our transgressions, have heartfelt remorse for them, and humbly call and beg our dear lord and father in heaven … for forgiveness and pardon in true, righteous, and genuine faith and trust in his bottomless grace and mercy."[141] The instructions were similar to those of earlier versions, with some subtle but important differences. In the 1562 version, residents still were urged to stay away from large gatherings of people, but the recommendation to stay away from church was dropped, leaving bathhouses as the only specifically mentioned place to avoid.[142] The heightened moral expectations in the 1562 edition of the *Ein kurtz Regiment* thus led to stricter religious guidance and a softened approach toward the church.

Hans Sachs in a poem dated 12 December 1563 described the actions taken by Nuremberg's council in great detail. He followed the flow of the 1562 plague ordinance, starting with the point that plague was caused by the wrath of God that was unleashed on humans because of their great sins, adding a list of transgressions common for the sixteenth century, such as "blasphemy, gluttony, adultery, pride, abusive usury, all kinds of fraud."[143] Sachs then described the nine measures mandated in the ordinance. He added information that was not part of the ordinance, in particular actions taken by the council on behalf of citizens. Sachs maintained that the council appointed physicians and hired barbers to assist the sick to provide the needed medicines. In addition, the city employed many men and women who took care of the sick in their homes. The city also provided medicines and priests (*Priester*) for the plague hospital, in addition to servants and maids, food and drink, and prayer robes. Sachs uncritically assumed the position of the city council while concealing public resistance and common non-compliance with the order. The contrast to Hans

Folz's position in 1482 could not be greater: while Folz urged his fellow citizens to look out for themselves, Sachs urged them to trust the council and to follow their orders.

The 1574 version of *Ein kurtz Regiment*, published at the onset of the serious 1574–75 plague outbreak, presented similar theological views but lacked the harsh moralistic tone of the 1562 text. Just one year later, a completely revised version appeared; at the same time, the 1562 plague ordinance was reprinted. The title page of the primer, again with the city's coat of arms, indicated that the text was "drafted by the appointed and sworn doctors of medicine of this city of Nuremberg," marking this text as an official communication. The preface returned to the brief and formulaic theological framework used in earlier versions and then focused on secular concerns: "Regarding human responses, however, humans being creations of God and his order, they should not be despised or disregarded, not just for the prevention of this cruel disease but also for its repudiation." This is why it was important to give a report to "common people and not to scholars" on how to respond in such times.[144]

In a radical departure from previous versions, the authors then complained about the ineffectiveness of past measures because people did not follow the ordinances and recommendations. The motivation for this report was that numerous infected people did not follow social distancing rules "because of the great disorder," much to the detriment of themselves and others. Both the 1582 and 1585 versions of the primer repeated these claims. Social distancing "is observed by few people if any at all. Daily experience shows sufficiently that such people who are afflicted with this cruel and horrible disease, or are recovering from it, nilly-willy encroach on others, eat and drink with them, and in addition sell all kinds of merchandise, like food and other things."[145] Furthermore, many were so daring as to use clothing and bed linen of those who died of plague without hesitation. "By doing that, they not only inflict ruin but also transfer the poison from themselves to others. This is why such people justly have to be considered double murderers." Likewise, public baths had become hot spots of infection "to which such poisoned people go without hesitation."[146] Noting that infected people could not be avoided, the text then transitioned to the standard points of how to protect oneself discussed in earlier versions of the text.

A look at the official texts issued by the Nuremberg council confirms a trend toward stricter plague regulations, which also is an indication that by the middle of the sixteenth century German cities had mature urban governments capable of formulating appropriate responses to new waves of plague. The trend toward introducing new rules to fight plague continued well into the seventeenth century. While health passes gained ground in northern Italy toward the end of the sixteenth century,[147] the city of Nuremberg introduced printed health passes only in November 1665.[148] Other measures taken elsewhere, however, like quarantine rules for new arrivals, never took hold in Nuremberg. The increasing interventions by urban authorities did not happen without friction, and moreover they opened up a number of moral and ethical issues. Urban pandemic management created conflicts between public and private interests that tied into a larger discussion regarding the contested relationship between common good and self-interest.

In 1625, the Nuremberg city physician Johann Heinrich Kirchberger (1580–1632) confirmed this trend toward increased interventions by the authorities and the corresponding growing public resistance in his *Aphorismi, Seu Canones Medicinales De Peste* (Aphorisms, or medical canons about plague). Here, Kirchberger gave advice specifically to three groups of authoritative figures who all played an official role in the management of plague outbreaks: health inspectors, caregivers for infected people, who also served as their guards, and practical surgeons. According to Kirchberger, infected residents concealing their health status was a significant problem, as the primers already had confirmed in the later sixteenth century.[149] For this reason, he developed strategies for inspectors to recognize disease and to deal with renitent residents. As integrity of the health inspectors was critical, they had to swear an oath, "namely that they would perform their duties faithfully and could not be bribed by money to help somebody conceal their illness."[150]

Conclusion

The investigation of plague texts between 1480 and 1580 allows us to arrive at the following conclusions.

(1) Early printed plague texts varied widely, taking on the author's individual perspective. After 1520, texts became increasingly homogenized and derivative, particularly the primers that focused on preventing and healing plague, some strictly theological texts forming an exception. Similarities include points and arguments made, the organization of texts, rhetorical strategies, poetic inclusions, and even specific formulations.

(2) Sixteenth-century plague texts were remarkably pragmatic, aside from some theological framing. They showed little interest in searching for scapegoats for the disease, including Jews, other than generally blaming the disease on the leading of sinful lives. Furthermore, plague texts rarely were confessionally marked.

(3) Plague presented an economic opportunity for printers who made money on printed plague texts. Plague contributed to the rapid expansion of vernacular print. As there was a big demand for these texts, many authors, mostly physicians, increasingly copied from other texts.

(4) Plague presented an economic opportunity for medical practitioners who published plague texts, raising their public and professional profiles, and who often promoted their own plague medicines.

(5) While earlier texts unreservedly recommended fleeing cities afflicted by plague, this option on a textual level was taken back after Luther's 1527 text and essentially disappeared after 1540. However, the actual practice of fleeing the city continued well into the seventeenth century.

(6) Early plague texts focused almost entirely on individuals and actions they could take to keep themselves safe from plague. In later texts, the focus shifted to the common good, with a focus on how governments could formulate public policy to protect the community. Furthermore, texts now discussed ethical obligations of individuals toward their families and communities. Hans Folz wrote as a citizen and as a barber-surgeon who reflected his own views. Hans Sachs, by contrast, fell in line with the position of council and promoted it in his text.

(7) The demand for an increased government role in the sixteenth century coincided with the rise of territorial and urban administrations around 1500 and the advancement of *Gute Policey*. It is in this context that governments were establishing regulatory frameworks. Inversely, the rise of plague also gave governments cause to advance the role of government in general. As German cities started to develop a civil service in the late fifteenth and early sixteenth centuries to manage growing cities with increasingly complex economies, as Italian cities had done before, they also created the capacity to effectively manage periodic outbreaks of plague.

Peter Hess is Professor Emeritus of German and European Studies at the University of Texas at Austin. From 2009 to 2018, he served as department chair. Recent publications are *Resisting Pluralization and Globalization in German Culture, 1490–1540: Visions of Nation in Decline* (De Gruyter, 2020) and *Violent First Contact in Venezuela: Nikolaus Federmann's Indian History* (Penn State University Press, 2021). He is currently working on a book on Ulrich Schmidel's service as a mercenary in the Río de la Plata region, 1534–54.

Notes

1. Bühl, "Die Pestepidemien," 123.
2. Jörg, *Teure, Hunger, Großes Sterben*, 147–51.
3. Belich, *The World the Plague Made*, 48–49.
4. Bühl, "Die Pestepidemien," 122–23.
5. Murphy, *A New Order of Medicine*, 45.
6. Hans Sachs mentioned in a poem dated 12 December 1563 that 9,256 people had died of plague in Nuremberg in 1562–63 (Sachs, *Sehr herrliche, schöne, und warhaffte Gedicht*, vol. 4, fol. Iv).

7. Dross, "'es flohen die reichen leud,'" 303–7.
8. Eckert, *The Structure of Plagues and Pestilences*, 22.
9. Seelbach, *In dieser harten und sterbenden Zeit*, 40.
10. For a comprehensive discussion of the rise of physicians in sixteenth-century Nuremberg, see Murphy, *A New Order of Medicine*.
11. Heinrichs, "The Plage Cures of Caspar Kegler," 425.
12. Kegler, *Eyn Nutzlichs vnd trostlichs Regiment*, fol. 15r. All translations are mine, unless stated otherwise.
13. Kinzelbach, "Seuchenkonzepte," 255.
14. Kruse, *Der Feind in der Stadt*, 29.
15. Eckert, *The Structure of Plagues and Pestilences*, 22.
16. Eckert, *The Structure of Plagues and Pestilences*, 22–23.
17. Bell, *Plague in the Early Modern World*, 174.
18. Anon., *Ein kurtz Regiment* (1520), sig. A2r.
19. Heinrichs, *Plague, Print, and the Reformation*, 5–11.
20. Kruse (*Der Feind in der Stadt*, 29) claims that about thirty plague regiments were printed in Nuremberg between the sixteenth and eighteenth centuries.
21. Spengler, *Wie sich eyn Christen mensch*, sig. B2v.
22. Kegler, *Eyn Nutzlichs vnd trostlichs Regiment*, fol. 5r–v; see Heinrichs, "The Plague Cures of Caspar Kegler," 431–32. On the nationalistic backlash against foreign influences, see Hess, *Resisting Pluralization and Globalization*, 289–307.
23. Translation by Rittgers, *The Reformation of Suffering*, 242.
24. Ulenbeck, *Ein schön und Christlich Gesprech*, sig. C6r–v.
25. Seitz, *Ain schöner Tractat*, sig. B2r.
26. Wolff, *Die Theorie der Seuche*, 87.
27. Luther, *Whether One May Flee from a Deadly Plague*, 130.
28. Conradinus, *KVrtze vnd nutze gegründte vnderricht*, sig. K4r.
29. Spengler, *Wie sich eyn Christen mensch*, sig. A3r.
30. Spengler, *Wie sich eyn Christen mensch*, sig. C3r.
31. Dietrich, *Der XCI. Psalm*, sig. A4r–v.
32. Anon., *Ein kurtz Regiment* (1520), sig. A2r; translation based on Heinrichs, *Plague, Print, and the Reformation*, 80. Frenzel ("Die Ordnung des Zorns," 45) documents this for an Ulm city ordinance from 1558.
33. Anon., *Ein kurtz Regiment* (1520), sig. A2r.
34. Link, "Wie sich ein Christen mensch," sig. A6r.
35. Osiander, *Wie vnd wohin ein Christ*, sig. b2r.
36. Osiander, *Wie vnd wohin ein Christ*, sig. a3r.
37. Slack, "Responses to Plague," 438–39.
38. Gasser, *Ainfeltiger vnd gegrünter bericht*, sig. a2v.
39. Oder, *Radt vnd Artzney*, sig. A3v.
40. Fenk, *Ain gut nützlich Regiment*, sig A3r.
41. Schweller, *Ein Christliche vnderricht*, fol. 20v.
42. Schweller, *Ein Christliche vnderricht*, fol. 20v–21v.
43. Schweller, *Ein Christliche vnderricht*, fol. 46v–47r.
44. Theodorus, *Gewisse vnnd erfahren Practick*, fol. 4v–5r.
45. Theodorus, *Gewisse vnnd erfahren Practick*, fol. 5r–5v. While Theodorus discussed the theme of divine punishment extensively here, his 1573 *Kurzer vnderricht vnd Rahtschlag* is entirely clinical in approach and free of theological references.

46. Anon., *Ains Erbern Raths der Stadt Nürmberg*, sig. A2r.
47. Anon., *Ains Erbern Raths der Stadt Nürmberg*, sig. A2r.
48. Folz, *Jtem von der pestilencz*, fol. 2r.
49. Folz published two plague tracts in 1482, one in prose, *Jtem von der pestilencz ein hübsch nüczlich vnd kurcz begriffes tractetlin*, and one in verse, *Jtem ein fast köstlicher spruch von der pestilencz*. For more on Folz, see Chapter 1 by Christopher Hutchinson in this volume.
50. Folz, *Jtem von der pestilencz*, fol. 2v.
51. Folz, *Jtem von der pestilencz*, fol. 2v. The text was reprinted in the anonymous anthology *Ein warhaftige Ertzney* in 1517. See also Seitz, *Ain schöner Tractat*, sig. B3r.
52. Murphy, "Decisions before Decision-Making," 203–4.
53. Heinrichs, *Plague, Print, and the Reformation*, 78, argues that Vadianus was the first plague writer not to rely on the intervention of saints, a trend that according to Heinrichs became the norm in the 1520s (*Plague, Print, and the Reformation*, 81).
54. Vadianus, *EJn kurtz vnd trüwlich vnderricht*, sig. B1v.
55. Seitz, *Ain schöner Tractat*, sig. B3r–v.
56. Kegler, *Eyn Nutzlichs vnd trostlichs Regiment*, fol. 4r.
57. Kegler, *Eyn Nutzlichs vnd trostlichs Regiment*, fol. 4r.
58. This view was also expressed in Veit Dietrich's 1544 sermon, *Der XCI. Psalm*, sig. A4v: "For medicine is a special gift from God."
59. Gasser, *Ainfeltiger vnd gegrünter bericht*, sig. a2v–a3r.
60. Kegler, *Eyn Nutzlichs vnd trostlichs Regiment*, fol. 2r.
61. Kegler, *Eyn Nutzlichs vnd trostlichs Regiment*, fol. 2v. See Heinrichs, *Plague, Print, and the Reformation*, 112.
62. See also Schnellenberg, *Experimenta*, sig. B4r.
63. Schnellenberg, *Experimenta*, sig. A3r.
64. Schnellenberg, *Experimenta*, sig. A2v.
65. For more on the rejection of imported herbs and the promotion of locally grown foods and herbs, see Hess, *Resisting Pluralization, and Globalization*, 308–27.
66. Strauß, *Haubtstuck*, fol. 2v (Thesis 20).
67. Strauß, *Haubtstuck*, fol. 2v (Thesis 18).
68. See Hess, *Resisting Pluralization and Globalization*, 324–27.
69. Luther, *Whether One May Flee from a Deadly Plague*, 131.
70. Examples: Fettich, *Ordenung vnd Regiment*, fol. 3r–7v; Anon., *Von der Pestilentz*, sig. A6r–B3r; Willich, *Von der Pestilentz*, sig. A4r–B2v; Gasser, *Ainfeltiger vnd gegrünter bericht*, sig. A2r–v.
71. Lonitzer, *Ordnung Für die Pestilentz*, sig A6r-v; similarly Anon., *Von der Pestilentz*, sig. B3r.
72. Fettich, *Ordenung vnd Regiment*, fol. 7v.
73. Copp, *Ein nutzlich Regiment*, fol. 6r.
74. Magenbuch, *Ain nützlichs vnd Bewärts gemains Regiment*, sig. A2v.
75. Murphy, *A New Order of Medicine*, 45.
76. Anon, *Ein kurtz Regiment* (1543), sig. a3r.
77. Boccaccio, *The Decameron*, 7.
78. Seitz, *Ain schöner Tractat*, sig. B3r.
79. Folz, *Jtem von der pestilencz*, fol. 11v. See also Folz, *Jtem ein fast köstlicher spruch*, fol. 3v, v. 56–59: "According to this old saying, flee soon, flee far, return late. These are the three healing herbs in distress for all pharmacists and physicians."
80. Wolff, *Die Theorie der Seuche*, 143.

81. Sudhoff, "*Pestschriften*," 92.
82. For instance Brunschwig, *Liber pestilentialis*, fol. 6r; Schweller, *Ein Christliche vnderricht*, fol. 46v; Conradinus, *KVrtze vnd nutze gegründte vnderricht*, sig. L1v–L2r.
83. Brelochs, *Eyn kurtzer gegründter vnderricht*, sig. A3v-A4r.
84. Luther, *Whether One May Flee from a Deadly Plague*, 120–24. This position was also favored by Schweller, *Ein Christliche vnderricht*, fol. 46r–v, and Ulenbeck, *Ein schön und Christlich Gesprech*, sig. E4r–F3r.
85. Leroux, *Martin Luther as Comforter*, 229.
86. Wolff, *Die Theorie der Seuche*, 113.
87. Luther, *Whether One May Flee from a Deadly Plague*, 130.
88. Leroux, *Martin Luther as Comforter*, 224.
89. Castner, *Wie man sich in Pestilentzischen sterbsleuffen*, sig. C3r.
90. Castner, *Wie man sich in Pestilentzischen sterbsleuffen*, sig. C3v.
91. Stromer, *Regiment Henrichen Stromers* (1533), sig. A4r.
92. Stromer, *Regiment Henrichen Stromers* (1533), sig. A4r.
93. Stromer, *Regiment Henrichen Stromers* (1533), sig. A4r.
94. Quoted in Bühl, "Die Pestepidemien," 127; translation mine.
95. Wolff, *Die Theorie der Seuche*, 127.
96. Bühl, "Die Pestepidemien," 130.
97. Castner, *Wie man sich in Pestilentzischen sterbsleuffen*, sig. C3v.
98. Dross, "'es flohen die reichen leud,'" 303.
99. Anon., *Ein kurtz Regiment* (1533), sig. A3r.
100. Rittgers, "Protestants and Plague," 140.
101. Osiander, *Wie vnd wohin ein Christ*, sig. b2r.
102. Osiander, *Wie vnd wohin ein Christ*, sig. a4v–b1r.
103. Osiander, *Wie vnd wohin ein Christ*, sig. b2v.
104. Bühl, "Die Pestepidemien," 159. Rittgers ("Protestants and Plague," 140–43) discusses numerous reprintings of the sermon in Nuremberg and other German cities, particularly in years of plague.
105. Sachs, *Sehr herrliche, schöne, und warhaffte Gedicht*, vol. 4, fol. Iv.
106. Sachs, *Sehr herrliche, schöne, und warhaffte Gedicht*, vol. 4, fol. IIv.
107. Sachs, *Sehr herrliche, schöne, und warhaffte Gedicht*, vol. 4, fol. IIIv.
108. In a different poem, "Das 13 capitel Osee, des propheten," dated 15 July 1563, Sachs elaborated on his understanding of suffering in times of plague and lamented the lack of faith in the Creator, who, in Sachs's view, looked after those who believed in him.
109. Eckert, *The Structure of Plagues and Pestilences*, 22.
110. Folz, *Jtem von der pestilencz*, fol. 9v–10r.
111. Folz, *Jtem von der pestilencz*, fol. 10r.
112. Copp, *Ein nutzlich Regiment*, fol. 4r.
113. Bulst, "Der Schwarze Tod," 62.
114. Mattausch, *Das Beerdigungswesen*, 68–69.
115. Mattausch, *Das Beerdigungswesen*, 61–68. See also Chapter 10 by Martin Christ on burial practices during plague in this volume.
116. Partial reprint in Mattausch, *Das Beerdigungswesen*, 158–63.
117. Mattausch, *Das Beerdigungswesen*, 68–85.
118. Porzelt, *Die Pest in Nürnberg*, 56–57.
119. Cited in Bühl, "Die Pestepidemien," 134. Translation mine. The 1562 plague ordinance was printed as well, with the same justification (Anon., *Ains Erbern Raths der Stadt Nürmberg*, sig. A2v).

120. Hahn, "Luft," 647.
121. Magenbuch, *Ain nützlichs vnd Bewärts gemains Regiment*, sig A2r.
122. Castner, *Wie man sich in Pestilentzischen sterbsleuffen*, sig. C3v.
123. Wolff, *Die Theorie der Seuche*, 121.
124. Newhouse, "The Mystery of the St. Sebastian Lazareth," 127–28.
125. Luther, *Whether One May Flee from a Deadly Plague*, 126.
126. Luther, *Whether One May Flee from a Deadly Plague*, 127.
127. Rittgers, "Protestants and Plague," 139–40.
128. Anon., *Ein kurtz Regiment* (1533), sig. a2r.
129. Rittgers, "Protestants and Plague," 138.
130. Anon., *Ein kurtz Regiment* (1533), sig. a2v.
131. Anon., *Ein kurtz Regiment* (1543), title page.
132. Rittgers, "Protestants and Plague," 132.
133. Anon., *Ains Erbern Raths der Stadt Nürmberg*, sig. A2v. This formulation first appeared in the ordinance of 9 November 1519.
134. Anon., *Ains Erbern Raths der Stadt Nürmberg*, sig. A2r.
135. Anon., *Ains Erbern Raths der Stadt Nürmberg*, sig. A2v.
136. Oder, *Radt vnd Artzney*, sig A6v–A7r.
137. Anon., *Ains Erbern Raths der Stadt Nürmberg*, sig. A2v–B1r. This was a common catalog of measures, described for instance in 1572 by Adam Lonitzer (Lonitzer, *Ordnung Für die Pestilentz*, sig. A6r–A7r).
138. Anon., *Ains Erbern Raths der Stadt Nürmberg*, sig. B1r–v.
139. Schweller, *Ein Christliche vnderricht*, fol. 46r–v.
140. Adam Lonitzer in 1572 proposed the outlawing of dance for the same reason; Lonitzer, *Ordnung Für die Pestilentz*, sig. A7r. Similalry, Anon., *Von der Pestilentz* (1563) sig. B1v.
141. Anon., *Ein kurtz Regiment* (1562), sig. A2r.
142. Anon., *Ein kurtz Regiment* (1562), sig. A4v.
143. Sachs, *Sehr herrliche, schöne, und warhaffte Gedicht*, vol. 4, fol. Ir.
144. Anon., *Ein kurtz Regiment* (1575), sig. A2v.
145. Anon., *Ein kurtz Regiment* (1575), sig. A3r.
146. Anon., *Ein kurtz Regiment* (1575), sig. A3v.
147. Bamji, "Health Passes," 441.
148. Bamji, "Health Passes," 459.
149. Kirchberger, *Aphorismi*, sig. B4r; Anon., *Ein kurtz Regiment* (1585), sig. A3r–v.
150. Kirchberger, *Aphorismi*, sig. B1r.

Bibliography

Primary Sources

Anon. *Ains Erbern Raths der Stadt Nürmberg/ vernewete Gesetz vnd Ordnung/ in gegenwertigen sterbsleufften diß M.D.LXII. Jars auffgericht*. Nuremberg: Valentin Geissler, 1562.

Anon. *Ein kurtz Regiment auß vil treffenlichen zůsamen geprachten tractaten verstendiger artzt gezogen/ wie sich zů zeiten der pestilentz zuhalten sey*. Nuremberg: Friedrich Peypus, 1520.

Anon. *Ein kurtz Regiment wie sich zu zeiten der Pestilentz zu halten sey*. Nuremberg: Johann Petreius, 1533.

Anon. *Ein kurtz Regiment/ wie sich zu zeiten der Pestilentz zu halten sey*. Nürnberg: Johann Petreius, 1543.

Anon. *Ein kurtz Regiment/ wie man sich in Zeit Regierender Pestilentz halten soll*. Nuremberg: Valentin Geyßler, 1562.

Anon. *Ein kurtz Regiment/ wie man sich in zeit Regierender Pestilentz halten soll*. Nuremberg: Dietrich Gerlach, 1574.

Anon. *Ein kurtz Regiment/ wie man sich in diesen gegenwertigen Sterbsleufften halten sol*. Nuremberg: Katharina Gerlach and Johann von Bergs Erben, 1575.

Anon. *Ein kurtz Regiment/ wie man sich in disen gegenwertigen Sterbsleufften halten soll*. Nuremberg: Katharina Gerlach and Johann vom Berg Erben. 1582.

Anon. *Ein kurtz Regiment/ wie man sich in disen gegenwertigen Sterbsleufften halten soll*. Nuremberg: Katharina Gerlach, 1585.

Anon. *Ein warhaftige Ertzney vnd Schatz des lebens wider die schwere vnd schnelle sucht der pestilentz*. Leipzig: Wolfgang Stöckel, 1517.

Anon. *Von der Pestilentz. Kurtzer nützlicher vnd einfältiger bericht/ wie sich ein jeder zu zeit der regierenden Pestilentz verhüten vnd halten soll*. Frankfurt am Main: Christian Egenolffs Erben, 1563.

Boccaccio, Giovanni. *The Decameron*, translated and with an introduction by Wayne A. Rebhorn. New York, London: W. W. Norton, 2013.

Brelochs, Anton. *Eyn kurtzer gegründter vnderricht/ vnnd erklerung einer geschwinden/ und überscharpffen seüchten*. Nuremberg: Jobst Gutknecht, 1529.

Brunschwig, Hieronymus. *Liber pestilentialis de venenis epidimie*. Strasbourg: Hans Grüninger, 1500.

Castner, Johannes. *Wie man sich in Pestilentzischen sterbsleuffen vor der vergifftung bewaren möge*. Nuremberg: Johann Petreius, 1542.

Conradinus, Balthasar. *KVrtze vnd nutze gegründte vnderricht/ für den gemainen Mann/ wie er sich in den geferlichen leüffen der Pestilentz halten sol*. Innsbruck: Ruprecht Höller, 1562.

Copp, Johann. *Ein nutzlich Regiment wie man sich halten sol das man gesunden leyb behalt/ vnd sunderlich vor die pestilentz*. Erfurt: Matthes Maler, 1521.

Dietrich, Veit. *Der XCI. Psalm. Wie ein Christ in sterbßleufften sich trösten soll*. Nuremberg: Johann vom Berg and Ulrich Neuber, 1544.

Fenk, Michael. *Ain gut nützlich Regiment/ wie man sich halten soll/ vor/ in/ und nach der zeit der erschröcklichen kranckhayt der Pestilentz*. Augsburg: Alexander Weissenhorn, 1533.

Fettich, Theobald. *Ordenung vnd Regiment/ sich vor der überscharpffen vnnd gifftigen kranckheit der Pestilentz zuenthalten*. Frankfurt am Main: Christian Egenolff the Elder, 1531.

Folz, Hans. *Jtem ein fast köstlicher spruch von der pestilencz vnd anfenglich von den zeichen die ein künfftige pestilencz beteuten*. Nuremberg: Hans Folz, 1482.

Folz, Hans. *Jtem von der pestilencz ein hübsch nüczlich vnd kurcz begriffes*. Nuremberg: Hans Folz, 1482.

Gasser, Achilles Pirmin. *Ainfeltiger vnd gegrünter bericht/ wie menigklich sich in Pestilentzischem vbergang/ mit artznyen/ vnd anderer lybs not/ halten/ bewaren/ vnd genören soll*. Nuremberg: Johann Petreius, 1544.

Kegler, Caspar. *Eyn Nutzlichs vnd trostlichs Regiment wider dy Pestilentz vnd Gifftigk Pestilentzisch Feber die Schweyssucht genant*. Leipzig: Valentin Schumann, 1529.

Kirchberger, Johann Heinrich. *Aphorismi, Seu Canones Medicinales De Peste. Das ist: Kurtze Erinnerungs puncten von der Pest*. Nuremberg: Balthasar Scherff, 1625.

Link, Wenzeslaus. *Wie sich ein Christen mensch im leyden trösten sölle.* Nuremberg: Jobst Gutknecht, 1528.
Lonitzer, Adam. *Ordnung Für die Pestilentz.* Frankfurt am Main: Christian Egenolffs Erben, 1572.
Luther, Martin. *Whether One May Flee from a Deadly Plague.* Translated by Carl J. Schindler. In *Luther's Works. American Edition*, edited by Gustav K. Wiencke, vol. 43, 119–38. Philadelphia: Fortress Press, 1968.
Magenbuch, Johann. *Ain nützlichs vnd Bewärts gemains Regiment/ vnd fürkommen des vergyfften luffts/ in der zeyt des Sterbens oder Regierung der Pestilentz.* Augsburg: Philipp Ulhart the Elder, 1530.
Oder, Hieronymus. *Radt vnd Artzney/ zu verhütung vnd zu rettung wider die Pestilentz.* Wittenberg: Veit Creutzer, 1550.
Osiander, Andreas. *Wie vnd wohin ein Christ die grausamen plag der pestilentz fliehen soll.* Nuremberg: Johann Petreius, 1533.
Rympffer, Johannes. *Ein kurtz Regiment wider die grausame plag der Pestilentz.* Nuremberg: Johann Petreius, 1538.
Sachs, Hans. *Sehr herrliche, schöne, und warhaffte Gedicht. Das vierdt Poetisch Buch.* Nuremberg: Leonhardt Heußler and Joachim Lochner, 1578.
Sachs, Hans. "Das 13 capitel Osee, des propheten." In *Werke*, edited by Edmund Goetze, vol. 15, 240–44. Tübingen: Laupp, 1885.
Schnellenberg, Tarquinius. *Experimenta. Von XX. Pestilentz Wurtzeln vnd Kreutern.* Frankfurt am Main: Weygand Han, 1546.
Schweller, Haimeran. *Ein Christliche vnderricht wie man sich zů den zeiten/ der trübsal vnnd plagen Gottes/ vnd sunderlich zůr zeit der Pestilentz/ halten soll.* Ingolstadt: Alexander Weissenhorn, 1550.
Seitz, Alexander. *Ain schöner Tractat von dem Saturnischen gschoß der Pestilenz.* Augsburg: Sylvan Otmar, 1521.
Spengler, Lazarus. *Wie sich eyn Christen mensch inn trübsal und widerwertigkayt trösten/ vnd wo er die rechten hilff vnd Ertzney derhalben suchen soll.* Nuremberg: Jobst Gutknecht, 1529.
Strauß, Jakob. *Haubtstuck vnd artickel Christenlicher leer wider den unchristlichen wůcher.* Augsburg: Heinrich Steiner, 1523.
Stromer, Heinrich. *Regiment Henrichen Stromers von Aurbach der ertzenney Doctors inhaltendt wie sich wider die pestilentz tzubewaren.* Leipzig: Melchior Lotter the Elder, 1516.
Stromer, Heinrich. *Regiment Henrichen Stromers von Aurbach der ertzney Doctors inhaltendt wie sich wider die Pestilentz zu bewaren.* Nuremberg: Friedrich Peypus, 1533.
Theodorus, Jacobus. *Gewisse vnnd erfahren Practick/ Wie man sich mit Göttlicher hülff/ vor der Pestilentz hüten vnd bewaren.* Heidelberg: Johannes Mayer, 1564.
Theodorus, Jacobus. *Kurzer vnderricht vnd Rahtschlag/ wie man dem jetzigen Pestilentzischen gifftigen vnd hitzigen Feber/ … begegnen vnd vorkommen.* Heidelberg: Johann Mayer, 1573.
Ulenbeck, Johannes. *Ein schön und Christlich Gesprech/ eines Jüngern vnd Meisters wie sich ein jeder Christ in sterbenden nöten/ auch zur zeit der Pestilentz halten sol.* S.l., 1556.
Vadianus, Joachim. *EJn kurtz vnd trüwlich vnderricht wider die sorgklich kranckeyt der Pestilentz.* Basel: Adam Petri, 1519.
Willich, Jodocus. *Vonn der Pestilentz ein nützlich Regiment/ auff diese zeit gestellet.* Frankfurt an der Oder: Johann Eichorn, 1550.

Secondary Sources

Bamji, Alexandra. "Health Passes, Print and Public Health in Early Modern Europe." *Social History of Medicine* 32, no. 3 (2019): 441–64.

Belich, James. *The World the Plague Made: The Black Death and the Rise of Europe*. Princeton: Princeton University Press, 2022.

Bell, Dean Phillip, ed. *Plague in the Early Modern World. A Documentary History*. London, New York: Routledge, 2019.

Bergdolt, Klaus. *Der schwarze Tod in Europa. Die große Pest und das Ende des Mittelalters*. Munich: Beck, 1994.

Bühl, Charlotte. "Die Pestepidemien des ausgehenden Mittelalters und der Frühen Neuzeit in Nürnberg (1483/84 bis 1533/34)." In *Nürnberg und Bern: Zwei Reichsstädte und ihre Landgebiete*, edited by Rudolf Endres, 121–68. Erlangen: Universitätsbund Erlangen-Nürnberg, 1990.

Bulst, Neithard. "Der Schwarze Tod. Demographische, wirtschafts- und kulturgeschichtliche Aspekte der Pestkatastrophe von 1347–1352. Bilanz der neueren Forschung." *Saeculum: Jahrbuch für Universalgeschichte* 30 (1979): 45–67.

Christ, Martin. "Preaching during Plague Epidemics in Early Modern Germany, c.1520–1618." *Studies in Church History* 58 (2022): 91–111.

Cohn, Samuel K., Jr. *Cultures of Plague: Medical Thinking at the End of the Renaissance*. New York, Oxford: Oxford University Press, 2010.

Dross, Fritz. "'es flohen die reichen leud alle auß der stat/ darinnen sturben 10345 Menschen.' Seuchen in der frühneuzeitlichen Stadt." In *Ingolstadt in Bewegung: Grenzgänge am Beginn der Reformation*, edited by Susanne Greiter and Christine Zengerle, 303–24. Göttingen: Optimus Verlag, 2015.

Eckert, Edward A. *The Structure of Plagues and Pestilences in Early Modern Europe: Central Europe, 1560–1640*. Basel: Karger, 1996.

Frenzel, Sebastian. "Die Ordnung des Zorns: Der Zorn Gottes in den Policeygesetzen der Reichsstadt Ulm (Gotteslästerung, Zutrinken und Unzucht, 1492–1630)." In *Göttlicher Zorn und menschliches Maß: Religiöse Abweichung in frühneuzeitlichen Stadtgemeinschaften*, edited by Alexander Kästner and Gerd Schwerhoff, 45–71. Konstanz und München: UVK Verlagsgesellschaft, 2013.

Hahn, Philip. "Luft—eine elementare Angelegenheit vormoderner Kommunalpolitik? Beobachtungen an einer deutschen Stadt vom 15. bis zum 19. Jahrhundert." *Geschichte in Wissenschaft und Unterricht* 67, no. 11–12 (2016): 637–55.

Heinrichs, Erik A. "The Plague Cures of Caspar Kegler: Print, Alchemy, and Medical Marketing in Sixteenth-Century Germany." *The Sixteenth-Century Journal* 43, no. 2 (2012): 417–40.

Heinrichs, Erik A. *Plague, Print, and the Reformation: The German Reform of Healing, 1473–1573*. London and New York: Routledge, 2018.

Hess, Peter. *Resisting Pluralization and Globalization in German Culture, 1490–1540: Visions of a Nation in Decline*. Berlin, Boston: De Gruyter, 2020.

Jörg, Christian. *Teure, Hunger, Großes Sterben: Hungersnöte und Versorgungskrisen in den Städten des Reiches während des 15. Jahrhunderts*. Stuttgart: Hiersemann, 2008.

Kinzelbach, Annemarie. "Seuchenkonzepte und frühneuzeitliche Gesellschaft: Deutungen von 'Pestilenzen' und städtischer Alltag." *Berichte zur Wissenschaftsgeschichte* 20, no. 2–3 (1997): 253–65.

Kruse, Christian, ed. *Der Feind in der Stadt: Vom Umgang mit Seuchen in Augsburg, München und Nürnberg*. Munich: Staatliche Archive Bayerns, 2016.

Leroux, Neil. *Martin Luther as Comforter. Writings on Death*. Leiden: Brill, 2007.

Mattausch, Hubert. *Das Beerdigungswesen der freien Reichsstadt Nürnberg 1219 bis 1806: Eine rechtsgeschichtliche Untersuchung an Hand der Ratsverlässe und der vom Rat erlassenen Leichenordnungen*. Würzburg: Dissertation Universität Würzburg, 1970.

Murphy, Hannah. *A New Order of Medicine. The Rise of Physicians in Reformation Nuremberg*. Pittsburgh: University of Pittsburgh Press, 2019.

Murphy, Hannah. "Decisions before Decision-Making: Concepts, Categories and Technologies in Sixteenth-Century German Medical Texts." In *Semantiken und Narrative des Entscheidens vom Mittelalter bis zur Gegenwart*, edited by Philip R. Hoffmann-Rehnitz, Matthias Pohlig, et al., 193–209. Göttingen: Vandenhoeck & Ruprecht, 2021.

Newhouse, Amy. "The Mystery of the St. Sebastian Lazareth: Mapping Place-Names and Contagious Disease Hospitals in Sixteenth-Century Nuremberg." In *Names and Naming in Early Modern Germany*, edited by Marjorie Elizabeth Plummer and Joel F. Harrington, 125–48. New York, Oxford: Berghahn Books, 2019.

O'Brien, Monica Catherine. "Practice and Power: The Rise and Disappearance of the Franzosenärzte, or Doctors of the French Pox, in Nuremberg, 1495–1560." *Journal of the Royal College of Physicians of Edinburgh* 51, no. 1 (2021): 91–97.

Porzelt, Carolin. *Die Pest in Nürnberg: Leben und Herrschen in Pestzeiten in der Reichsstadt Nürnberg (1562–1713)*. St. Ottilien: EOS Verlag, 2000.

Rittgers, Ronald K. "Protestants and Plague. The Case of the 1562/63 Pest in Nürnberg." In *Piety and Plague from Byzantium to the Baroque*, edited by Franco Mormando and Thomas Worcester, 132–55. Kirksville: Truman State University Press, 2007.

Rittgers, Ronald K. *The Reformation of Suffering: Pastoral Theology and Lay Piety in Late Medieval and Early Modern Germany*. Oxford, New York: Oxford University Press, 2012.

Seelbach, Kirsten Renate. *In dieser harten und sterbenden Zeit. Maßnahmen gegen die Pest 1620–1750*. Marburg: Tectum-Verlag, 2007.

Slack, Paul. "Responses to Plague in Early Modern Europe: The Implications of Public Health." *Social Research* 55, no. 3 (1988): 433–53.

Sudhoff, Karl. "Pestschriften aus den ersten 150 Jahren nach der Epidemie des 'schwarzen Todes' 1348. XIV. Pesttraktate aus Süddeutschland in der 2. Hälfte des 15. Jahrhunderts." *Archiv für Geschichte der Medizin* 14, no. 3–4 (1923): 79–105.

Wolff, Katharina. *Die Theorie der Seuche: Krankheitskonzepte und Pestbewältigung im Mittelalter*. Stuttgart: Franz Steiner Verlag, 2021.

CHAPTER 3

Fighting Plague and Heresy in Bavaria

The Confessionalization of Bavarian Plague Literature, 1521–1650

ERIK A. HEINRICHS

Introduction

Early modern struggles against plague left enduring monuments visible today in Bavaria, most notably in Munich's central square, Marienplatz. Here in 1638 Bavarian authorities erected the Mariensäule, a baroque column topped with a statue of the Virgin Mary, to commemorate deliverance from the Swedish occupation and plagues of the Thirty Years' War. Most importantly, this column counts heresy among the scourges of the era. Among the striking statuary on the Mariensäule are four monsters representing war, plague, famine, and heresy, depicted on the verge of defeat by four putti holding swords and spears.[1] As this monument demonstrates, the struggle against plague during premodern times was never merely a struggle against a physical sickness, as modern thinking would have it. Plague counted among a set of threats, all of which were ultimately explained in terms of divine will and therefore laden with spiritual meaning. The fight against plague was therefore intimately linked to the struggle against sin and, in an age of intense religious disputes, to the struggle against heresy. This chapter explores the background of this dramatic scene on the Mariensäule by examining how Bavarian physicians and political leaders came to treat plague and heresy as interrelated problems between the Reformation and the end of the Thirty Years' War. It pursues these connections in physicians' printed plague advice as well as in the public plague mandates enacted by city and territorial leaders. What this investigation reveals is how medical, religious, and political goals mixed among Bavarian authorities as they sought to manage plague and new religious disputes in a public way for the first time.

Recent work has shown that responses to plague were central to the Protestant Reformation in German-speaking lands, as physicians and clerics used their printed plague advice to reform religious piety and strengthen the social authority of university-trained physicians.[2] The case of ducal Bavaria allows historians to assess how this trend played out within a Catholic context and within one early modern state. This approach allows for demonstration of how plague policies fit into the broader goals of political authorities, including a preoccupation with establishing religious orthodoxy during an era of religious dispute. What emerges from this study is a broader view of the historical process that Reformation historians call confessionalization. This is an historical term with its own long history, but in this case describes how authorities of church and state united after the Reformation to establish a particular religious confession as the state religion, with the broader goal of promoting social order and unity.[3] This study highlights the role that public plague mandates played within this process of confessionalization, and recounts the history of how Bavarian physicians sometimes aided the Catholic revival through their printed plague advice literature. One major narrative pursued here is the decline and revival of the saints and other forms of Catholic piety within printed plague advice. Overall, the Catholic revival in plague literature and policy represents a lesser-known chapter of the Catholic Reformation in Bavaria.[4]

Bavaria here means the lands ruled by the dukes of Bavaria, one branch of the noble Wittelsbach family. Despite the dukes' success in expanding their territory in the early modern period, ducal Bavaria was much smaller than today's German state. It was mostly rural and situated between the bishopric of Eichstätt to the north, Passau and Bohemia to the east, Tyrol and Salzburg to the south, and Swabian lands across the river Lech to the west. Large and powerful imperial cities, such as Nuremberg, Augsburg, and Regensburg, were independent of the Bavarian dukes, and thereby reduced the dukes' political and cultural power in the region. Although none of the towns in ducal Bavaria matched the great population centers of the Holy Roman Empire, they included Landshut, Straubing, the university town of Ingolstadt, and the residence of the ducal family, Munich. The present investigation of Bavarian plague literature and plague mandates considers only the works that originated within ducal Bavaria or that were composed for a Bavarian patron or audience. Most Bavarian plague literature appeared on presses in Munich or Ingolstadt, although a minority appeared in Landshut or Augsburg.[5]

Munich city records show that epidemics threatened the city and region nearly every decade between 1500 and the end of the Thirty Years' War: 1506, 1520–21, 1533–36, 1541, 1547–48, 1562–63, 1572–73, 1586–90, 1598–99,

1607–8, 1628–29, 1634–35, 1649–51.[6] The dukes of Bavaria issued public plague mandates for the entire territory in the years 1585, 1592, 1596, 1599, 1606, 1613, 1625, 1634, and 1649.[7] Although this list reveals the grave dangers of the time, Bavaria fared rather well compared to surrounding lands. Bavaria experienced fewer plagues than other parts of the Holy Roman Empire, especially the territories along the rivers Rhine, Main, Neckar, and Elbe, as well as the northern coasts.[8] After the mid-seventeenth century, plague became somewhat rare, but still loomed in neighboring Salzburg and the more distant Habsburg lands. The major epidemics that devastated Vienna and Prague in 1679 and 1713 bypassed much of Bavaria.[9]

The Decline of the Saints in Bavaria

To appreciate the renewal of Catholic piety in Bavaria during the later sixteenth century one must understand how it first dimmed and came under dispute during the first half of the century. Protestant sentiment spread in Bavaria at the outset of the Reformation as criticism of the cult of the saints and other traditional aspects of Christianity began to circulate broadly.[10] The effect of these messages is apparent by 1521 within physicians' plague advice literature. Among all German plague publications written by physicians throughout German-speaking lands, 1521 marks the sudden and nearly complete disappearance of saints. Out of sixteen plague treatises written by German physicians and published in 1521, only two mention a saint, representing a steep decline compared to earlier.[11] For reform-minded authors, this moment represents the start of a broader reform of healing that unfolded during the Reformation, since Protestant critics had rejected many aspects of Catholic spiritual healing, including the intercession of saints.[12] Of course not all physicians acted out of Protestant inspiration in 1521 when composing plague advice. Physicians' willingness to omit any mention of saints may also stem from the long history of competition between spiritual and natural healing or, rather, between clerics and physicians, that existed since the Middle Ages. One Bavarian example comes from a 1497 miracle book that promotes the Marian pilgrimage to Altötting, one of Bavaria's premier pilgrimage sites. The author depicts the Virgin Mary as a doctor whose exceptional healing powers place her above all other doctors.[13] Such views certainly challenged university-trained physicians as they sought to spread their views of natural medicine to a broad population in a new era of vernacular print.

In 1521 Alexander Seitz, the city physician of Munich, offered a response to such cultural trends that prioritized saints over physicians. Indeed, his plague treatise of that year attempts to limit the appeal of the Virgin Mary. When discussing why more people from St. Peter's parish in Munich were dying from the plague compared to the parish of Our Lady (Frauenkirche), Seitz dismisses the notion that the Virgin Mary provides special protection to her own parish. He instead points to a physical cause, the air, to explain the difference in mortality. Seitz explains that the area of St. Peter's parish receives the dangerous midday winds first, while the area of Our Lady's parish is more prone to receive the healthier winds of midnight.[14] This and other surprising statements certainly drew controversy. While Seitz had been a city physician in Munich since 1519, and served the city well during the plague of 1520–21, he eventually fled Munich for Protestant territories at some point during or after 1521. Seitz distinguished himself in his career as a free thinker on medical and religious matters, and left behind many writings, including letters exchanged with the Swiss reformer Ulrich Zwingli.[15]

The First Stirrings of Catholic Revival

Despite the example of Seitz, and despite the broader trend away from saints in physicians' plague writing, the saints played a more prominent role in Bavarian plague literature than in any other German-speaking land. Indeed, Bavaria provides the few exceptions to the disappearance of saints and traditional Catholic piety within physicians' plague treatises after 1521. The treatises by the Ingolstadt medical professors Michael Fenckh (1533) and Johann Bosch (1562) demonstrate that not only did Catholic piety survive in this genre, but some Bavarian physicians and magistrates were speaking out against Protestantism even before the Council of Trent concluded in 1563.[16]

The plague treatise by the medical professor Michael Fenckh (d. 1538) represents an early attempt to support traditional spiritual healing during the early years of the Protestant Reformation. Fenckh composed his plague advice in 1533, addressing it to the city council and common man of Ingolstadt.[17] It hews closely to the late medieval genre of plague *consilia*, focused as it was on natural medicine but prefaced with brief discussion of plague's spiritual aspects. Here Fenckh's spiritual advice stands out for its unambiguous Catholic piety. To counter the plague's origin as a divine punishment, Fenckh recommends that one should appeal to the saints every day and singles out St. Sebastian in particular.[18] Later he also recommends seeking aid from Sts. Sebastian, Gaian, Roch, and Job, and especially the Virgin Mother of God and St. Moritz, who enjoyed special devotion in Ingolstadt. In an unusual move, Fenckh supports his Catholic measures against plague by appealing to the authority of Avicenna (ca. 980—1037). Although aware that this physician of the Islamic Golden Age was not Christian, Fenckh hails his use of natural understanding to recognize that prayer, sacrifice, litanies, processions, pilgrimages, and similar good works are helpful during plagues.[19] Fenckh's statement on confession is also unusual, since the saints play a role in his description of the practice. The first step of confession includes being God fearing and placing the saints before one's eyes. Particularly Catholic instructions for confession follow, including doing penance for one's sins.[20]

Fenckh's context at the University of Ingolstadt suggests that his advice is not merely a holdover of traditional religion but represents an effort to encourage it in the face of the Protestant challenge. At this time the university became known for harboring defenders of Catholicism. Most famously, it was the home of Johannes Eck (1486–1543), Martin Luther's arch-rival in theological debates. Furthermore, Ingolstadt repelled Protestant scholars while attracting Catholic ones during the first decades of the Reformation. The medical humanist Leonhart Fuchs (1501–66) twice left the Ingolstadt medical faculty for religious reasons. Others were drawn to Ingolstadt for its Catholic affiliation, such as Veit Amerbach (1503–57), a professor who traded Wittenberg for Ingolstadt in 1543 after his disputes with Luther and Melanchthon.[21]

As Fenckh was writing in Ingolstadt, city leaders in Munich were busy devising their first comprehensive plague mandates for the epidemic of 1532–33 in an attempt to manage the city's physical and spiritual response. Reflecting an atmosphere of increased religious tensions, these mandates emphasize peace and a common understanding of the Bible, while also encouraging traditional Catholic piety. Furthermore, Munich's plague mandates of 1532/33 may be the first German plague mandates that were also printed, reflecting an effort to embrace the new vernacular print media to publicize the new rules for plague. Neighboring imperial cities were the first to develop a civic plague policy and issue plague mandates, including Nuremberg in ca. 1520 and Augsburg in 1521.[22] But it is unclear if civic magistrates in these cities also printed their mandates, as happened in Munich by 1533.[23] In 1532 the city of Munich paid an anonymous book printer to produce fifty copies of this single-leaf broadside.[24]

Munich's plague mandates of 1532/33 lay out the city's spiritual and physical measures against the plague, ranging from rules on isolating the sick, washing bedding, as well as the need to bring the sacraments to those affected. Their first point is the most pertinent for this investigation since it establishes weekly processions in each parish as an important part of the spiritual solution. Here city fathers sought to appease divine anger and to promote love of neighbor, all while emphasizing a concordant (*ainhelligem*) understanding of the holy scriptures. Through such processions and spiritual change, city fathers saw themselves as working against the archenemy of the Christian faith (the Devil) as they sought both "peace and concord in all Christendom" as well as a "blessed, healthy air" free of poisonous influences.[25] Similar statements that work against divisions within Christianity appear in other plague treatises from Catholic lands at the time, including Caspar Kegler's popular 1529 pamphlet from Leipzig.[26]

Building a Confessional State amid Plague after 1560

After 1533 no plague literature written by physicians appeared from Bavarian presses until the 1560s, when a widespread plague began. By the time physicians published again, the political and religious landscape in Bavaria had become even more polarized between Catholics and Protestants. Duke Albrecht V (r. 1550–79) had joined the anti-Protestant cause in response to swelling Protestant sentiment in his lands and surrounding imperial cities. The years around 1560 saw the height of a Protestant resurgence among nobles and urban dwellers within Bavaria as well as the lowest point in a steady decline of pilgrimage to saints' shrines. The lenience that Duke Albrecht had shown earlier to Protestant factions changed as Protestant nobles appeared to threaten ducal power. When Albrecht sensed a rebellion forming in 1563, he moved forcefully against the Protestant faction, increasing his control over religious practice and the Bavarian estates. Strict ordinances against Protestant worship and Protestant literature soon followed, culminating in 1570 when the duke mandated that Protestants should renounce their belief or leave Bavaria.[27]

It is no coincidence that strong action against Protestant factions in Bavaria came after the final session of the Council of Trent, which ended in 1563. The council's conclusion supplied Catholic rulers and clergy with the moral authority and intellectual basis to move against heresy and heterodoxy. The single most important trend that strengthened Catholicism in Bavaria, however, was the growing cooperation between the Bavarian duchy and the Jesuit order, beginning during Duke Albrecht's reign. In his survey of south German literature, Dieter Breuer singles out 1565 as a key year in Bavarian history as the duchy allied itself with the Jesuits, each party recognizing their mutual interests. The duchy sought greater political and social unity by promoting a specifically Catholic confessional culture, while the Jesuits sought to counter Protestant influence in the region.[28]

A more intense confessional climate engulfed the faculty of the University of Ingolstadt during the 1560s as well. Professors' beliefs were placed under greater scrutiny and after 1568 all graduates were required to profess the Tridentine faith.[29] The 1562 plague treatise by the medical professor Johann Lonäus Bosch (Boscius) (1515–85) reflects the mounting tensions. Unlike Fenckh's 1533 text, Bosch's work features a general denunciation of heresies of the time, including fatalism and medical passivity. After dedicating his work to the city council of Ingolstadt, Bosch opens with: "Among all the heresies going on in these dangerous times, not the least of them that derive from an evil understanding of the Holy Scriptures, is the belief that life and death have a predetermined time which can neither be shortened nor lengthened."[30] Bosch views this heresy as dangerous to earthly affairs, since it dismisses the possibility of meaningful action by physicians and public leaders, and dangerous to the soul, since it contradicts the Bible itself. To demonstrate that human actions, medical and spiritual, can lengthen or shorten human lives, Bosch cites King David's successful repentance and the fig poultice that Isaiah ordered for King Hezekiah's sickness.[31] By the 1560s, medical passivity had long been a target among both Catholic and Protestant authors, among them Martin Luther. Luther feared those who preached that "faith alone" meant that natural medicine was unnecessary or unbiblical.[32] Although Bosch and Luther could agree on the danger of medical passivity, Bosch's references to "all the heresies" and "evil understandings of the Holy Scriptures" certainly reveal his willingness to call out divergent religious beliefs by the 1560s.

Bosch's personal history suggests that he was acting to revive Catholicism at the University of Ingolstadt as he wrote in 1562, forming an early step in the Bavarian Catholic Reformation. Bosch came to Ingolstadt from Louvain in 1558, possibly upon the request of the duke, and led a revival of Catholic piety within the Ingolstadt medical faculty with his colleague Adam Landau.[33] He distinguished himself as a professor of medicine and for supervising the acquisitions of the university library until his death in 1585. A sign that the Bavarian duchy trusted and supported him is that Duke Wilhelm V (r. 1579–97) honored Bosch's service posthumously by promising to care for his widow and four children. A broad assessment of Bosch's medical thought shows that learning at Ingolstadt was not tradition bound, since he was open to the new medical ideas of the "Neoterici" and praised the anatomist Andreas Vesalius (1514–64) especially. As a fellow Catholic from the Low Countries, Bosch had much to admire in Vesalius.[34]

Further evidence that a new spirit was present at the University of Ingolstadt comes in the unusual martial tone of Bosch's writing. Although Bosch does not aim to create soldiers of God as the Jesuits would, his 1562 plague treatise urges his audience to stand firm in the face of plague like a soldier, since cowardly and lazy conduct does not please God. Bosch closes his pamphlet by saying that in the war of this world a man must stick to his battle orders and hold the battleground until God, the highest general and emperor, calls him from it.[35] That Bosch and the Jesuits shared a martial tone and an emphasis on obedience is likely no coincidence. There was much contact between Jesuits and Ingolstadt professors after 1549 when Duke Wilhelm IV (r. 1508–50) called the Jesuits to Ingolstadt to support Catholicism at the university.[36] Bosch's example shows that the struggle against plague was becoming more closely connected to the broader trends of the Catholic Reformation in Bavaria.

Most telling of a new Catholic Reformation spirit at Ingolstadt is the support that Bosch received in publishing his work from the new rector of the university, the theologian and preacher Martin Eisengrein (1535–78). In his preface Bosch thanks the rector for the opportunity to translate his lecture on plague and publish it within three months of first delivering it to students.[37] Although Eisengrein had converted to Catholicism only a few years prior to becoming rector, he distinguished himself in subsequent years as one of the most energetic Catholic reformers in southern German lands. Eisengrein attracted the attention of Duke Albrecht for his purge of Protestants at the University of Vienna after his conversion there in the late 1550s. During his tenure in Bavaria, Eisengrein advised Duke Albrecht on church matters, led anti-Lutheran efforts through his sermons and writings, and bolstered the reforming impulse at Ingolstadt.[38]

Trends that encouraged Catholic piety in plague literature only grew in the coming decades, as a new era of Catholic confessionalism in print began to flourish with the founding of Adam Berg's press in Munich in 1565. Since Duke Albrecht V sought to promote orthodox printed literature in his territory, he welcomed and supported Berg when he moved to Bavaria. In the coming decades, Berg became one of the most important printers of the Catholic Reformation in Europe, producing everything from popular literature to costly editions of important religious works.[39] Berg's press came to Munich just as a new audience was forming that could access the printed literature of Catholic reform. Bavaria, and especially Munich, had a growing class of literate elites, comprised of ducal officials, the clergy, influential burghers, and students at local church schools.[40] Berg is a key figure in the story of the Bavarian struggle against plague and heresy, since he published nearly all of Bavaria's medical plague pamphlets printed between 1572 and the end of the sixteenth century. His plague publications demonstrate the emerging alliance between the dukes, physicians, clerics, and printers in Bavaria.[41]

The Confessional State Grapples with Plague and Heresy, 1579–1651

The Catholic revival gained even greater impulse in Bavaria when Duke Wilhelm V came to power in 1579. Deeply pious and educated by Jesuits since youth, Duke Wilhelm accelerated the political and religious trends that promoted and enforced a specifically Catholic culture. In this effort, Wilhelm continued the work of his father, Albrecht V, and maneuvered successfully to acquire more power over religion and domestic politics. In 1583 the duchy signed the Bavarian Concordat with the Catholic Church, which gave the dukes greater control over the discipline and morals of the clergy and laity. In historian David Lederer's view, this constitutional agreement provided the basis for Duke Wilhelm, and later his son Maximilian I, to build and enforce a "penitential regime" that aided political modernization and had lasting effects on Bavarian religion and culture.[42] Duke Wilhelm and his successors justified their incursions on the traditional privileges of the church and city with the new concept of the *Landesvater*. The father of the land had to rule with a strong and loving hand to ensure peace and prosperity among his subjects.[43] An important duty of the *Landesvater* in an era of war, plague, famine, and heresy was to guide morals and to protect right religion to prevent divine punishments.

Only after expanding power over church and state did Duke Wilhelm turn his attention to Bavaria's first plague policy at the territorial level. Compared to Munich's earlier civic mandates, Duke Wilhelm's are much more extensive and urge an even more regimented religious practice. These are dated 1 October 1585 and appeared on Berg's press later that year as a prologue to a plague treatise by the physician Theobald Fettich (fl. 1530). Berg added his own introduction as well as Catholic prayers to the end of Fettich's text.[44] The duke opens his mandates by connecting the punishment of plague to mankind's great sins and discusses the importance of caring for the body and soul of his subjects.[45] While Duke Wilhelm seeks to maintain earthly order during epidemics, he seems to prioritize the health of the soul by basing his earthly mandates on the argument that taking care of the body is necessary for the health of the soul.[46] Because Christ says that one must strive for God's kingdom above all else, Duke Wilhelm commands that each person attend church services and turn to God with more reverence than before. A Catholic expression of confessing sins appears within the duke's command that his subjects confess their sins, show regret, and do penance. Rare for plague mandates of the era, Duke Wilhelm identifies specific sins that have aroused divine wrath, including "all kinds of punishable vices, such as blasphemies, swearing, immoderate consumption, obscenity, unreasonable complaints against neighbors, and other misdeeds by young and old."[47] To carry out these spiritual mandates, the duke enlists the aid of the various clerics throughout the land, commanding that they institute weekly processions or church services for this spiritual work, as well as use the pulpit to bolster attendance. In a later passage, Duke Wilhelm mandates that the clergy urge their flock from the pulpit to go to confession and receive the holy sacrament once every week or two. He also adds a quasi-apocalyptic reference to support this spiritual regimen—so that when the Lord comes, the people are not found sleeping.[48]

Duke Wilhelm's mandates represent an intensification of Catholic practices fitting of the broader Catholic revival of the early modern era, known for its emphasis on regular and frequent reception of the sacraments. Perhaps because the duke had already successfully suppressed Protestantism by 1585 there is no specific mention of heresy. In general, it seems that by 1585 Bavarian authorities were less focused on fighting heresy than they were on maintaining or intensifying specifically Catholic practices among the population, such as processions and confession with penance. This represents a shift away from the impulse of the Counter Reformation of the early to mid-sixteenth century and towards a broader Catholic revival that would define the next century of Bavarian history. Most importantly, these plague mandates were long lasting in form and content in Bavaria. Duke Wilhelm, and later Duke Maximilian I, reissued them multiple times with few or no changes to the spiritual content through the Thirty Years' War—1592, 1596, 1599, 1606, 1613, 1625, 1634, and 1649.[49] Overall, such plague mandates were important instruments of instilling religious order and discipline, and deserve more attention from historians of religion.

Adam Berg's 1585 edition of the texts by Duke Wilhelm V and Theobald Fettich also features appended prayers that give the first direct rhetorical attack on Protestant sects and that bring the saints' aid back into Bavarian plague pamphlets. Such references to saints were not present in prayers that Berg added to the end of Fettich's text in an earlier 1572 edition.[50] Berg described this three-page prayer as useful to read from the pulpit and in the home. It recognizes God's majesty and enumerates human sins, including the lack of prayer, fasting, alms giving, and good works. Themes of repentance, spiritual renewal, and divine protection dominate. A clear Counter-Reformation voice comes through in the request that God lift the current division within Christianity and destroy all harmful groups and sects. And, in a final Catholic touch, Jesus and the saints appear as sources for divine aid.[51]

The physical and medical aspects of Duke Wilhelm's mandates do not stand out among contemporary plague mandates but are worth mentioning for their level of detail, which was new for Bavaria. Here Duke Wilhelm promotes cleanliness, free care for the poor, and the regulation of surgeons. He takes greater efforts to regulate malodorous waste in cities and towns, banning discarded blood, dung, overripe fruit in markets, and the keeping of pigs and birds within towns. The last two points reveal more attention to the problems of bureaucracy, as the duke informs that officials must perform their assigned duties and that should a public servant fall sick, no effort will be spared to help them regain health.[52] With God's grace and a skilled doctor, the duke believes that one could recover from the plague (*Pestilentz*) if infected.[53]

While printers like Berg were reviving the cult of the saints in printed literature by 1585, it is important to note that Bavarian physicians did not participate in this trend as authors for another few decades, likely due to the long-standing competition between physicians and clerics. Some Bavarian physicians eventually overcame any lingering hostility towards the cult of the saints during the seventeenth century and began to vouch for saints' miracles.[54]

The first example of saints reentering physicians' plague treatises comes in 1607 in the work of Bonifacius Sauter, who wrote for the Bavarian town of Wasserburg. Sauter opens his text with a discussion of divine punishment and offers spiritual medicines to appease divine wrath. Daily prayers to the Holy Mother Mary and the Holy Martyr St. Sebastian appear here, including the standard lines of true regret, repentance, and firm faith in Jesus.[55] Other physicians in the region soon followed by incorporating other traditional aspects of Catholicism into their plague advice. The most striking example comes in the 1612 plague pamphlet by the Tyrolean physician Hippolytus Guarinonius (1571–1654), published in Ingolstadt.[56] This self-described "worldly Jesuit" describes the Eucharist in terms of the philosopher's stone, presenting it as the greatest weapon against plague. Mocking the alleged Calvinist disciples of Paracelsus, Guarinonius boasts that he has discovered the true philosopher's stone as a Catholic and Galenist physician. He goes on to argue that the philosopher's stone is the Eucharist itself, a "complete and eternal balsam, superior in its virtue, eternal and ineffable in its being."[57] This treatment of the Eucharist as a healing medicine was also not unique among later Bavarian plague literature.[58]

Considering both religious and medical works, much plague literature in Bavaria was "confessionalized" to varying degrees by the mid-seventeenth century. Two pamphlets published in 1649, one by a physician and one by a priest, demonstrate the extent to which plague literature acquired confessional messages by the end of the Thirty Years' War. The work of the Munich city physician Malachias Geiger contains a direct reference to specific Bavarian relics and saints. At the end of his thirty-one-page pamphlet, Geiger recommends the intercession of the most holy Virgin Mother of God and, especially, the patrons of plague protection Sts. Sebastian, Benno, Cosmas and Damian, whose relics rest in Bavaria.[59] Such pious elements in seventeenth-century plague pamphlets, however, did not signal a lack of interest in natural medicine on the part of physicians. Geiger's appreciation of natural medicine is apparent on his title page, which shows two ancient medical figures standing over the Munich skyline, in places where one might expect saints in more pious artwork. To one side stands Andromachus holding a jar marked "THERIACA" while Mithridates stands to the other side with "MITHRIDATIUS." Geiger's broader interest in secular antidotes for physical poisons is also reflected in a 1657 Latin tract that describes his experience using unicorn horn to fight poisons.[60] Equally striking are the unusual illustrations that supplement Geiger's 1649 pamphlet. These six large illustrations depict the layouts of various plague hospitals in Europe, including the lazarettos of Paris and Milan, and reflect Geiger's interest in the architectural aspects of managing plague. Geiger states that he made the illustrations himself in 1634, possibly drawing on his own experience in France and Italian lands.[61]

However, a very different picture of plague prevention appears in a 1649 pamphlet from Altötting, the site of a Marian pilgrimage of the utmost importance to the dukes of Bavaria.[62] This seventeen-page sermon reprints the dramatic words delivered by the Jesuit Christoph Camerer before an assembled plague procession. Seeking protection from a plague epidemic in neighboring Austria, the Jesuits planned to process with the "wonder-working image of the most worthy Virgin Mary of Altötting," departing from the church of Sts. Jacob and Philip on the feast day of St. Carlo Borromeo.[63] Camerer's rousing speech uses rhetorical questions, short sentences, and exclamations to present a persuasive argument for the superiority of divine love over death and plague. Most noteworthy is the revival of the late medieval theme that holds Mary as a doctor above all others. According to Camerer, asking God for mercy is not enough. One must also turn to the most dependable doctor, the Virgin Mary—"When all doctors forsake you, this doctor to the world (*Weltartztin vnnd Doctorin*) in Altötting does not."[64]

The 1649 pamphlets by Geiger and Camerer illustrate two ways that the Catholic Reformation affected vernacular plague literature towards the end of the reign of Maximilian I. According to categories formulated by historians Ute Lotz-Heumann and Matthias Pohlig, Camerer's pamphlet was confessionalized in a strong sense, since its primary goal was to program specific religious behavior in accordance with the goals of authorities. Geiger, on the other hand, probably did not intend his pamphlet primarily to reform Catholics but was focused on providing useful natural medicines to protect oneself from plague. Geiger's work was therefore confessionalized in a weak sense, since its Catholic messages emerged because Geiger was embedded in a confessionally defined cultural context that encouraged appealing to saints and visiting relics.[65] It is significant, however, that the religious context affected how physicians wrote about plague at all. The struggle against plague was more than a struggle against physical poisons but became closely connected to the war on sin and heresy during Bavaria's Catholic Reformation.

Up to 1651, promoting spiritual medicines for plague and heresy, or, rather, encouraging Catholic religious practices, were important political goals of the Bavarian dukes Albrecht V, Wilhelm V, and Maximilian I. The burial plan that Duke Maximilian devised for his own death reflects this intense devotion to saints among Bavaria's reforming elite. Soon after his death in 1651 Maximilian's heart was removed and stored in a special cardiotaph in the chapel to Our Lady of Mercy in Altötting. At this time officials found a pact that Duke Maximilian had written in his own blood and left at the chapel near the start of his reign in 1598, dedicating himself to the Virgin Mary.[66] It should be no surprise, then, that Maximilian commissioned the Mariensäule that one sees in Munich's central square today to commemorate his victory over war, plague, famine, and heresy. By 1651 Maximilian's cultural project had reached critical importance as rulers, physicians, clerics, and printers worked to revive Catholic piety, overlapping with the public fight against plague. Such efforts enabled a full revival of Catholicism that had an impact on Bavaria for centuries to come.

Erik A. Heinrichs is Professor of History at Winona State University (Minnesota). He is a historian of late medieval and early modern Europe and earned his PhD from Harvard University. His work on German plague literature includes his recent book *Plague, Print, and the Reformation: The German Reform of Healing, 1473–1573,* part of the History of Medicine in Context Series at Routledge (2018).

Notes

1. Heimers, *Krieg, Hunger, Pest und Glaubenszwist,* 48–55, pictures on pages 52–55.
2. Heinrichs, *Plague, Print, and the Reformation.*
3. For a recent history of the term confessionalization and for treatment of confessionalization in Bavaria, see Fisher, *Music, Piety, and Propaganda,* 13–15.
4. I use the term Catholic Reformation when discussing these historical trends within German-speaking lands and use it with the hope that it captures the various trends of the movement—sometimes attempting to counter Protestant influence, sometimes seeking to simply renew Catholicism, but within a time and place marked by struggles against the Protestant Reformation. On the complexities of such attempts to label the Catholic Reformation or Early Modern Catholicism, see O'Malley, "Was Ignatius Loyola a Catholic Reformer?"
5. Augsburg presses attracted Bavarian authors, especially during the early sixteenth century, since there were relatively few presses in Bavarian towns at the time. Such is the case with the 1533 pamphlet by the Ingolstadt medical professor Michael Fenckh as discussed below.
6. Stahleder, *Chronik der Stadt München,* Vol. 2, 15–556.
7. This list of plague mandates is compiled from Hoffmeister and my own research, although I have not seen the 1599 and 1625 mandates that Hoffmeister mentions. Similarly, Hoffmeister does not mention the 1585 and 1634 mandates. Hoffmeister, *Das Medizinalwesen im Kurfürstentum Bayern,* 100.
8. For example, epidemics during the 1580s outright bypassed most regions of ducal Bavaria by moving directly from the Main River valley to Bohemian towns. Eckert, *The Structure of Plagues and Pestilences,* 99. Eckert speculates that Bavaria's dispersed settlement, particular building styles, and various biological factors contributed to this resistance. See 146.
9. Eckert, "The Retreat of Plague from Central Europe," 1–28. Öhler, *Die Pest in Salzburg.*
10. Soergel, *Wondrous in His Saints,* 44–73.
11. For the broader context of plague publications circa 1521: Heinrichs, *Plague, Print, and the Reformation,* 80–86.
12. Heinrichs, *Plague, Print, and the Reformation,* 75–82.
13. Assion, "Geistliche und Weltliche Heilkunst in Konkurrenz," 10–16.

14. Seitz, *Ain schöner Tractat von dem Saturnischē gschoß der Pestilentz*, C3r–v.
15. Schottenloher, *Doktor Alexander Seitz und seine Schriften*, 10–15; Linder, "Doktor Alexander Sytz," 224–32.
16. Since the process of defining Catholic orthodoxy at the Council of Trent was not complete until 1563 it is notable to find authors using plague literature to criticize Protestant positions before then.
17. Fenckh graduated from the University of Ingolstadt as a doctor of medicine in 1510 and served as a medical professor there between 1531 and his death in 1538. Although Fenckh's name is spelled "Fenck" and "Fengk" and "Fencken" in the source, I am adopting the spelling used by Leonore Liess, who provides the sole recent biography. Liess, *Geschichte der medizinischen Fakultät in Ingolstadt*, 130–31.
18. Fencken, *Ain gut nützlich Regiment*, A3v.
19. Here Fenckhen, *Ain gut nützlich Regiment*, A8v draws on Avicenna's Metaphysics.
20. Fenckhen, *Ain gut nützlich Regiment*, C8r–v.
21. On Fuchs, see Liess, *Geschichte der medizinischen Fakultät in Ingolstadt*, 128. On the confessional nature of Ingolstadt: Helm, "Religion and Medicine," 53.
22. Porzelt, *Die Pest in Nürnberg*, 168–71. Horanin, "Die Pest in Augsburg um 1500," 128–49.
23. Physicians and printers in Nuremberg and Augsburg released a number of works on plague for this epidemic, but any attempt by magistrates to publicize their own mandates in print is unknown to me.
24. Stahleder, *Chronik der Stadt München*, Vol. 2, 89.
25. Stadtarchiv München, Gesundheitsamt 3, "Sterbenns leüffen Ordnung" 1532/33? Various exempla of this print, as well as manuscript notes on the city's plague policy of 1532/33, are also held under Gesundheitsamt 63. All translations are mine.
26. At the time Duke Georg I of Saxony, Leipzig's overlord, was a noted enemy of the Protestant Reformation. Kegler, *Eyn Nutzlichs vnd trostlichs Regiment*, A5r–v.
27. Soergel, *Wondrous in His Saints*, 69–77.
28. Breuer, *Oberdeutsche Literatur*, 99–101.
29. Helm, "Religion and Medicine," 53.
30. Boscius, *Rathschlag*, A2r.
31. Boscius, *Rathschlag*, A2r–v. The Hezekiah story appears in Isaiah 38: 1–8.
32. Heinrichs, *Plague, Print, and the Reformation*, 90–93.
33. Helm, "Religion and Medicine," 63–66.
34. Liess, *Geschichte der medizinischen Fakultät in Ingolstadt*, 139–42. See also Helm, "Religion and Medicine," 63.
35. Boscius, *Rathschlag*, C4v.
36. Soergel, *Wondrous in His Saints*, 75. The Jesuit Peter Canisius served as vice-chancellor of the university between 1549 and 1552. See also Lederer, *Madness, Religion and the State*, 63.
37. Boscius, *Rathschlag*, A3r.
38. Soergel, *Wondrous in His Saints*, 105–7. Soergel devotes chapter 4 to Eisengrein's efforts to revive the cult of the saints and local shrines in Bavaria.
39. Breuer, *Oberdeutsche Literatur*, 101–10. An important treasure volume that Berg printed includes Matthias Rader's *Bavaria Sancta et Pia* of 1615.
40. Soergel, *Wondrous in His Saints*, 104–5 and Breuer, *Oberdeutsche Literatur*, 122.
41. Berg published four medical plague pamphlets between 1572 and 1589, as the presses of Ingolstadt ceased to publish plague literature in the later sixteenth century.

42. Lederer, *Madness, Religion and the State*, 59.
43. Strasser, *State of Virginity*, 17.
44. Fettich, *Ordnung Vnd Regiment*, 1585. The fact that Duke Wilhelm's 1585 mandates were published as a prologue is unusual. There is also no reference to Duke Wilhelm on the titlepage, which may have kept this text hidden from historians over time. Alexander von Hoffmeister seems to have overlooked this source, since he lists 1592 as the first printed plague mandate for the territory of Bavaria. Hoffmeister, *Das Medizinalwesen im Kurfürstentum Bayern*, 100. It is striking that the duke would sanction his mandates being published as a prologue to Fettich's work and suggests that this text sold well and had a broad distribution. The mandates presumably were publicized in other ways as well, such as read from pulpits.
45. On the character of *Policeyordnungen* changing from supporting traditional customs in the Middle Ages to being motivated by a leader's duties to care for his people and issue new laws in the early modern period: Wüst, *Die "gute" Policey*, 75.
46. Fettich, *Ordnung Vnd Regiment*, A4r.
47. Fettich, *Ordnung Vnd Regiment*, A6r–v.
48. Fettich, *Ordnung Vnd Regiment*, B5r. This is a reference to Matthew 25.
49. There are only slight changes to the content over time within the parts devoted to the soul and clergy.
50. Fettich, *Ordnung Vnd Regiment*, 1572.
51. Fettich, *Ordnung Vnd Regiment*, 1585, H3v–4r.
52. Fettich, *Ordnung Vnd Regiment*, B5–B8.
53. Fettich, *Ordnung Vnd Regiment*, A8r.
54. Habermas, "Wunder, Wunderliches, Wunderbares," 38–66.
55. Sauter, *Regiment / verhütung vnd Curation*, A2r.
56. Gemert, "Tridentische Geistigkeit und Moraldidaxis," 45–63 and Dörrer et al., eds, *Hippolytus Guarinonius (1571–1654)*. Guarinonius came from a Trent family, was educated at the courts of Emperors Maximilian II and Rudolf II in Vienna and Prague, and practiced medicine for fifty-six years in Tyrol's Inn valley.
57. Guarinonius, *Pestilentz Guardien*, 27–53 (on the Eucharist), 277–79 (worldly Jesuit).
58. *Wolbewehrte MItl wider die vergiffte Pest*, 48–49.
59. Geiger, *Kurzer Underricht vnd Güetachten*, 28–29. Geiger wrote his pamphlet upon the request of the ducal court and the Munich city council. At the time he was a Munich city physician and oversaw the Kurfürst's hospitals as well.
60. Unicorn horn was a traditional antidote against poison. Kobolt, *Ergänzungen und Berichtingungen*, 108–9.
61. Geiger studied medicine in Paris and Montpelier. Kobolt, *Ergänzungen und Berichtingungen*, 108–9.
62. Much of Soergel's work deals with Our Lady of Altötting, but see especially 25–27 and 41–42 for the shrine's late medieval rise to prominence among Bavarian elites. Soergel, *Wondrous in His Saints*, 25–27 and 41–42.
63. Camerer, *Predig Vmb gnädige Abwendung der Pest*.
64. "Wann dich schon alle Doctor vnd Leibarztet verlassen / so verlaßt dich doch dise Weltartztin vnnd Doctorin in zu AltenOeting nit." Camerer, *Predig Vmb gnädige Abwendung der Pest*, 14.
65. Lotz-Heumann and Pohlig, "Confessionalization and Literature in the Empire," 44–45.
66. Lederer, *Madness, Religion and the State*, 101–4. Lederer provides images of these documents.

Bibliography

Archival Sources

Stadtarchiv München Gesundheitsamt 3, "Sterbenns leüffen Ordnung" ca. 1532/33.

Gesundheitsamt 63, "Sterbenns leüffen Ordnung" ca. 1532/33.

Primary Sources

Boscius, Johann Lonaeus. *Rathschlag. Wie man sich zů disen gefährlichen zeiten / vor der Pestilentz hütten Vnd Wie dieselbig so sie eingerissen / wider zů vertreiben / vnd zů curieren sey*. Ingolstadt: Alexander and Samuel Weyssenhorn, 1562.

Camerer, Christoph. *Predig Vmb gnädige Abwendung der Pest / vor der Procession, vnd herumbtragung deß wunderthätigen Bildt der glorwürdigisten Jungkfrawen MARIAE zu Alten Oetingen*, 1649.

Fencken, Michael. *Ain gut nützlich Regiment / wie man sich halten soll / vor / in / vnd nach der zeyt d erschröcklichē kranck hayt der Pestilentz / durch Michaelem Fencken / der Artzney Doctoren / diser zeyt Ordinarien der löblichen Vniuersitet zů Ingoldstat*. Augsburg: Alexander Weyssenhorn, 1533.

Fettich, Theobald. *Ordnung Vnd Regiment / wie man sich vor der scharpffen vnd gifftigen kranckheit der Pestilentz bewaren sol: Auch wie denen / so darmit begriffen / zuhelffen sey. Sampt den natürlichen vrsachen des Englischen Schwaiß*. Munich: Adam Berg, 1572.

Fettich, Theobald. *Ordnung Vnd Regiment / wie man sich vor der scharpffen vnd gifftigen Kranckheit der Pestilentz bewahren soll: Auch wie denen / so darmit begriffen / zuhelffen sey. Sambt den natürlichen vrsachen des Englischen Schwaiß*. Munich: Adam Berg, 1585.

Geiger, Malachias. *Kurzer Underricht vnd Güetachten Wie mann sich bey ietzigen sterbens Läuffē Praeseruieren vnnd Da iemand inficiert würde Curieren solle Sambt Ainer Instruction für die Wündartzt vnd Warter auch anderen welche sich bey dergleichen Kranckhen brauchen lassen*. Munich: 1649.

Guarinonius, Hippolytus. *Pestilentz Guardien / Für allerley Stands Personen / mit Säuberung der inficierten Häuser / Beth-Leingewandt / Kleider / etc Durch drey sonders außerlesneste Pest Waffen / darunder der wahre Philosophische Stein*. Inglostadt: Andreas Angermayr, 1612.

Kegler, Caspar. *Eyn Nutzlichs vnd trostlichs Regiment wider dy Pestilentz vñ Gifftig Pestilentzisch Feber die Schweyssucht genannt / vnd sust mācherley gifftig vñ tödlich kranckheit / Durch Casparū Kegler / der ertzney Doctorn / zwsamen gebracht / vornewt vñ mit vil trostlichen experimentē gebessert / Die zuuor heymlich gehalten / vnd an den tag nyhe gegebē seyn. Anno 1.5.2.9. auß gegangen*. Leipzig: Valten Schumann, 1529.

Sauter, Bonifacius. *Regiment / verhütung vnd Curation, der erschröcklichen Kranckheit der Pestis. Zu Nutz vnd Nachrichtung / Den Edlen / Ehrnvesten / ...* Munich: Nicolaus Henricus, 1607.

Seitz, Alexander. *Ain schöner Tractat von dem Saturnischē gschoß der Pestilentz mit ettlichen klügen fragstucken / dariñ der vngelert man sich irret / zü gferlichem abbruch seins lebens / ee zeit / alles durch den hochgelerten philosophum Alexander Seitzen von Marckbach Doctor zü München, auß menschlicher lieb trewlich beschriben / vnd verantwurt*, 1521.

Stahleder, Helmuth. *Chronik der Stadt München*. Vol. 2: Belastungen und Bedrückungen Die Jahre 1506–1705. Ebenhausen, Hamburg, Munich: Dölling und Galitz Verlag, 2005.

Von Gottes Gnaden, Wir Maximilian, Pfaltzgraf bey Rhein, Hertzog in obern vnd nidern Bayrn, [et]c. Deß H: Röm: Reichs ErtzTrucksäß vnd Churfürst. Embieten allen vnd jeden vnsern LandtHofmaistern, HofrathsPraesidenten, Vitzthomben, Hauptleuthen ... vnsern Gruß vnd Gnad zuvor, vnd fügen denselben zuwissen, nach dem sich die Sterbläuff, vnd fürnem[m]lich die erschröcklich abschewlich Sucht der Pestilentz, an vilen orthen im Heil: Reich, ohne zweifel von Gott dem Allmächtigen ... geschickte Straff erzaigt vnd eingerissen ... : Geben vnder vnserm fürgetruckten Secret, in vnser Statt München, den 19. MonatsTag August, Anno 1634. [1634].

Wolbewehrte MItl wider die vergiffte Pest. Zu disen gefährlichen Läuffen sehr nutz vnd nothwendig. Durch ein trewhertzige vnd in vnderschidlichen Sterbsläuffen wolpracticierte Person Menigklich zu nutz vnd gutem in Truck geben. Munich: Cornelio Leysserio, 1634.

Secondary Sources

Assion, Peter. "Geistliche und Weltliche Heilkunst in Konkurrenz." *Bayerisches Jahrbuch für Volkskunde* (1976/77): 7–23.

Breuer, Dieter. *Oberdeutsche Literatur 1565–1650. Deutsche Literaturgeschichte und Territorialgeschichte in frühabsolutischer Zeit.* Munich: Beck, 1979.

Dörrer, Anton et al., eds. *Hippolytus Guarinonius (1571–1654).* Innsbruck: Universitätsverlag Wagner, 1954.

Eckert, Edward A. "The Retreat of Plague from Central Europe, 1640–1720: A Geomedical Approach" *Bulletin of the History of Medicine* 74 (2000): 1–28.

Eckert, Edward A. *The Structure of Plagues and Pestilences in Early Modern Europe. Central Europe, 1560–1640.* Basel: Karger, 1996.

Fisher, Alexander J. *Music, Piety, and Propaganda. The Soundscapes of Counter-Reformation Bavaria.* Oxford: Oxford University Press, 2014.

Gemert, Guillaume van. "Tridentische Geistigkeit und Moraldidaxis in Guarinonius' 'Greweln.' Der Arzt als geistlicher Autor." In *Hippolytus Guarinonius im interkulturellen Kontext seiner Zeit. Acta der Tagung Neustift 1993*, edited by Elmar Locher, 45–63. Bozen: Edition Sturzflüge, 1995.

Habermas, Rebekka. "Wunder, Wunderliches, Wunderbares. Zur Profanisierung eines Deutungsmusters in der Frühen Neuzeit." In *Armut, Liebe, Ehre. Studien zur historischen Kulturforschung*, edited by Richard van Dülmen, 38–66. Frankfurt: Fischer Taschenbuch Verlag, 1988.

Heimers, Manfred Peter. *Krieg, Hunger, Pest und Glaubenszwist. München im Dreißigjährigen Krieg.* Munich: Buchendorfer Verlag, 1998.

Heinrichs, Erik A. *Plague, Print, and the Reformation. The German Reform of Healing, 1473–1573.* London, New York: Routledge, 2018.

Helm, Jürgen. "Religion and Medicine: Anatomical Education at Wittenberg and Ingolstadt." In *Religious Confessions and the Sciences in the Sixteenth Century*, edited by Jürgen Helm and Annette Winkelmann, 51–68. Leiden/Boston/Cologne: Brill, 2001.

Hoffmeister, Alexander von. *Das Medizinalwesen im Kurfürstentum Bayern.* Munich: Werner Fritsch, 1975.

Horanin, Mariusz. "Die Pest in Augsburg um 1500. Die soziale Konstruktion einer Krankheit." PhD thesis. Georg-August-Universität Göttingen, 2011.

Kobolt, Anton Maria. *Ergänzungen und Berichtingungen zum Baierischen Gelehrten-Lexikon.* Landshut: Franz Seraph Storno, 1824.

Lederer, David. *Madness, Religion and the State in Early Modern Europe.* Cambridge: Cambridge University Press, 2006.

Liess, Leonore. *Geschichte der medizinischen Fakultät in Ingolstadt von 1472 bis 1600.* Munich: Münchner Vereinigung für Geschichte der Medizin, 1984.
Linder, Gottlieb. "Doktor Alexander Sytz. Ein Lebensbild aus der Reformationszeit." *Zeitschrift für Allgemeine Geschichte, Kultur-, Literatur-, u. Kunstgeschichte* 3 (1886): 224–32.
Lotz-Heumann, Ute, and Matthias Pohlig. "Confessionalization and Literature in the Empire." *Central European History* 40 (2007): 35–61.
Öhler, Leopold. *Die Pest in Salzburg*. Salzburg: Verlag Anton Pustet, 2013.
O'Malley, S. J., John W. "Was Ignatius Loyola a Catholic Reformer? How to Look at Early Modern Catholicism." *The Catholic Historical Review* 77, no. 2 (1991): 177–93.
Porzelt, Carolin. *Die Pest in Nürnberg. Leben und Herrschen in Pestzeiten in der Reichsstadt Nürnberg (1562–1713)*. St. Ottilien, Germany: EOS Verlag, 2000.
Schottenloher, Karl. *Doktor Alexander Seitz und seine Schriften. Ein Kleinbild aus dem Münchner Ärtzeleben des XVI. Jahrhunderts*. Munich: Verlag der Münchner Drucke, 1925.
Soergel, Philip M. *Wondrous in His Saints: Counter-Reformation Propaganda in Bavaria*. Berkeley: University of California Press, 1993.
Strasser, Ulrike. *State of Virginity. Gender, Religion and Politics in an Early Modern Catholic State*. Ann Arbor: University of Michigan Press, 2004.
Wüst, Wolfgang. *Die "gute" Policey im Bayerischen Reichskreis und in der Oberpfalz*. Berlin: Akademie Verlag, 2004.

PART II

Political Strategies: Rulers and City Councils Responding to Plague

CHAPTER 4

Contagion and Control

City Councils and the French Pox in Frankfurt am Main and Nuremberg, 1495–1510

MONICA C. O'BRIEN

Introduction

In August 1495, Germany, along with much of continental Western Europe, was coming to terms with the pandemic "pösen plattern" (evil pox).[1] Those infected suffered with a range of symptoms, including severe pains in the joints and limbs and the outbreak of pustules, boils, and other "festering or hardened eruptions of the skin."[2] In its most horrific form the disease would rot the skin and bones of its living victims, devouring, amongst other things, noses, penises, and leg bones.[3] One contemporary witness (and, later, victim) of the disease, Joseph Grünpeck, a secretary to the Holy Roman Emperor Maximilian I, recorded that the pain was so great, those infected "wished to die as soon as possible."[4]

The epidemic had begun its spread early in 1495, as Charles VIII of France and his forces returned from their siege of Naples. When the soldiers and mercenaries on both sides travelled home within Italy, Spain, France, Scotland, and elsewhere, contemporaries began to comment on the appearance of this strange sickness.[5] Some believed the pox was a new disease, while others thought it was known by the classical medical authorities.[6] The pandemic spread rapidly, reaching Scotland by 1497, India by 1498, Russia by 1500, and China by 1505.[7]

Across the globe the disease became known by a variety of names.[8] In the Italian and German lands, it was commonly called "the French pox" (or slight variations thereof, such as "French disease"). This designation came to be recognized across Europe, although different names were common elsewhere, such as the "Great pox" in France and "grandgore" in Scotland. Many historians, including Claude Quétel and Robert Jütte, have used the term "syphilis" to refer to the disease that pervaded in Europe during the period 1495–1510.[9] In contrast, following historians such as Claudia Stein and Jon Arrizabalaga, John Henderson, and Roger French, this chapter uses an early modern term, "French pox," because it accurately represents the language of my primary sources, while the term "syphilis" (although occasionally used during the early modern period) did not come into common usage until the twentieth century. Moreover, as Stein argues, a disease is a "socio-cultural construct specific to a particular scientific and socio-cultural setting at a given time."[10] For example, the medical frameworks of the late fifteenth and early sixteenth centuries, within which the individuals in this chapter understood the French pox, are vastly different from current concepts of syphilis founded in the laboratory medicine that isolated the bacterium *Treponema pallidum* subspecies *pallidum* in 1905. Therefore, a contemporary name more accurately reflects both the sources and their authors' thinking.

The French pox arrived in the free imperial cities of Frankfurt am Main and Nuremberg in the late summer of 1496. Nuremberg was a thriving city in its golden age, with one estimate placing its population at twenty thousand.[11] The city was prospering and there was a profusion of artistic, humanist, and scientific production; Albrecht Dürer and Wilibald Pirckheimer, among others, worked there. Frankfurt was also a large city for Germany in this period, with an estimated population of ten thousand.[12] It was thriving financially; sitting on the intersection of vital trade routes on the Main River, most of its profits were generated through commerce and banking.[13]

Both cities were governed by a *Rat* (city council). In Nuremberg, the council consisted of the *Größere Rat* (Greater Council) and the *Innere Rat* (Inner Council). The former was comprised mostly of men from "respectable businesses" and a small number of craftsmen; it held little power and met only when convened by the *Innere Rat*, to approve new taxes or discuss issues like war.[14] All of the power lay with the Inner Council. Here, men of the city's forty-three patrician families, socio-economically powerful merchants and manufacturers, held thirty-four of the forty-two seats, with the rest going to craftsmen, who were barred from occupying the positions of authority. Most of the power was concentrated in the Seven Elder Gentlemen, who "made all the important decisions, knew almost every secret, and deliberated on serious or very discreet matters before the rest of the Small Council was informed."[15] Therefore, where this chapter refers to Nuremberg's "council," this indicates the *Innere Rat*. Frankfurt's *Rat* consisted of three benches; the first two had fourteen members each and were occupied by the aldermen and the "community" (nobles, academics, wealthy merchants). The third had fifteen members drawn from nine of the city's guilds; they were largely subordinate and excluded from positions of power, which were held by the city's forty-five elite families.[16]

This chapter explores how these governments understood and responded to the French pox between 1495 and 1510. To contextualize the municipal authorities' thinking, it introduces contemporary medical understandings of the disease's transmission in the publications of medical practitioners. The main focus and core sources for this investigation are the records of the councils' meetings, kept in Frankfurt's *Bürgermeisterbücher* (Mayor's Books) and Nuremberg's *Ratsverlässe* (Council Decisions). The Frankfurt council met twice weekly, while in Nuremberg the council met at least three times a week; these sources record issues raised and decisions taken at these meetings. Importantly for this study, they document the orders issued by the councils to control the spread of the pox and to care for its victims, providing vital insights into how the municipal authorities reacted to the disease. Unfortunately, these records do not detail debates, differing perspectives, and influences that conditioned the decisions taken. Instead, the councils are portrayed as responding with a single voice. Moreover, we cannot fully assess the efficacy of the pox measures from these sources and, indeed, it is beyond the scope of this chapter to attempt this. Nevertheless, looking at the decisions on the disease in these records from 1495 to 1510 and beyond it is clear that many, if not most, of the actions ordered were taken. Nuremberg's records, for example, continue to chart their decisions on the pox up to at least 1700 and contain recurring entries charting the development of topics like hiring new practitioners, the movement of patients, and decisions on hospital budgets for the poxed.[17]

To investigate the place of the councils' pox measures in the development of municipally controlled health care in these cities, this study contextualizes the municipal authorities' decisions against their previous responses to epidemics and compares the responses of Frankfurt and Nuremberg with those of governments elsewhere in Western Europe.

This investigation demonstrates that theories of non-sexual transmission deeply influenced measures enacted by these city councils. These measures, moreover, illustrate the councils' growing control over municipal health care and, indeed, their cities. Although valuable scholarship has been devoted to the sexual transmission of the French pox, until now the prevalence of non-sexual notions of transmission has received little attention in the historiography. Looking at the records of southern German free imperial cities, Annemarie Kinzelbach has argued that there is little evidence that the pox was perceived as an exclusively sexually transmitted disease until at least the early seventeenth century. Samuel Cohn extends this argument to the late eighteenth century.[18] Much more work is needed, however, as the municipal records for the cities at the center of Kinzelbach's studies make only sporadic mentions of the epidemic during its earliest years.[19] Meanwhile, Cohn's work focuses on published texts from across Western Europe. Therefore, by investigating municipal sources, this chapter will provide new insight into early modern German understandings of the pox (or at least its perception) as a disease transmitted sexually and non-sexually. Importantly, it shows the significant influence of these perceptions on early responses to the pandemic in two major free imperial cities.

Contagion in Medical Minds

Before turning to the responses of the city councils, medical practitioners' understandings of the French pox's transmission need to be examined. The municipal authorities of Frankfurt and Nuremberg looked to local physicians for advice and relied on their publications. From the start of the pandemic in 1495, many European medical practitioners believed that the French pox had sexual and non-sexual forms of contagion. That said, not all medical texts on the pox discussed transmission and some focused solely on sexual transmission. This section considers sixteenth- and seventeenth-century works that address both forms of transmission.

Franz Renner, a surgeon who practiced in Nuremberg's Franzosenhaus (French pox hospital), published his *Handtbüchlein* (Handbook/Little Handbook) on the French pox in the mid-sixteenth century.[20] This work, which expounds the virtues of guaiacum treatment over mercury, was commissioned by the city, showing that they valued Renner's views.[21] Renner believed the pox spread through sexual and non-sexual routes. In his chapter on "How this sickness travels through external things," he argued that the disease spread through various non-sexual routes such as sharing a bed, clothes, or eating and drinking utensils, as well as in municipal baths and through surgeons using the same instruments on infected and healthy individuals.[22] However, he maintained that the disease spread most frequently through sexual intercourse and, in that form, was a punishment from God for sexual immorality.[23]

Similarly to Renner, the Ferrarese physician Rostinio, whose *Tractat* was first published in Italian in 1565 and translated into German in 1620, emphasized frequent transmission through sexual contact. Nevertheless, like Renner, he devoted considerable attention to non-sexual transmission,[24] asserting that sharing a bed, plate, glass, or hand towel with a poxed individual facilitated the spread of infectious matter which entered through the mouth or was absorbed into the body through the skin.[25] He also presented a case of a child who, Rostinio maintained, contracted the pox because he absorbed the infected matter from the bed that he shared with his mother or from close physical proximity to her.[26] Indeed, Rostinio believed that the disease could be so contagious that one could contract it simply through touching the hand or body of an infected individual.[27] For Renner and Rostinio, non-sexual transmission, while not as widespread as sexual transmission, was a medical fact and posed a threat to healthy individuals.

My research shows that non-sexual theories endured in medical texts published in Germany until at least the second half of the seventeenth century.[28] For example, in 1620 Tobias Knobloch, a city physician of Ansbach and the personal physician of the princess of Brandenburg, wrote that the disease spread through sexual and non-sexual routes. His section on the latter is extensive. He believed that children could contract it through the infected milk of nurses and that it could spread through the preparation of food by infected persons, through money changing hands, through drinks and drinking vessels, beds, and surgical instruments.[29]

In 1667 Joseph Schmid, a *Stadt-* and *Wundarzt* (city surgeon and surgeon) in Augsburg, argued that the disease was God's judgment on those who pursued *Unzucht* (sexual immorality) and on prostitutes.[30] However, he also maintained that "honest persons" were at risk from non-sexual transmission, which usually occurred when infected individuals ate with the healthy and shared their tableware. Moreover, it could spread through sweat when an infected person shared a bed with a healthy individual.[31]

For published medical practitioners, there were varied levels of concern with non-sexual transmission of the pox. Although practitioners believed sexual transmission was most prevalent, non-sexual contagion remained a medical fact into at least the late seventeenth century and, as we shall see, similar theories influenced the medical and municipal practitioners of Frankfurt and Nuremberg between 1495 and 1510.

Frankfurt

On 9 August 1496, the Frankfurt authorities penned their first entry on the French pox in their *Bürgermeisterbücher*. They stated that the city's doctors recommended that, because "the pox" was now "visible" in Frankfurt, a list of those with the disease should be drafted and given to the council to separate the infected from the healthy.[32] This measure was to be publicly announced the following day, and all of the infected were to proceed to the "fare porte," one of the city's gates.[33] Two days later, the master of the Heilig-Geist Spital was ordered to prepare the *Pestilenzhaus* (plague house) and to employ female staff to receive the pox victims.[34] This move to quarantine was reminiscent of European measures during times of plague, a disease perceived as highly contagious and believed to spread through various mechanisms, including via the air and infected goods. These actions imply that, from the outset, the council believed and greatly feared that the pox spread through airborne or other non-sexual forms of contagion.

This legislation and provision of institutional care for pox victims reflected the council's expanding control of municipal health care, much of which had been overseen by religious groups in the preceding centuries. During the late fifteenth century, before the arrival of the pox, Frankfurt's authorities had already begun taking greater control of the care and regulation of the city's lepers, who resided in the *Gutleuthof* (leper house), which, overseen by a Christian brotherhood, had been in operation since at least 1283.[35] Severe plague epidemics struck Frankfurt in 1461, 1482, and 1493.[36] Despite these outbreaks and discussion of creating a plague hospital, the city did not, however, establish a *Pestilenzhaus* until 1492–93.[37] The Frankfurt council's response to the pox and its provision of institutions for the sick was more rapid and comprehensive than its earlier responses to plague. Along with concerns surrounding the contagiousness of the pox, another important factor motivating Frankfurt's haste was the contemporaneous efforts of councils across Germany to expand their power over their cities and health care.[38] These endeavors increased their control over their populations and their city's finances.

In 1497, Frankfurt's council ordered a building called the Ritterhaus (knight's house) to prepare to receive poor persons infected with the French pox, and they were to reside beside the Bockenheim Gate until the house was ready.[39] It is unclear whether these individuals were being moved from the plague house or whether they represented an additional group of patients. In contrast to orders in 1496, which legislated that all the infected should be isolated, the *Ritterhaus* was specifically for the poor. A year's experience with the disease had likely proved that it brought fewer fatalities than plague, and faith in its curability may have been increasing. By focusing on those who could not afford private treatment, the council could limit its spending on the disease, while protecting the healthy population from infection transmitted by the sick poor. Moreover, treatment for the poor could prevent serious illness, lasting debilitating effects, and possibly death of breadwinners, thereby saving the council further expenses in the future. These efforts to develop and control municipal health care and poor relief continued into the early sixteenth century, witnessed not only in provisions of institutional spaces for the poxed but also in the proliferation of orders regulating the infected.

In 1496, the municipal authorities ordered two male pox victims, Georgen Reisen and Hansen Thomas, to quarantine themselves. There is no suggestion that they were to be sent to the plague house. Instead they could stay in their residences, perhaps reflecting their socio-economic status and ability to pay for their medical care. The order warned that no one was to have direct contact with the men; all communications were to be made by letter.[40] The same practice was seen with leprosy. While some lepers went to the leprosaria or *Gutleuthäuser*, others remained in their homes, under strict conditions that they did not mix with the unafflicted.[41]

The strict quarantine of Reisen and Thomas illustrates Frankfurt's fear of a non-sexual spread of the pox. However, on the same day in 1496, the authorities also ordered that the *Dirne* (a prostitute or a young, usually unmarried, woman) who had infected the two men was to be banished from city.[42] This suggests a sexual theory of contagion, as, since the Middle Ages, the term was frequently used to describe women who engaged in extramarital sex. It is also probable that she did not have residency rights, as Frankfurt's statutes ordered the expulsion of non-native pox victims.[43] Similarly, in 1498, the council expelled two pox-infected "old whores," who were also likely non-natives.[44] Perhaps, like the authors Renner and Schmid, the council viewed these individuals as immoral because of their sexual behavior, and therefore felt justified in expelling rather than aiding them. Prostitutes were often expelled in times of plague, not because of fears of sexual transmission but as part of the authorities' efforts to make their cities pleasing to God. Moreover, the exclusion of non-native itinerant beggars was justified by the concepts of "deserving" and "undeserving" poor, which became increasingly embedded in German municipal policy from the fifteenth century onwards.[45] Beggars in the latter category were portrayed as immoral persons who preyed on the charity of good citizens.[46] Poxed non-native itinerants' status as an infection risk further legitimated the council's actions, allowing them to deny access to their city and their relief systems.

Native victims' movements were also restricted. On 28 June 1498, the council ordered an investigation into whether Clansen Schellen had been afflicted with the French pox, likely connected with the diagnosis of his wife and child a little over six months previously.[47] He was ordered to remain away from both the council and the Fahrtor, the city's most important gate located between the center and the port, until his results were known.[48] This recalled plague measures: when a Frankfurt inhabitant died of plague, household members were ordered not to visit the city council for four weeks, a practice that began in the fifteenth century and was enshrined by statute in 1502.[49] In 1507, those with the French pox were ordered to quarantine and abstain from contact with society.[50] Of course, orders such as this may have been intended to prevent sexual transmission of the disease, but the emphasis on the need to remove oneself completely from society supports the notion of the significance of non-sexual theories of transmission.

In addition to individuals, the council also took measures against businesses. Between July 1497 and February 1502, the Frankfurt council ordered periodic closures of the Rote Badestube (Red Bathhouse). Located in a populous and relatively central area of the city, it was linked with several pox cases.[51] Bathhouses were popular public spaces, and the council routinely closed them in times of plague.[52] As noted above, Renner identified bathhouses as places where the pox could spread through non-sexual routes. Annemarie Kinzelbach has also identified further early modern anxieties surrounding the spread of the pox through shared bathing.[53] On the other hand, bathhouses were routinely associated with illicit sexual activity. Nevertheless, the council's beliefs on the particular form, or forms, of contagion in the bathhouse remain unclear. Nowhere in the city's *Bürgermeisterbücher* from 1495 to 1510 is the pox explicitly linked with sexual transmission. Further, Frankfurt never took sweeping action on brothels, sex workers, or other bathhouses because of the pox.

In Frankfurt, many of the council's orders were driven by a belief in and concern with non-sexual transmission of the French pox. While not openly acknowledged in the *Bürgermeisterbücher*, anxieties surrounding sexual contagion also likely played a role, motivating orders such as the expulsion of the "dirne." The council's rapid response illustrates their determination to extend their control and develop a sophisticated municipal health care system. Further, the threat of contagion, combined with the growing stigmatization of the undeserving poor, also served the council in their efforts to expand their control and expel undesirable individuals from their city.

Nuremberg

On 2 September 1496, an entry in Nuremberg's *Ratsverlässe* recorded that "the French sickness" was "to be cared for" by the city's "learned" doctors.[54] As in Frankfurt, Nuremberg's council turned to its local medical authorities for advice and support. Indeed, the contagiousness of the disease had already been discussed by Nuremberg's physicians three days previously, when they concluded that any person or clothes infected by the pox's "contagious vapors" should be avoided, especially in enclosed spaces.[55] Their belief in non-sexual transmission of the pox was unambiguous and recalled theories surrounding the transmission of plague.

However, despite the physicians' warnings, and in contrast to Frankfurt's rapid isolation of the sick, Nuremberg's council did not act for a further four weeks. In this interim, they sought additional advice on the disease. On 30 September they wrote to the authorities of Bamberg, their neighbor fifty-seven kilometers to the north, inquiring about the pox and its management, and how to deal with it.[56] On 4 October they ordered that those with the "French evil" were to be contained in the Heilig Kreuz (Holy Cross) hospital, located outside the city walls.[57] In further contrast to the first Frankfurt order, the poxed were not explicitly compelled to go to this institution. However, by 20 October, the Nuremberg council issued more stringent rules, ordering all infected "citizens or inhabitants" to the Heilig Kreuz. Located on an arterial road outside the city, this hospital had been established in 1354 to provide one or two nights' accommodation to pilgrims and certain non-native itinerants.[58] While the hospital normally excluded those with contagious diseases such as leprosy, it had been used to house plague victims during the 1494–95 epidemic.[59] The Heilig Kreuz had thirty-eight beds, approximately eight of which were for staff. Initially, only one room was given to pox patients, but a second soon followed as the hospital became increasingly dedicated to the treatment of this disease.[60] Patients with non-contagious illnesses were moved to the general hospital, the Heilig-Geist (Holy Ghost), while the poxed were moved in the opposite direction.[61] The move to quarantine the infected outside of the city walls echoed Frankfurt's pox measures as well as plague and leprosy procedures in Western Europe. Clearly, Nuremberg's medical and municipal authorities were concerned with the contagiousness of the pox.

By January 1497, the Heilig Kreuz had surpassed its capacity. The council began to send patients to the extramural leper hospitals along with the Siechhauß, a hospital which was located inside the walls and accommodated hundreds of lepers during the *Lepraschau*, an annual festival during Holy Week when the city provided charity for non-native lepers.[62] The latter was not in use outside of festival time. To minimize contagion, it was built by the outflow of the river to ensure potentially contagious waste left the city.[63]

Although rates of leprosy were declining in Europe by the fifteenth century,[64] the council wished to cease using the leper institutions as overflow facilities. Sometime between 1506 and 1507, the council designated a hut or, more likely, huts to house the poxed by the Schleifersteg footbridge on the Pegnitz River within the city walls.[65] It is not wholly clear whether the poxed remained at these locations or were moved, because in 1509 some male poxed poor were sent to huts in the Saumarkt area, within the walls but away from the majority of inhabitants' homes, on a small island in the river.[66] The council had these huts constructed specifically for the poxed. They consisted of a single room and a kitchen with a hole to allow smoke to escape, but with few windows. Human waste and water from the huts were not emptied directly into the river and instead had to be taken nightly to the outflow at the wall.[67] These specifications demonstrate a fear of non-sexual contagion through the air and pollution and, evidently, the council believed that their prophylactic measures would neutralize this threat. As with lepers who entered the city during the *Lepraschau*, the poxed could dwell within the walls once their conditions were tightly controlled. In 1510, the guardian of the Heilig Kreuz stated that the institution would no longer accept pox patients.[68] Consequently, the Saumarkt huts became their principal accommodation until the construction of the extramural Franzosenhaus (French pox hospital), which began accepting poor patients by 1543.[69] This sustained use of extramural and specific contagious disease strategies for the poxed poor demonstrates the council's belief in non-sexual transmission.

Before the arrival of the French pox, the Nuremberg council's interventions in health care were inconsistent. In 1365 they began taking control of leper institutions, when the St. Johannes leper house, overseen by the Teutonic Knights since at least 1234, came under their administration.[70] From around the time of the Black Death (1347–51) onwards, plague appeared regularly in the city, on average every eleven years, until the seventeenth century.[71] Nevertheless, the council made no serious attempt to combat plague until the late fifteenth century. The city's earliest known plague decrees were religious measures passed by the council in 1483. The first attempt to halt the spread of plague through regulations on any public spaces failed to arise until 1494–95, with, for example, a suspension of court sessions.[72] In 1490 Konrad Toppler, a local patrician, left a bequest of 160 gulden to found a plague hospital, but the donation was insufficient and the council did not complete the St. Sebastian hospital until 1528. As in Frankfurt, the Nuremberg council's relatively swift and comprehensive response to the French pox represents an important early stage in its quest to take greater control of municipal health care, poor relief, and the city.

Beyond bringing the poxed to specially designated locations, the council took further measures to control the spread of the disease. In October 1496 they wrote again to the municipal authorities of Bamberg to inquire if anyone had contracted the disease from pig meat.[73] Increasingly concerned about the pox's mechanisms of contagion, the Nuremberg authorities ordered an interrogation and inspection of the pig keepers.[74] During the medieval and early modern period, pigs and pork caused considerable concern during epidemics because these animals were seen as unsanitary and their meat harmful to the sick body. Therefore, in times of plague the council ordered that pigs be driven from Nuremberg.[75] In 1497 Johannes Widmann, Professor of Medicine at the University of Tübingen, wrote that cases of the French pox had been discovered in pigs.[76] Similarly, field reports published in 1549 from Alessandro Benedetti, a Venetian military physician, raised concerns that eating poorly cured pork had caused the pox to develop among French troops in 1495.[77] The Nuremberg physicians' concern with vapors and the council's worries about pigs again demonstrate prevailing concerns with non-sexual contagion among Nuremberg's medical and municipal authorities in the early years of the epidemic.

As in Frankfurt, legislation also regarded infected individuals but was indifferent to those in the sex trade. The poxed were banned from the city's baths.[78] Surgeons would face a fine of ten gulden if they used the same instruments on the poxed and their other patients.[79] Like in Frankfurt, Nuremberg's council did not issue any French pox regulations for brothels or sex workers, and the municipal brothel remained open until 1561–62.[80] Moreover, the *Ratsverlässe* did not clearly link the disease with sexual transmission until 1632.[81] Among those admitted to the Heilig Kreuz in 1496 were a female sex worker and a male brothel servant.[82] The former could enter only after making her penance at church for taking up sex work.[83] Nevertheless, neither of these cases were explicitly linked to sexual transmission, and no action was taken against the brothel.

While infected citizens were required to proceed to the Heilig Kreuz, the council decided that any infected non-native itinerant beggars were to be expelled.[84] In 1497 the council decided that those sick with the French pox should be removed from its bridges and streets.[85] Later that year, the council ordered that persons with the pox "should not be allowed to enter the city and the same for beggars coming from plague-infected areas."[86] This association between pox and plague was repeated in a subsequent order barring those with either disease from Nuremberg.[87] Overall, the decisions to remove and exclude the sick from the public realm suggest that the council was convinced about the non-sexual spread of the disease. The legislation regarding the poor and non-natives also demonstrates how the pox provided the opportunity for the council to increase its control over the civic sphere.

Despite orders forbidding admission of the poxed poor, the non-native sick maintained a persistent presence in the city.[88] The municipal authorities had to contend with those who broke their regulations, who were sometimes very sick non-native individuals. For example, in 1497 Nuremberg's council ordered a non-native male be removed from the Obstmarkt (fruit market), a central point in the city, to the Heilig Kreuz for treatment. This was to be done "in der stille" (quietly), arguably so the council would not be seen to contradict its own orders against non-natives.[89] In 1499 the council revised its policies on poxed non-natives, specifying that if they were too sick to walk they would be provided with some medical care until they were well enough to leave the city.[90] While compassion for the very ill may have played a role in the development of this law, it was also a practical move to ensure that the very sick individuals would not pose a hazard to Nuremberg's healthy population.

At the close of the fifteenth century, concerns surrounding transmission of the pox through the air and close physical proximity seem to have eased in Nuremberg. From January 1499 to December 1500, the council gave permissions to native poxed individuals to beg in the city,[91] as with "a poor woman" suffering from the French disease and with four children, who was permitted to beg before the Church of Our Lady.[92] However, I have not uncovered any permissions granted to poxed beggars after 1500. Moreover, the 1522 *Armenordnung* (Poor Order) forbade lepers and the poxed to beg in the city.[93] Through the early years of the pox, the council adapted its regulations on movement to embrace often conflicting concerns between contagion and civil responsibilities toward the poor.

In Nuremberg, concerns over the non-sexual transmission of the French pox significantly influenced municipal legislation, from the placement of the sick in buildings designed to control contagious diseases to strict legislation on the presence of the poxed in the municipal sphere. While the council faced challenges, including overflowing hospitals and the persistence of the non-natives who defied the authorities and entered the city, their response to the French pox expanded their municipal health care system and their control of the civic sphere.

Placing Frankfurt and Nuremberg in the Wider German and European Contexts

Much research remains to map German and European municipal authorities' understandings of and responses to the French pox's contagion mechanisms. Nevertheless, the present state of research demonstrates that concerns and measures regarding non-sexual contagion were not unique to Frankfurt and Nuremberg, while some regions offer important contrasts which indicate the complex histories of the French pox.

Frankfurt and Nuremberg's municipal responses to the pox marked an important moment in the development of councils' control of health care and their cities. This reflected a broader pattern in late medieval and early modern Germany and Western Europe, where municipal authorities were becoming increasingly involved in health care and poor relief.[94] In the fifteenth and sixteenth centuries cities, for example Ulm, Augsburg, and urban areas in Lower Saxony, began developing comprehensive plague measures and institutions.[95] Meanwhile, Jütte shows that fourteen German cities developed pox hospitals or wards between 1495 and 1510.[96] The city governments' growing involvement in health care was prompted by a number of factors, including desire for greater control of the municipal sphere and the need to control increasing numbers of the poor and sick.[97] Peer Friess maintains that traditional institutions of relief, "based on the fundament of personal charity," were unable to cope with these rising numbers.[98] Consequently, municipal governments were forced to protect and develop their civic spheres. Overall, regarding health care, this movement for greater control has been mostly studied in relation to plague. However, as this chapter and the works of Stein and Kinzelbach demonstrate, researching the pox offers new insights into the development of municipal governments' power in early modern Germany.[99]

In contrast to many German cities, Italian states who had been the pioneers of plague legislation and hospitals developed new institutions for the poxed at a slower rate during pandemics' early years. Confraternities rather than municipal authorities led the establishment of *incurabili* (incurables), hospitals for the poxed, who were excluded from other hospitals because of their contagious illnesses, as in Genoa in 1497 and Bologna in 1500.[100] No further *incurabili* were established until the period 1515–26, which saw the foundation of seven such hospitals and at least three specialized wards.[101] New research is needed to understand these differences between German and Italian institutions, and to compare pox hospitals across Europe. I hypothesize that among other influences, politics was a major factor; many German municipal authorities were highly invested in their pursuit of direct control, while in Italy the turmoil of the Italian wars impeded many municipal governments.

Along with new institutions, German cities outside of Frankfurt and Nuremberg also introduced legislation to curb the spread of the French pox, particularly its non-sexual spread. Kinzelbach provides important insights in her study of upper German imperial cities in the sixteenth and seventeenth centuries. She found that municipal authorities forbade the sick from attending community events or public institutions during their treatment and for half a year thereafter. Further, during isolation, the sick could not go to the butchers, markets, or even to church.[102] In Hildesheim, the council ordered those with the pox to remain in their homes for six weeks.[103] In late sixteenth-century Überlingen, the council ordered that the clothes and bedding of the sick were not to be washed by the sick or the regular washerwomen but by specially designated laundresses.[104] In 1581 this city also passed a pox ordinance, stipulating that the infected could not leave their houses until they were examined and declared healthy by one of the city's physicians.[105]

Belief in non-sexual contagion also influenced legislation beyond Germany. In 1497, King James IV's "Grandgore Act" ordered all of Edinburgh's pox victims to be quarantined on the island of Inch Keith in the Firth of Forth. Those who failed to comply were to be branded with a hot iron and banished.[106] In Aberdeen, the burgh council initially treated the disease as a sexual one and commanded all female sex workers to cease practicing the "syne of venerie," to inhibit the spread of the pox.[107] However, further investigation of the Aberdeen records reveals that the council's understanding of the disease changed over time. On 8 October 1507 a statute ordered an inquisition to identify all poxed persons for the safety of the town. Infected persons were ordered to quarantine themselves in their houses and were forbidden from frequenting public places, including areas where food was prepared, such as the premises of butchers, bakers, and brewers—to avoid infecting their neighbors.[108] To repeat, belief in and measures to curb the non-sexual spread of the pox were not unique to Frankfurt, Nuremberg, or even Germany.

Along with Aberdeen, Zurich offers a contrast to Frankfurt and Nuremberg's lack of measures directly related to the sexual transmission of the disease during the early years of the pox. There, in 1496, it was decided that "loose" women and prostitutes were to be banned from the city.[109] Like Aberdeen, Zurich also legislated to control the non-sexual spread of the disease in public spaces. In 1496 the municipal authorities ordered all those with the pox to remain in their houses and banned them from public places including the streets, places of business, baths, and surgeons' practices.[110]

The evidence of the influence of sexual and non-sexual contagion theories indicates a fruitful and important area for research. Future studies will illuminate the full extent of these theories' influence and may also help to identify reasons for variations in regional responses and the explicit recognition of sexual transmission in some places and not in others.

Conclusion

From 1495 to 1510, the city councils of Frankfurt and Nuremberg understood the French pox as possessing multiple mechanisms of contagion, and many of these were unconnected to sex. Indeed, the majority of their regulations and actions to control this disease concerned non-sexual forms of transmission, while sexual behavior was never explicitly discussed or regulated. The understanding of non-sexual mechanisms, the spread of the disease through food, shared items, non-sexual touch, and close physical proximity, drove the careful regulation and hospitalization of the infected.

The pox responses of both Frankfurt and Nuremberg were extensive, surpassing their actions in previous pandemics and epidemics. The arrival of the pox enabled and motivated these councils to expand their power over municipal health care. Combined with the concept of the undeserving poor, contagion theories legitimated the exclusion of non-natives, furthering the councils' authority over their cities. The early years of the French pox in Frankfurt and Nuremberg were a time of trying to control contagion, but also of using contagion to develop control.

Monica (Mona) O'Brien is an Effective Learning Adviser at the University of Glasgow, where she uses her experience as a historian to develop students' academic literacies through designing courses including Theory for the Terrified and History of Argument. Her ongoing research explores the social, emotional, and medical histories of the French pox. She held fellowships with the Herzog August Bibliothek and Northern Network for Medial Humanities. Monica received her PhD from the University of Glasgow. In 2019 she won the McCarthy Award for History of Medicine Research (Royal College of Physicians of Edinburgh) for her work on Nuremberg's French pox doctors.

Notes

The research in this chapter was funded as part of a Leverhulme Trust "Collections" Doctoral Scholarship (2015–19) at the University of Glasgow (History).

1. Maximilian I, "Mandat gegen Gotteslästerung," 273. All translations are mine, unless noted otherwise.

2. Stein, *Negotiating the French Pox*, 35.
3. Stein, *Negotiating the French Pox*, 34–39, 44–57; Arrizabalaga et al., *The Great Pox*, 25–27.
4. Grünpeck, "A Neat Treatise," in Moore and Solomon "Joseph Grünpeck," 9.
5. A small number of primary sources suggest that the pox had appeared in Spain before its pandemic spread after the siege of Naples. Quétel, *History of Syphilis*, 42–44.
6. Cohn, *Epidemics*, 98–100.
7. Cohn, *Epidemics*, 95.
8. Cohn, *Epidemics*, 96–126.
9. In certain places the use of the term "syphilis" is an accurate representation of contemporary sources, for instance when discussing Fracastoro's sixteenth-century *Syphilis sive Morbus Gallicus*.
10. Stein, *Negotiating the French Pox*, 4. See also, Kinzelbach, "'Böse Blattern,'" 43–52.
11. Strauss, *Nuremberg in the Sixteenth Century*, 36. Murphy, "Reforming Medicine in Sixteenth Century Nuremberg," 23, n. 1, references a higher estimate of 22,000–40,000.
12. Jütte, *Obrigkeitliche Armenfürsorge*, 50.
13. Huppert, *After the Black Death*, 52.
14. Christoph Scheurl, "Concerning the Polity and Government of the Praiseworthy City of Nuremberg" (1516). Cited and translated in Strauss, *Nuremberg in the Sixteenth Century*, 59.
15. Fleischmann, *Rat und Patriziat*, Vol. 1, 62, 78–81.
16. Jütte, *Obrigkeitliche Armenfürsorge*, 50. Huppert, *After the Black Death*, 45.
17. O'Brien, "Practice and Power," 91–97; O'Brien, "Contagion, Morality, and Practicality."
18. Kinzelbach, "'Böse Blattern,'" 49; Cohn, *Epidemics*, 96.
19. Kinzelbach, "'Böse Blattern,'" 53.
20. Proksch (*Die Litteratur*, Vol. 1, 17) dates the first publication to 1554. Stein (*Negotiating the French Pox*, 20) dates the first edition to 1548.
21. Newhouse, "Outside the Walls," 106.
22. Renner, *Handtbüchlein*, 4r–v.
23. Renner, *Handtbüchlein*, 4r–v.
24. On Rostinio, see Cohn, *Epidemics*, 118–19.
25. Rostinio, *Tractat*, 38–40.
26. Rostinio, *Tractat*, 40–41.
27. Rostinio, *Tractat*, 41.
28. O'Brien, "Contagion, Morality, and Practicality," 163–68.
29. Knobloch, *Die lue venere*, 17–21.
30. Schmid, *Kurtzer Jedoch eigentlicher Bericht*, i(v).
31. Schmid, *Kurtzer Jedoch eigentlicher Bericht*, ii(r)–ii(v), 139–40.
32. Institut für Stadtgeschichte, Frankfurt am Main (hereafter: ISG), *Bürgermeisterbuch* No.66 (hereafter: BB.number) (1496), f.32v.
33. ISG, BB.66 (1496), f.32v.
34. ISG, BB.66 (1496), f.33v.
35. This can be traced through entries in the *Bürgermeisterbücher*, for example: ISG, BB67 (1497), f.88v, f.124r; BB68 (1498), f.8v, f.49r; BB69 (1499), f.35v, f.40v, f.109r; BB70 (1500–1501), f.2r, f.4r, f.6v; f.7r, f.11r, f.37r, f.74v, f.82v; f.110r. Moritz, "Die bürgerlichen Fürsorgeanstalten," Vol. 1, 69–70. Stricker, *Die Geschichte der Heilkunde*, 145.
36. Moritz, "Die bürgerlichen Fürsorgeanstalten," Vol. 1, 106.
37. Moritz, "Die bürgerlichen Fürsorgeanstalten," Vol. 1, 107.
38. Ribbentrop, *Pest und Policey*, 29–30.

39. ISG, BB.67 (1497), f.56v.
40. ISG, BB.66 (1496), f.56r.
41. Meteling, "Gesundheitsfürsorge," 484.
42. ISG, BB.66 (1496), f.56r. Daumen, "Städtische Prostitution," 330.
43. Sudhoff, "Anfänge der Syphilisbeobachtung," 101–2.
44. Sudhoff, "Anfänge der Syphilisbeobachtung," 114.
45. Stein, *Negotiating the French Pox*, 75–76.
46. Jütte, *Poverty and Deviance*, 159.
47. ISG, BB.67 (1497), f.82v; Sudhoff, "Anfänge der Syphilisbeobachtung," 111.
48. ISG, BB.68 (1498), f.19r.
49. Moritz, "Die bürgerlichen Fürsorgeanstalten," 106.
50. ISG, BB.77 (1507), f.108v.
51. ISG, BB.67 (1497), f.27r, f.54v, f.89v.; BB.67 (1498), f.106r, f.116r; BB.70 (1500), f.81v, f.106r; BB.71 (1501), f.34r; Medicinalia 187 (14 August 1498).
52. ISG, Heilig-Geist Spital 2626 Nr. 4–5 (August 1625), Nr. 23 (February 1635).
53. Kinzelbach, "'Böse Blattern,'" 49.
54. Staatsarchiv Nürnberg (hereafter: StAN), *Ratsverlässe* No. 335 (hereafter: RV.number) (1496), f.10r.
55. Sudhoff, "Die ersten Maßnahmen der Stadt Nürnberg," 3.
56. StAN, RV.336 (1496), f.5r.
57. StAN, RV.336 (1496), f.7v.
58. Dross, "Patterns of Hospitality," 19; Haller "Die Geschichte," 41.
59. Dross, "Patterns of Hospitality," 25.
60. Haller, "Die Geschichte," 43; StAN, RV.336 (1496), 7v. Jütte ("Syphilis and Confinement," 110) estimates that most pox hospitals had the capacity to house between five and thirty patients at one time. See also StAN, RV.338 (1496), f.5v; Sudhoff, "Die ersten Maßnahmen der Stadt Nürnberg," 9.
61. StAN, RV.339 (1497), f.9r; StAN, RV.348 (1497), 4v.
62. StAN, RV.340 (1497), f.4r; Sudhoff, "Die ersten Maßnahmen der Stadt Nürnberg," 14–15; Newhouse, "Outside the Walls," 60–70.
63. Newhouse, "Outside the Walls," 66–68.
64. Hays, *The Burdens of Disease*, 27.
65. Newhouse, "Outside the Walls," 112; Mummenhof, "Die öffentliche Gesundheits- und Krankenpflege," 304.
66. Mummenhoff, "Die öffentliche Gesundheits- und Krankenpflege," 104; Newhouse, "Outside the Walls," 112. StAN, RV.509 (1509), f.4v. The Saumarkt is now known as the Trödelmarkt. Newhouse, "Outside the Walls," 113.
67. StAN, RV.509 (1509), f.4v.
68. StAN, RV.525 (1510), f.8v.
69. Newhouse, "Outside the Walls," 114.
70. Newhouse, "Outside the Walls," 49.
71. Porzelt, *Die Pest*, 37.
72. Mummenhoff, "Die öffentliche Gesundheits- und Krankenpflege," 25.
73. StAN, RV.336 (1496), f.9r.
74. StAN, RV.336 (1496), f.9r.
75. Stadtarchiv Nürnberg (hereafter: StadtAN), B19 Nr. 418 [1562].
76. Sudhoff, "Die ersten Maßnahmen der Stadt Nürnberg," 6.

77. McGough, *Gender, Sexuality, and Syphilis*, 1.
78. StAN, *Ratsbuch* No.6 (hereafter RB.number) (1496–1497), f.222r; Sudhoff, "Die ersten Maßnahmen der Stadt Nürnberg," 17.
79. StAN, RB.6 (1496–1497), f.197r.
80. Kriegk, *Deutsches Bürgerthum im Mittelalter*, Vol. 2, 293.
81. StAN, RV.2142 (1632), ff.64r–65r; O'Brien, "Contagion, Morality, and Practicality," 169–74.
82. StAN, RV.339 (1496), f.11r; RV.340 (1497), f.4r; RV.348 (1497), f.7v.
83. StAN, RV.339 (1496), f.11.r.
84. StAN, RV.337 (1496), f.1r.
85. StAN, RV.341 (1497), f.8v.
86. StAN, R.350 (1497), f.2v.
87. StAN, RV.350 (1497), f.6v.
88. Some examples of general orders to expel non-native beggars can be found in StAN, RV.337 (1496), f.1r; RV341 (1497), f.8v; RV.352 (1497), f.2v. Examples of expulsions of specific individuals and groups can be seen in StAN, RV.357 (1498), f.3v; RV.360 (1498), f.3v; RV.416 (1502), f.6v.
89. StAN, RV.350 (1497), f.19v.
90. Haller, "Die Geschichte," 43.
91. StAN, RV.366 (1499), f.16v; RV.371 (1499), f.5r; RV.374 (1499), f.9r; RV.378 (1499), f.13v; RV.388 (1500), f.14r, 15v; RV.396 (1500), f.10v.
92. StAN, RV.378 (1499), f.4v.
93. Sudhoff, "Die ersten Maßnahmen der Stadt Nürnberg," 9–10. This order aimed to halt all begging in the city. Winkelmann, "Die Armenordnung von Nürnberg," 251.
94. Safley, *The Reformation of Charity*, 193.
95. Ribbentrop, *Pest und Policey*, 37; Stein, *Negotiating the French Pox*, 82; Kinzelbach, *Gesundbleiben, Krankwerden, Armsein*, 250–53, 378–81.
96. Jütte, "Syphilis and Confinement," 102.
97. Frohman, *Poor Relief*, 26; Hammond, "Contagion," 94; Heinrichs, *Plague, Print and the Reformation*, 138–39.
98. Friess, "Poor relief," 77.
99. Stein, *Negotiating the French Pox*; Kinzelbach, "'Böse Blattern,'" 43–70; Kinzelbach, *Gesundbleiben, Krankwerden, Armsein*.
100. Arrizabalaga et al., *The Great Pox*, 147, 150.
101. Arrizabalaga et al., *The Great Pox*, 153.
102. Kinzelbach, "'Böse Blattern,'" 53–54.
103. Sudhoff, "Vorsorge für die Syphiliskranken," 1434.
104. Kinzelbach, ""Böse Blattern,'" 55.
105. Friess, "Poor Relief and Health Care," 81.
106. Edinburgh City Archive, Edinburgh Town Council Minutes, SL1/1/1 1456, ff. 33–34.
107. Aberdeen City and Aberdeenshire Archives (hereafter: ACA), Aberdeen City Council Register, Vol. 7 (1487–1501), CA/1/1/7.
108. ACA, Aberdeen City Council Register, Vol. 8 (1501–11), CA/1/1/8.
109. Gall et al., "Quarantine as a Public Health Measure," 4.
110. "Abscheid 25 May 1496, Stadt Zürich." In Gall et al., "Quarantine as a Public Health Measure," Appendix, 3.

Bibliography

Archival Sources

Aberdeen City and Aberdeenshire Archives (ACA)
Edinburgh City Archive (ECA)
Institut für Stadtgeschichte, Frankfurt am Main (ISG)
Staatsarchiv Nürnberg (StAN)
Stadtarchiv Nürnberg (StadtAN)

Primary Sources

Fracastoro, Girolamo. *Syphilis sive Morbus Gallicus*. Verona: [Micolini da Sabbio, Stefano et fratelli], 1530.

Grünpeck, Joseph. "A Neat Treatise on the Origin of the French Evil," translated by Merrill Moore and Harry C. Solomon. In Merrill Moore and Harry C. Solomon, "Joseph Grünpeck and his Neat Treatise (1496) on the French Evil: A Translation with a Biographical Note," *British Journal of Venereal Diseases* 11, no. 1 (1935): 1–27.

Knobloch, Tobias. *Die lue venere, von Frantzosen kurtzer Bericht*. Giessen: Nicolaus Hampel, 1620.

Maximilian I. "Mandat gegen Gotteslästerung." In *Regesta Imperii XIV:I. Ausgewählte Regesten des Kaiserreiches unter Maxi Böhmer, Johann Friedrichmilian I. 1493–1519*, edited by Johann Friedrich, Hermann Wiesflecker, et al., 273–74. Vienna: Böhlau Verlag, 1990.

Renner, Franz. *Ein new wolgegründet nützlichs und haylsams Handtbüchlein*. Nuremberg: Gabriel Hain, 1559.

Rostinio, Pietro. *Newer außführlicher unnd nutzlicher Tractat von den Frantzosen*. Frankfurt am Main: Ludwig von Hörnigk, 1626.

Schmid, Joseph. *Kurtzer Jedoch eigentlicher Bericht von denen drey abscheulichen ererblichen ansteckenden Seuch- oder Kranckheiten; Als die Pest Frantzosen und Scharbock*. Augsburg: Johann Wehe and Johann Schultes, 1667.

Secondary Sources

Arrizabalaga, Jon, John Henderson, and Roger French. *The Great Pox: The French Disease in Renaissance Europe*. New Haven: Yale University Press, 1997.

Cohn, Samuel Kline, Jr. *Epidemics: Hate and Compassion from the Plague of Athens to AIDS*. Oxford: Oxford University Press, 2018.

Cohn, Samuel Kline, Jr. *Cultures of Plague: Medical Thinking at the End of the Renaissance*. Oxford: Oxford University Press, 2010.

Coy, Jason Philip. "Beggars at the Gates: Banishment and Exclusion in Sixteenth-Century Ulm." *The Sixteenth Century Journal* 39, no. 3 (2008): 619–38.

Daumen, Arndt. "Städtische Prostitution." In *Spätmittelalter am Oberrhein: Alltag, Handwerk und Handel 1350–1525*. Vol. 2: Essay Volume, edited by Sönke Lorenz and Thomas Zotz, 329–334. Stuttgart: J. Thorbecke, 2001.

Diefenbacher, Michael. "Nürnberg, Reichstadt: Verwaltung." In *Historisches Lexikon Bayerns* (2010). Retrieved 28 June 2021 from https://www.historisches-lexikon-bayerns.de/Lexikon/Nürnberg,_Reichsstadt:_Verwaltung.

Dross, Fritz. "Patterns of Hospitality: Aspects of Institutionalisation in 15th and 16th Centuries Nuremberg Healthcare." *Hygiea Internationalis* 9, no. 1 (2010): 13–34.

Fleischmann, Peter. *Rat und Patriziat in Nürnberg: Die Herrschaft der Ratsgeschlechter vom 13. bis zum 18. Jahrhundert*, Vol. 1–4. Neustadt an der Aisch: Verein für Geschichte der Stadt Nürnberg, 2008.

Friess, Peer. "Poor Relief and Health Care Provision in South-German Catholic Cities during the Sixteenth Century." In *The Reformation of Charity: The Secular and the Religious in Early Modern Poor Relief*, edited by Thomas Max Safley, 76–91. Boston: Brill, 2003.

Frohman, Larry. *Poor Relief and Welfare in Germany from the Reformation to World War I*. Cambridge: Cambridge University Press, 2008.

Gall, Gabriella Eva Cristina, Stephan Lautenschlager, and Homayoun C. Bagheri. "Quarantine as a Public Health Measure against an Emerging Infectious Disease: Syphilis in Zurich at the Dawn of the Modern Era (1496–1585)." *GMS hygiene and infection control* 11 (2016). Retrieved 28 August 2025 from https://pmc.ncbi.nlm.nih.gov/articles/PMC4899769/.

Haller, Helmut Frhr. von. "Die Geschichte der Heilig-Kreuz Stiftung." In *Das Pilgrimspital zum Heiligen Kreuz vor Nürnberg*, by Helmut Frhr. von Haller and Ernst Eichhorn. Nuremberg: Verein für Geschichte der Stadt Nürnberg, 1969.

Hammond, Mitchell Lewis. "Contagion, Honour and Urban Life in Early Modern Germany." In *Imagining contagion in early modern Europe*, edited by Claire L. Carlin, 94–106. Basingstoke: Palgrave Macmillan, 2005.

Harvey, Katherine. "The Pustulent Penis: Searching for STDs in the Centuries before Syphilis," *Notches: (Re)marks on the History of Sexuality* (2016). Retrieved 28 June 2021 from https://notchesblog.com/2016/06/02/the-pustulent-penis-searching-for-stds-in-the-centuries-before-syphilis/.

Hays, J. N. *The Burdens of Disease: Epidemics and Human Response in Western History*. London: Rutgers University Press, 2003.

Heinrichs, Erik A. *Plague, Print and the Reformation: The German Reform of Healing, 1473–1573*. Abingdon: Routledge, 2019.

Henderson, John. "Coping with Epidemics in Renaissance Italy: Plague and the Great Pox." In *The Fifteenth Century XII: Society in an Age of Plague*, edited by Linda Clark and Carole Rawcliffe, 175–94. Woodbridge: Boydell Press, 2013.

Huppert, George. *After the Black Death: A Social History of Early Modern Europe*. Bloomington: Indiana University Press, 1998.

Jillings, Karen. "Plague, Pox and the Physician in Aberdeen, 1495–1516." *Journal of the Royal College of Physicians of Edinburgh* 40 (2010): 70–76.

Jütte, Robert. *Poverty and Deviance in Early Modern Europe*. Cambridge: Cambridge University Press, 2001.

Jütte, Robert. "Syphilis and Confinement: Hospitals in Early Modern Germany." In *Institutions of Confinement: Hospitals, Asylums, and Prisons in Western Europe and North America, 1500–1950*, edited by Norbert Finzsch and Robert Jütte, 97–115. Cambridge: Cambridge University Press, 1997.

Jütte, Robert. *Obrigkeitliche Armenfürsorge in Deutschen Reichsstädten in der Frühen Neuzeit: Städtisches Armenwesen in Frankfurt am Main und Köln*. Cologne: Böhlau, 1984.

Kinzelbach, Annemarie. "'Böse Blattern' oder 'Franzosenkrankheit': Syphiliskonzept, Kranke und die Genese des Krankenhauses in oberdeutschen Reichsstädten in der frühen Neuzeit." In *Neue Wege in der Seuchengeschichte*, edited by Martin Dinges and Thomas Schlich, 43–70. Stuttgart: Steiner, 1995.

Kinzelbach, Annemarie. *Gesundbleiben, Krankwerden, Armsein in der frühneuzeitlichen Gesellschaft: Gesunde und Kranke in den Reichsstädten Überlingen und Ulm, 1500–1700*. Stuttgart: Steiner, 1995.

Kriegk, Georg Ludwig. *Deutsches Bürgerthum im Mittelalter*, Vol. 2. Frankfurt am Main: Sauer et Auvermann, 1969.

Lindberg, Carter. *Beyond Charity: Reformation Initiatives for the Poor*. Minneapolis: Fortress Press, 1993.

McGough, Larua J. *Gender, Sexuality, and Syphilis in Early Modern Venice: The Disease that Came to Stay*. Houndmills: Palgrave Macmillan, 2011.

Meteling, Wencke."Gesundheitsfürsorge." In *Spätmittelalter am Oberrhein: Alltag, Handwerk und Handel 1350–1525*. Vol. 2: Essay Volume, edited by Sönke Lorenz and Thomas Zotz, 481–89. Stuttgart: J. Thorbecke, 2001.

Moritz, Werner. "Die bürgerlichen Fürsorgeanstalten der Reichsstadt Frankfurt im späten Mittelalter." Vol. 1. PhD thesis. Johann Wolfgang Goethe Universität zu Frankfurt am Main, 1977.

Mummenhoff, Ernst. "Die öffentliche Gesundheits- und Krankenpflege im alten Nürnberg." In *Festschrift zur Eröffnung des Neuen Krankenhauses der Stadt Nürnberg*, edited by Carl Distler and Gottlieb Merkel, 1–122. Nuremberg: Städtischen Kollegien, 1898.

Murphy, Hannah Saunders. "Reforming Medicine in Sixteenth Century Nuremberg." PhD thesis. University of California, Berkeley, 2012.

Newhouse, Amy Melinda. "Outside the Walls: Civic Belonging and Contagious Disease in Sixteenth-Century Nuremberg." PhD thesis. University of Arizona, 2015.

Newhouse, Amy. "The Mystery of the St. Sebastian Lazareth: Mapping Place-Names and Contagious Disease Hospitals in Sixteenth-Century Nuremberg." In *Names and Naming in Early Modern Germany*, edited by Marjorie Elizabeth Plummer and Joel F. Harrington, 125–148. Afterword by Randolph C. Head. New York, Oxford: Berghahn Books, 2019.

O'Brien, Monica C. "Practice and Power: The Rise and Disappearance of the *Franzosenärzte*, or Doctors of the French Pox, in Nuremberg, 1495–1560." *Journal of the Royal College of Physicians of Edinburgh* 51, no. 1 (2021): 91–97.

O'Brien, Monica C. "Contagion, Morality, and Practicality: The French Pox in Frankfurt am Main and Nuremberg, 1495–1700." PhD thesis. University of Glasgow, 2019.

Porzelt, Carolin. *Die Pest in Nürnberg: Leben und Herrschen in Pestzeiten in der Reichsstadt Nürnberg (1562–1713)*. St. Ottilien: EOS-Verlag, 2000.

Proksch, Johann Karl. *Die Litteratur über die venerischen Krankheiten: von den ersten Schriften über Syphilis aus dem Ende des fünfzehnten Jahrhunderts bis zum Jahre 1889*, Vol. 1. Bonn: P. Hanstein, 1889.

Quétel, Claude. *History of Syphilis*, translated by Judith Braddock and Brian Pike. London: Polity Press, 1990.

Ribbentrop, Sonja. *Pest und Policey im norddeutschen Raum: Die Entwicklung der Pest im Kontext von Wirtschaft, Administration und Policey*. Hamburg: Hamburg Diplomica-Verlag, 2014.

Safley, Thomas Max, ed. *The Reformation of Charity: The Secular and the Religious in Early Modern Poor Relief*. Boston: Brill, 2003.

Stein, Claudia. *Negotiating the French Pox in Early Modern Germany*. Farnham: Ashgate, 2009.

Strauss, Gerald. *Nuremberg in the Sixteenth Century: City, Politics and Life between Middle Ages and Modern Times*. Bloomington: Indiana University Press, 1976.

Stricker, Wilhelm. *Die Geschichte der Heilkunde und der verwandten Wissenschaften in der Stadt Frankfurt am Main*. Frankfurt am Main: Kessler, 1847.
Sudhoff, Karl. "Vorsorge für die Syphiliskranken in Würzburg und Augsburg zu Ende des 15. bis ins zweite Viertel des 16. Jahrhunderts." *Dermatologische Wochenschrift* 97 (1933): 1431–1445.
Sudhoff, Karl. "Anfänge der Syphilisbeobachtung Und Syphilisprophylaxe Zu Frankfurt a. Main. 1496–1502." *Dermatologische Zeitschrift* 20, no. 2 (1913): 95–116.
Sudhoff, Karl. "Die ersten Maßnahmen der Stadt Nürnberg gegen die Syphilis in den Jahren 1496 und 1497." *Archiv für Dermatologie und Syphilis* 118 (1913): 1–30.
Sudhoff, Karl. "Sorge für die Syphiliskranken und Luesprophylaxe zu Nürnberg in den Jahren 1498–1505." *Archiv für Dermatologie und Syphilis* 118 (1913): 285–318.
Winkelmann, Otto. "Die Armenordnung von Nürnberg (1522), Kitzingen (1523), Regensburg (1523) und Ypern (1525)." *Archiv für Reformationsgeschichte* 10, no. 3 (1913): 242–58.

CHAPTER 5

Tracing Sixteenth-Century Infection Chains in Central Germany

THOMAS WOZNIAK

Introduction: Preconditions and Initial Structural Situation

The region around the low mountain range of the Harz, between the Weser and the Elbe rivers, was far from literary consideration in Roman times, for it was uncultivated landscape. During late antiquity in the sixth and seventh centuries, however, it seems to have taken on a central function.[1] At the beginning of the tenth century this function, which has hardly been researched yet, led to it becoming a central place of the Ottonian dynasty, where, on the one hand, the important Christian Easter Feast was celebrated and, on the other hand, King Henry I (876–936) and Queen Mathilde (896–968) found their burial place. A convent for ladies was established in order to permanently secure the *memoria* with prayers; it existed until the nineteenth century and its heads, the abbesses, were the descendants of ruling families. North of this convent, a market was established at the end of the tenth century, around which the Old Town (Altstadt) was formed. With later rulers' relocation of their residences, the importance of the place decreased. To counteract this slow process, the abbesses founded a New Town (Neustadt) to the west of the Old Town in the twelfth century. The two towns, which were originally separated both structurally and legally, increasingly grew together in the thirteenth century, and from about 1330 they formed a double town that appeared as a single unit from the outside. Half of the council was made up of councilors from the Old Town and half from the New Town. There were always at least two mayors, one each from the Old and New Towns, and for a time even four.[2] The Old Town consisted of three parishes (Sts. Blasii, Benedikti, and Aegidii) but four quarters, called "Huden." St. Nikolai church was the parish church for the New Town, which consisted of two "Huden."[3] According to an early tax list from 1310–30, there were 750 households at that time. By 1461, this number had increased to 1,024, but it decreased to 723 by 1525. Thereafter, with interruptions from plague epidemics, it increased to over 1,100 households by about 1600. However, by the Thirty Years' War (1618–48) the number of households had fallen again to about eight hundred, and then increased more or less continuously until the nineteenth century.[4]

Of the 2,119 half-timbered houses systematically recorded in 2012, over 95 percent had not yet been built in 1550.[5] Although the city has one of the best-preserved old towns in Germany, most of the buildings extant today did not exist at that time.

Medical care was not yet well developed. A doctor, i.e. a university-trained physician, was employed by the city only in exceptional circumstances. Although there were several hospitals, these seldom served to cure illnesses but, rather, performed the function of today's retirement homes and long-term care facilities. In cases of dental problems, open wounds, broken bones, or similar external injuries, the services of barbers could be used. The most important location for a barber was at the intersection of Breite Strasse and Bockstrasse. Across the street was the municipal council pharmacy (*Ratsapotheke*). However, it did not carry many medicines. To gain a picture of the epidemic situation in Quedlinburg in the sixteenth century, it is necessary to briefly consider the available historical sources.

Historical Sources

Our historical knowledge of Quedlinburg before 1450 is based almost exclusively on charters and chronicles. Many council records have survived from this time onward. In the second half of the sixteenth century the preservation of serial sources begins, which allows for a much more detailed picture. For the following study, five sources in particular were used: (a) chronicles, (b) tax registers, (c) lists of new citizens in the town account ledgers, (d) death lists of the parishes, and (e) funerary inscriptions. The advantage of using parallel sources is that the individual sources can be checked against each other for reliability and consistency. What could we reconstruct if we had only one of these sources? What typical errors could arise?

Chronicles have a long tradition in Quedlinburg, the oldest preserved examples being the Quedlinburg Annals from the tenth and eleventh centuries.[6] Various chronicles were also written during the sixteenth century. These are often infused with a Protestant perspective and must be examined accordingly. Taxes were collected from the thirteenth century onward, but tax records have survived only sporadically. The oldest surviving list for the entire city dates from 1310 to 1330 and is one of the earliest surviving examples in Central Europe.[7] From 1480 and 1520 onward, tax lists are preserved at irregular intervals, and from 1700 on they are preserved in their entirety for each year. An edition of all surviving Quedlinburg tax registers before 1600 is to be published soon.[8] New citizens were also recorded by the town clerk, since they had to pay a fee. These lists of new citizens have been preserved as a component of the council accounts (*Ratsrechungen*), some of which have survived in Quedlinburg from 1454.[9] With the Reformation, lists of baptisms, weddings, and burials began to be kept in Quedlinburg. From about 1600 onward, these are preserved to a greater extent. Especially for the year 1598–99, the burial list of St. Nikolai church has been preserved and allows an accurate insight into the progression of the number of deaths in that year. In the churches of Quedlinburg, some epitaphs and funerary inscriptions have been preserved from the end of the sixteenth century that refer directly to the plague epidemics. They have been included here for comparison.

Question and Methodology

All citizens as well as the council were subordinate to the abbess as the sovereign ruler. Particularly in emergency situations, all those involved were dependent on each other.

Three epidemics that occurred in the second half of the sixteenth century will be examined in detail: the epidemics of 1566–67, 1577, and 1598–99. First of all, the chronological course of the epidemics, their spread, and the topographical spread are examined. Furthermore, the options of the abbess for containing their spread and attempts by the leading economic classes to contain such measures are investigated. This short study ends with an assessment of the long-term handling of plague by the abbess and the city, and the future need for research based on additional sources.

Not All "Plagues" Are the Same

Epidemic caesurae, which had an impact on the source data of the Quedlinburg tax registers, are understood here as various epidemic diseases, especially plague, which occurred in regular cycles.[10] Before modern times, the term *pestis* (Latin for "plague") was not used to designate a disease *sui generis*, such as bubonic plague. Contemporaries used terms such as pestis, pestilence, pestilential fever, holy fire, or *ignis St. Antonii* to refer collectively to different diseases, epidemic diseases per se, which they did not precisely separate conceptually.

Such epidemic diseases could have been smallpox, plague, dysentery, measles, English sweat, syphilis, typhus, influenza, anthrax, and others, but also ergot poisoning.[11] In a figurative sense, however, famines and war campaigns could also be called "plague."[12] Leprosy, as an exception, was already recognized in contemporary perception and presented as such in the sources. However, it rarely spawned epidemic spread. A much-cited sentence from the late antique physician Galen makes clear what was understood by pestis "when at the same time many fall ill and the greater part of the sick perish."[13] Using comparative chronological studies and evidence from contemporaries, individual diseases can be identified as more likely for epidemics of different times.[14] Smallpox epidemics seem to have occurred since ancient times.[15] While it occurred in ancient times, plague (*Yersinia pestis*) had not been seen in Europe since the cessation of the Justinian Plague before the fourteenth century. After 1348–51, various forms of plague were added that occurred on average every eight to eleven years. Other epidemic diseases, such as dysentery, measles, or the so-called English sweat, appeared from the fifteenth century, without being reliably distinguished from the plague (*Yersinia pestis*) in sources.[16] It was not until the sixteenth century that a stronger differentiation of the diseases began, however without a reliable conceptual delimitation in the death registers or even the tax record.

The Regional Epidemic until 1550

When the plague first appeared in Quedlinburg, it was a very significant event for the city. It took almost 350 years until an effective countermeasure against the regularly recurring waves of plague was found in 1680, with the establishment of a plague hospital outside the city walls. In recent years, several detailed studies on plague have been presented for northern Germany, focusing on Hildesheim, Bremen, and the cities of the Ruhr region. A similar study was presented in southern Germany for Nuremberg.

In Hildesheim and Bremen, the results of the studies are presented at the level of the city quarters. As an example, some streets in Hildesheim are analyzed, with the qualification that the topographical spread of the epidemic over time can be reconstructed only imprecisely, since a precise determination of the locations of the dwellings is lacking.[17] A precise temporal subdivision of the data would be possible for such an analysis, due to the exceptional source materials offered by the Hildesheim Plague Book (1597–1623).[18]

A similar regret has been expressed by one author about the 1577 plague in Venice: "Today, unfortunately, from our knowledge of the topography of the city, we can no longer draw any conclusions regarding the course and spread of plagues of the past."[19] A parcel-by-parcel mapping was successfully attempted for the so-called plague of 1611–12 in Innsbruck, which was actually a typhus epidemic. However, the temporal course was not analyzed there.[20]

As was common in the second half of the sixteenth century all over Central Europe, plague waves raged relatively regularly in Quedlinburg and the surrounding area, as in 1566–67, 1577 and 1598–99. Remarkably, within very short periods of about eight years, the number of households was not only replenished but exceeded pre-pandemic levels. The increase in population due to immigration exceeded the shrinkage due to epidemics. While in the fourteenth and fifteenth centuries the surrounding villages served as reservoirs to replenish the town's population, it is not clear where the new inhabitants came from in the late sixteenth century, when only one of the former fourteen surrounding villages remained. During the period of the Thirty Years' War, the extinct households were probably replenished by war refugees from other regions, although this cannot be proven with certainty.

The next plague in northern Germany is not documented until 1547–48.[21] An outbreak in Quedlinburg in 1547–48 is mentioned in 1828 by the local historian Johann Heinrich Fritsch, who writes that "in 1547 and later in 1565 plague-like diseases raged and caused a great death, which also among others completely depopulated the Wiperti and Münzenberg monasteries."[22] Whether there was an epidemic in Quedlinburg during this period is questionable, because according to the tax registers the number of households decreased by only 4 percent, from 860 to 825, and because the decrease is limited to the New Town.[23]

According to the chronicles, more than 2,500 Quedlinburg citizens died in the largest epidemic, in 1566–67,[24] and almost half as many, 1,215, died in the second epidemic, in 1577.[25] The third epidemic, in 1598–99, could not be avoided either, despite the timely orders by Abbess Anna III, who banned the fairs in October 1598 and February 1599, against the protests of the council.[26] The large number of deaths is clearly reflected in the tax registers.[27] Two sources form the basis of the following description: the death registers of the parishes of St. Nikolai and of St. Benedikti.

The Epidemic of 1566–67

The tax register from 1567 is a unique source. The scribe marked the households affected by the plague with crosses or wrote the word "tot" ("dead") instead of a cross.[28] This peculiarity allows for graphic mapping of the households affected by the 1566–67 plague in the entire Old and New Town (Figure 5.1). With the help of this plague mapping, some qualitative statements about the plague can be verified quantitatively with a concrete case study.[29] Overall, in the 1567 tax register the names of 31 percent of the entries, or 309 out of 990 households,

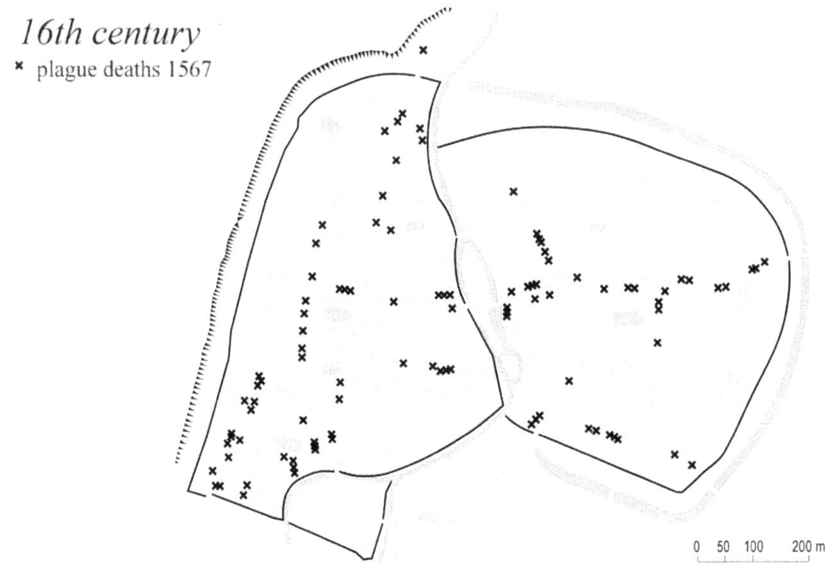

Figure 5.1. Plague deaths in 1567 in St. Benedikti and St. Nikolai parishes. © Thomas Wozniak

are marked with crosses. The crosses seem to mark all those households where the plague appeared, regardless of who died. For only 10 ten percent of the households can it be shown that the head of the household died of the plague. The number of household heads as a percentage of the total number of plague victims in a year was 10 to 12 percent. The total of 2,500 plague deaths during the 1566–67 plague wave, as recorded in the chronicles, is fairly accurate. The percentage of plague victims (one third of the total population) is in the average range for the number of plague deaths determined for Central Europe.[30]

In the New Town, 34 percent (132 of 390) of households were affected by one or more deaths, slightly more than in the Old Town with 30 percent (177 of 600). Klink Street in the Old Town was particularly badly affected, in both absolute and relative terms, with 56 percent (fourteen out of twenty-five households).

In absolute terms, the most inhabitants were lost in the Old Town in Hohe Strasse, Pölle, Stieg, and Kramerstrasse (Table 5.1). In the New Town, absolute mortality was highest in the outer part of Weberstrasse, followed by Nobben. Relative mortality was above average in three small streets: Im Hirtenhause (now Kaiserstrasse/Pölkenstrasse), close to the Pölkentor gate, at 100 percent, in Beginenstrasse at 75 percent, and in the street "In der Gasse beÿ Veith Romel" at 67 percent. The least affected streets in the Old Town were In

Table 5.1. The mortality in selected streets during the 1567 plague. © Thomas Wozniak

Streetname	Town	Percentage	Households Affected	Households Total
Uffem Grase	New	0%	0	6
Steinweg	New	17%	6	36
Reichenstrasse	New	17%	2	12
Stieg	Old	24%	12	48
Pölle	Old	25%	12	49
Nobben	New	28%	12	43
Weberstrasse	New	34%	16	47
Hohe Strasse	Old	37%	29	78
Kramerstrasse	Old	44%	12	27
In der Gasse beÿ Veith Romel	New	67%	4	6
Beginenstrasse	New	75%	3	4
Im Hirtenhause	New	100%	6	6

den Hoken, Dovenstrasse, and the peripheral street "In den Gropern vor dem Thore," with 10 percent. The least affected in the New Town were Steinweg, and Reichenstrasse, and the street "Uffm Grase." Because of the high number of 309 affected households, the number of new citizens admitted in 1568 increased significantly from an average of 26 earlier in the sixteenth century to 57.[31] During this plague wave the mayor, Jacob Seifart, also died.[32]

The 1577 Epidemic

According to Winningstedt's chronicle, in 1576 a violent thunderstorm caused flooding and a plague-like death of 1,215 people in the town of Quedlinburg.[33] This plague year also occurred elsewhere and is well described and researched for Bremen and Venice.[34] During this plague cycle in Quedlinburg, the physician Magister Caspar Bucha distinguished himself in particular; he was appointed town physician in 1579 in recognition of his achievements.[35]

For the year 1577, the death register of St. Benedikti parish has survived.[36] The figure of 1,215 is found at the end of the record for that year, but, according to the scribe, one must subtract "those who would have died because of old age,"[37] i.e. the thirty-eight dead who would have died even without the influence of the plague must be deducted from this figure. The preserved church book of

Table 5.2. The deceased of the year 1577 in the Quedlinburg parishes (Kirchspiel). © Thomas Wozniak

Parish	Plague Victims		Other (Age, Accidents)		Total	
	Deceased	Share	Deceased	Share	Deceased	Share
St. Nikolai	395	34%	0	0%	395	33%
St. Wiperti/St. Spiritus	334	28%	10	26%	344	28%
St. Benediki	268	23%	20	53%	288	24%
St. Ägidii	122	10%	1	3%	123	10%
St. Blasii	58	5%	7	18%	65	5%
Total	1,177	100%	38	100%	1,215	100%

Source: Evangelisches Kirchen-Archiv Quedlinburg, Sterberegister St. Benedikti 1577.

St. Benedikti church records a total list of deaths in the city for 1577, containing 268 plague deaths and twenty old-age deaths.[38] According to this list, most of the deaths were in the three quarters of the Old Town, with 38 percent, followed by the New Town with exactly one third and the extramural suburbs with the remaining 28 percent. Accordingly, 1,177 people died of the plague. These were distributed among the five parishes of Quedlinburg as shown in Table 5.2.

The high number of deceased in the suburbs of St. Wiperti and St. Spiritus is irrelevant for the evaluation of the tax registers, because they do not contain any data about the suburbs. In order to determine the number of deceased inhabitants of the Old and New Towns recorded in the tax registers without the inhabitants of the suburbs, 334 victims must be subtracted from the total of 1,177. In 1577, 843 people died of the plague in the Old and New Towns.

In the temporal development of the number of victims, it is striking that many plague victims died in October 1577, i.e. in the fall (Figure 5.2). The first plague victim of 1577 died in April, according to the recorder of the death register. However, a sharp increase can be observed from the end of August, with a clear rise at the end of September and a peak in the number of deaths in October. Toward the end of the year, the number of victims dropped, without disappearing completely. It was not until mid-February 1578 that the last plague victims of this period were recorded.

The scribes of the death registers recorded the date, the name of the head of the household, and the nature of the deceased person's relationship to him, as well as the first name. Children were identified by gender as daughter (*filia*) or son (*filius*) (Table 5.3). The 288 deceased in St. Benedikti parish correspond

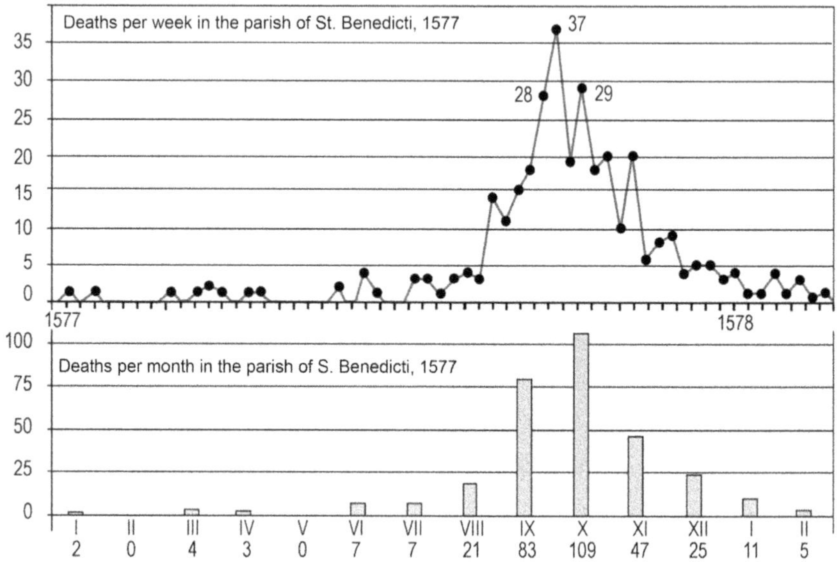

Figure 5.2. Deceased of the plague epidemic 1577 in St. Benedikti parish, Quedlinburg. © Thomas Wozniak

to about one third of the 843 people who died in total in the Old and New Towns. Of this one third, only 11 percent are heads of households, and only their deaths were documented in the tax registers. The recorder of the death registers also provided the age at death for 184 of the 208 children who died. Thus, for about 90 percent of the children, the age at which they died is known.

About one third of the children were under five years old, another third under ten, and the remaining third between ten and twenty years. From the analysis of their ages at death, it is clear that in 1577 at least 42 percent of all plague victims in St. Benedikti parish were under ten years old, best seen in the spike of week 40 (Figure 5.3). The absolute highest susceptibility to die of the plague was among children up to the age of two.

If the data are grouped in five-year increments, the following results are obtained: the under-fives are most susceptible to dying from the epidemic, and the under-tens only slightly less so (Figure 5.4). The susceptibility of those aged ten to fifteen years is reduced by one third compared to the highest group, and it decreases by almost three-quarters for those aged fifteen to twenty years and by more than 80 percent for those aged twenty to twenty-five years, always in relation to those aged under five. The documentation of the ages of the victims is unique in Quedlinburg; in other places a statistically useful data set can rarely be found.

By contrast, the church register of St. Benedikti for 1577 contains almost no occupational data on those who died of the plague. There is a remarkable

Table 5.3. Group-specific mortality in St. Benedikti parish in 1577.[39] © Thomas Wozniak

•* = Designation in the death register			
		Deceased	**Percentage**
Mann	Husband	31	11%
(Ehe) Frau	(Married) wife	25	9%
Witwen	Widows	8	3%
Sohn*	Son	87	30%
Tochter*	Daughter	113	39%
Knecht*	Servant	1	0.3%
Magd*	Maid	14	5%
Lehrjunge*	Apprentice	1	0,3%
Schüler*	Pupil	7	2%
Geselle*	Journeyman	1	0.3%
Number of children		208	72%
Total		288	100%

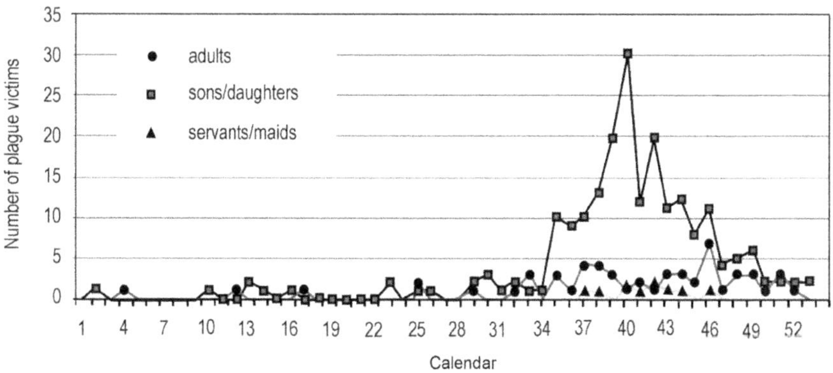

Figure 5.3. Seasonal group mortality in 1577 in the St. Benedikti parish of Quedlinburg. © Thomas Wozniak

addition to the church register for the parish of St. Blasii, whose death register has not survived. To the left of the rear entrance of St. Blasii church, on the church wall outside is a gravestone of the Lüders family, which bears an inscription testifying to the plague of 1577.

The inscription states that the father, Andreas Lüder, died on 15 September, his son Michael on 25 November, the son Andreas Lüder the Younger on 28

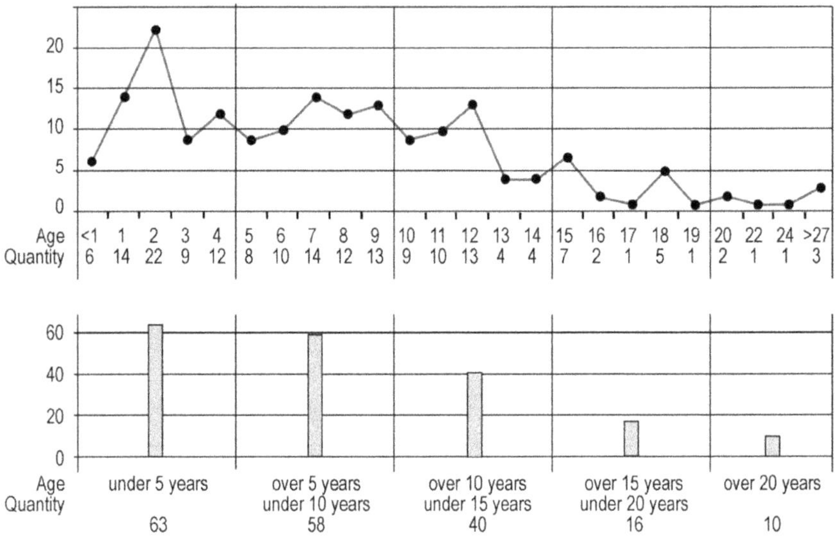

Figure 5.4. Child mortality in 1577 in St. Benedikti parish (n=184/208).
© Thomas Wozniak

November, Matthias Lüder on 26 January, and (another) Andreas Lüder on 8 November.[40] The death dates that are later in the year coincide with the shift in the plague pattern mentioned above, due to the relatively mild weather in 1577. It is striking that these are all male family members, four sons and the father, who died of the plague in 1577. The family lived in Pölle Street.[41]

The 1598–99 Epidemic

The chronicles of Quedlinburg's history describe a great plague epidemic at the end of the sixteenth century, in 1596 or 1598, that is said to have claimed three thousand[42] or four thousand[43] lives. This fits in with the fact that a plague wave is documented in Hildesheim and Bremen in the period 1597–98.[44]

While older research believed the report as such,[45] regional historian Nagel wrote: "In 1598–99 and 1681, the invasion of the plague in Quedlinburg was prevented by rigorous isolation measures."[46]

There is doubt about the occurrence of plague at the end of the sixteenth century on the basis of several preserved plague decrees issued by Abbess Anna III for the years 1598 and 1599. When the abbey area was threatened by the plague in 1598, she forbade the holding of the Martini Market on 11 November and similar events. The council objected to this, saying that the citizens would suffer a "great loss of their food" through the absence of the market. The abbess replied in a letter of 30 October 1598 that she would "not throw a goose egg after a pigeon egg," and that "more consideration must be given to most of the crowd than to a shock of traders," especially as "the loose-minded often visit the market more than those who wish to invest money."[47] In a quantitative analysis of the tax registers, the plague of 1566–67 described above was immediately and clearly noticeable in the data set, due to the drop in the number of taxpayers. For the years between 1596 and 1604, however, the data show no obvious irregularities with regard to the number of the *Schosszahler* (taxpayers), the total number growing continuously, with no outliers. The tax registers alone indicate that there was no plague with high numbers of victims. The supposed success of the abbess's decrees and the continuous growth in the number of households liable to pay tax, as shown in the tax registers, seem to confirm that Quedlinburg was spared the plague in 1598. The qualitative and quantitative results seem to confirm each other.

For two parishes, St. Benedikti and St. Nikolai, the death registers have survived. In 1597 these registers show an average of about four deaths per month in the two parishes. According to what has been said, we would expect that the death rates for 1598 would not show any unusual features. It is therefore noteworthy that the figures increase rapidly in 1598, when the number of deceased in both parishes was 1,274. The graph in Figure 5.5 illustrates the distribution over time, with a clear peak in August.

The two death registers, which subsume the deceased under the heading "Pestis," show that the plague certainly found victims in Quedlinburg in 1598. In the St. Benedikti quarter, the disease apparently began in May and subsided

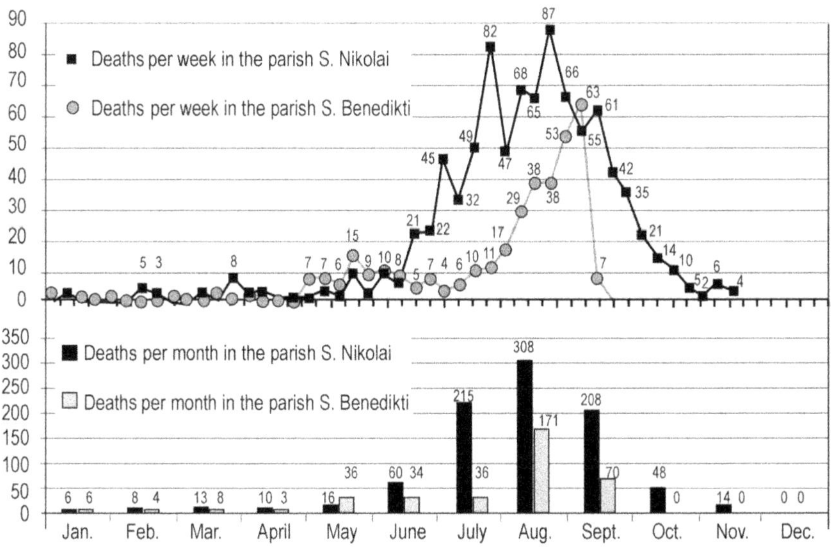

Figure 5.5. Plague epidemic of 1598 in the parishes of St. Benedikti and St. Nikolai. © Thomas Wozniak

again before October, while in the St. Nikolai quarter an increase in the number of deaths became visible only in June and continued into October.

The scribe[48] of the deaths register recorded the date, the name of the head of the household, and the relationship of the deceased person to the head of the household. Children were identified as daughter, son, and child.[49] Unfortunately, age groups are not indicated, although the scribe also recorded entries such as "Söhnlein" (little son) or "Medlein" (little girl), which suggests small children.[50] As a special feature, the scribe in St. Nikolai quarter also recorded the first names of deceased people who were closer to him. The largest proportion of the dead, over 70 percent, are children (Table 5.4).

The proportion of household heads in the total number of deceased is 13 percent. In 1598 there were 502 households in Quedlinburg's Old Town and 390 in the New Town, making a total of 892. In addition, there were 208 servants and 52 temporary members of households. Quedlinburg's New Town was (and still is) congruent with the St. Nikolai parish, so the 117 heads of household out of 390 households in the New Town gives a proportion of exactly one third of deceased heads of household. The high proportion of children in the number of deaths is striking, at over 70 percent. Similar to the plague pathogen (*Yersinia pestis*), the smallpox pathogen (*Variola*) also claims many children among its victims. Smallpox also has a mortality rate of one third in the absence of treatment. However, the chronological course of the epidemic in 1598, which is considered typical of the course of plague in Europe, beginning in spring and ending in autumn, speaks against smallpox as the cause of the epidemic. Apart from the age structure of the deceased, few statements can be made about the social structure, because the occupational details of only some of them are listed in the church records of 1598. In the parish of St. Benedikti, two town messengers, a cook, a brush maker, two blacksmiths, a redsmith, two painters, a pond digger, a lamp maker, a donkey driver, a guardian, a leather tanner, a tanner, and a pig herder are named.[51] In the parish of St. Nikolai there are a shoemaker, a table maker, a horse trader, a needle man, two magistrates, and a swineherd.[52] A former mayor, Ambrosius Grashof, his wife, and his daughter also died of the plague, as did the relatives and servants of thirteen chamberlains;[53] the town clerk, Johannes Balcke, also died of the plague.[54] In addition, in the 1598 council accounts there are six acting councilors who died of the plague.[55] Likewise, Doctor Bodtger was "buried in front of the castle."[56] The municipal doctor Rekeleben first had two of his daughters die before he himself passed away, and the deacon Samuel Hahnenberg also died of the epidemic in 1598.[57] In addition to the age and occupational structure, the topographical locations for about a quarter of the deceased of St. Benedikti parish can be traced with parcel accuracy. Concentrations can be identified in the area of western Klink Street, eastern Stieg, and Pölle, as well as at the south-eastern end of the market. For example, two households (Schulstrasse

Table 5.4. Group-specific mortality in St. Benedikti and St. Nikolai parishes in 1598. © Thomas Wozniak

•* = Designation in death register		St. Benedikti		St. Nikolai		Total	
		Deceased	**Percentage**	**Deceased**	**Percentage**	**Deceased**	**Percentage**
Mann	Husband	26	12%	117	13%	143	13%
(Ehe)Frau	(Married) wife	29	14%	89	10%	117	11%
Sohn*	Son	27	13%	95	11%	122	11%
Tochter*	Daughter	53	25%	93	10%	144	13%
Kind*	Child	65	31%	447	50%	514	46%
Tochter Kind*	Daughter's child	0	0%	5	1%	5	0,5%
Knecht*	Servant	4	2%	13	2%	16	1%
Magd*	Maid	8	4%	22	3%	29	3%
Lehrjunge*	Apprentice	1	0,5%	0	0%	1	0,1%
Schüler*	Pupil	0	0%	2	0,2%	2	0,2%
Geselle*	Journeyman	0	0%	3	0,3%	3	0,3%
unspecified		0	0%	16	2%	24	2%
Total children		145	68%	640	71%	785	71%
Households				390	30%	892	
Sum total		213	100%	898	100%	1,111	100%

Source: Evangelisches Kirchen-Archiv, Sterberegister St. Benedikti and St. Nikolai.

Table 5.5. Epidemic situation in Schulstrasse 12 and Klink 2 in 1598. © Thomas Wozniak

	Family	Relation	Date	Address
1	Allermunds	Child	25.03.1598	Schulstr. 12
2	Allermunds	Daughter	03.04.1598	Schulstr. 12
3	Dörings	Child	24.06.1598	Klink 2
4	Dörings	Child	09.07.1598	Klink 2
5	Allermunds	Child	20.07.1598	Schulstr. 12
6	Dörings	Men	24.07.1598	Klink 2
7	Allermunds	Child	03.08.1598	Schulstr. 12
8	Allermunds	Child	05.08.1598	Schulstr. 12
9	Allermunds	Child	06.08.1598	Schulstr. 12
10	Dörings	Women	11.08.1598	Klink 2

Source: Evangelisches Kichen-Archiv Quedlinburg, Sterberegister St. Benedikti 1598.

12 and Klink 2) stand out with four and six deaths, respectively (Table 5.5 and Figure 5.6). A topographical observation that can be made here is that the properties back directly onto each other.

For 1598 it remains to be noted that an epidemic occurred in Quedlinburg in which at least 143 heads of household (13 percent) and a total of at least 1,266 people died in both towns and in the extramural suburbs. However, the households that became vacant were replenished within such short periods of time that no gaps can be observed in the tax register records. The point in time at which a household became vacant seems to be when the head of the household, then his widow, and then his direct heirs had died. If their heirs were still minors, a relative would be appointed as guardian, or a servant of the council in cases where there were no relatives. In the tax registers the orphans are recorded in a separate additional list. The epidemic is confirmed by the list of new citizen admissions in the council accounts; on average, twenty-six new citizens are recorded each year here in the sixteenth century. In 1599 the figure of ninety-seven is almost four times higher, and the fifty-nine new citizens in 1602 still were more than double the average. The households that had died out thus were replenished within a very short time. The decision to admit a larger number of new citizens to the town seems to have been taken as early as 1598, for when the council account book was compiled five pages remained empty, reserved for new citizen admissions.[58] To register an average of twenty-six new admissions, only a single page was necessary. The deterrent created by the high risk of contagion could explain why only nine new citizens were admitted in 1598. Another indication that the plague occurred is a wooden

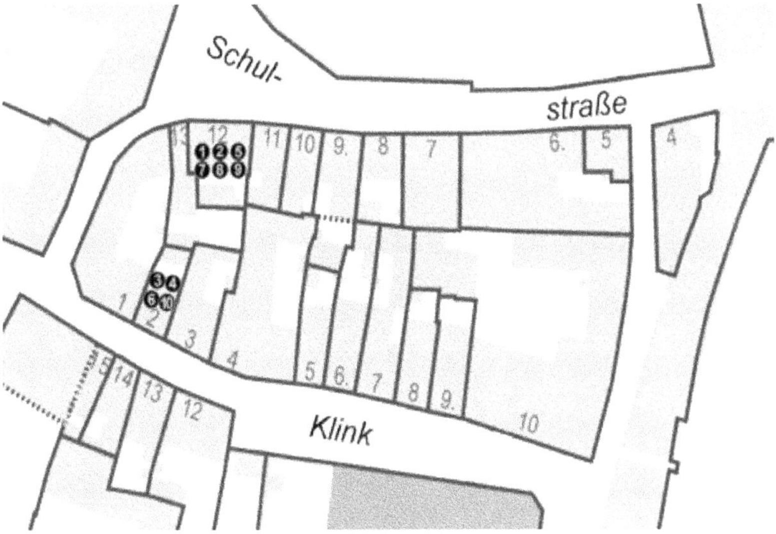

Figure 5.6. Epidemic situation in Schulstrasse 12 and Klink 2 in 1598. © Thomas Wozniak

relief in the Marktkirche which the council had erected for the school rector, Magister Heinrich Faber, who was carried off on 27 August 1598 along with fifty-three others.[59]

Chronological observation suggests that the abbess's tightened quarantine measures were implemented from mid-September 1598, and thus the number of epidemic victims in the St. Benedikti quarter dropped from sixty-six per week to zero within two weeks. These measures were maintained until February 1598 and thus further infections were prevented. In the lists of new citizens, the last admissions date to 1 July 1598, and the first admissions after the plague outbreak to 14 February 1599.[60] Apparently, after the many deaths of the epidemic in the autumn of 1598, it was expected that the vacant households would be filled up very quickly. However, the intake of new citizens proceeded more slowly than planned and the five pages in the tax register remained empty. Overall, it is instructive to note that although the qualitative and quantitative observations from chronicles and tax registers suggest that a more severe epidemic had been successfully averted, an epidemic did occur nonetheless. However, this could only be proven by the death registers, the lists of new citizens, and grave inscriptions.

For the period from 1572 to 1598, the death registers of St. Benedikti parish have been preserved. They show that a total of 2,045 people died in this parish during the twenty-seven-year period (the page for 1585 is blank).

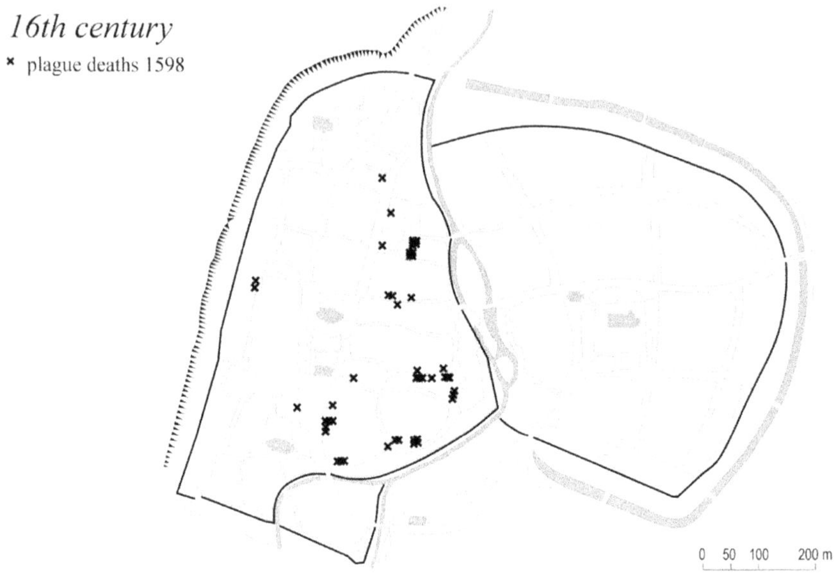

Figure 5.7. Plague deaths in St. Benedikti parish 1598. © Thomas Wozniak

This corresponds to an annual average of seventy-nine persons. The two epidemics of 1577 and 1598 clearly stand out in the data set (Figure 5.8). If one excludes the plague victims, a total of 1,410 people died, which corresponds to an annual average of about fifty-six. The maximum number of deaths outside a plague year was 108 in 1575, and the lowest numbers in 1579 and 1596 were 38 and 32, respectively.

Brief Excursus: Blame and Harsh Consequences

In the death register of 1598 there is a revealing entry: "Andreas Mittlach was executed in prison on Tuesday and burnt with fire on the Schindergruben the following Wednesday because of his sorcery."[61] Little is known of Andreas Mittlach; he is mentioned in the tax registers from 1589 to 1594 as a "housemate" in the New Town, and in 1594 the designation "Wechter" (guardian) is added. Whether or how he was associated with the plague is unclear. However, it is striking that at a time when many innocent sick people were dying, a man was burned for sorcery. What accusations were made against him could perhaps be seen in the council minutes of those years, which, however, could not be used for this study, due to current construction work and reorganization of the city archive.

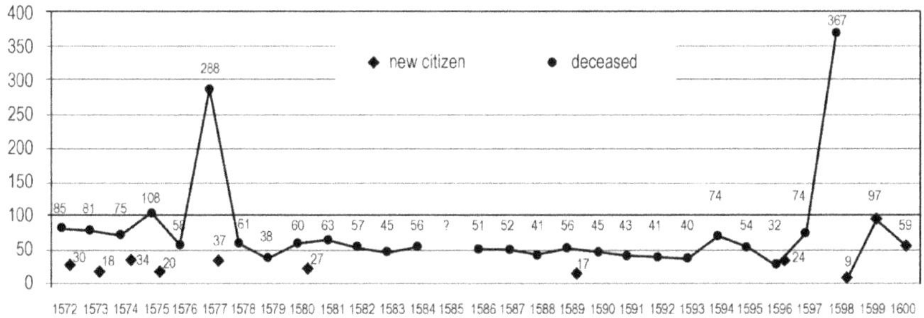

Figure 5.8. Deceased persons in St. Benedikti parish and new citizens, from 1572 to 1600. © Thomas Wozniak

Subsequent Epidemics

Since the following plague epidemics extend too far beyond the time frame of this research, the evaluation of the death registers available in the Protestant church archives is reserved for another study; only a brief overview is outlined here.

Even during the tenure of the thirty-third abbess, Dorothea Sophie (r. 1617–45), it was not possible to prevent the plague. The city history by Hermann Lorenz states about the plague of 1626–27: "Raging of the plague in the city, in the St. Nikolai parish alone 2,374 people die from Easter to Advent."[62] This plague seems to have affected only the New Town of Quedlinburg. In the same year, the plague is also documented in Hildesheim. In the council accounts, Kleemann found an entry recording that the market master and other council servants received four thalers "because they can earn little due to the rampant plague and have had a lot of running around at the present time."[63] In an original letter from Abbess Dorothea Sophie dated 1 October 1633, she ordered travelers to stay away from the abbey: "Since the plague is said to be quite rampant in Leipzig, it is ordered that anyone travelling from the Abbey of Quedlinburg to Leipzig abstain from Quedlinburg's messengership for at least four weeks after his departure from Leipzig."[64] Of the further precautions to keep the plague away, which consisted mainly in the description of the "Präservatifmittel" (prophylactic medicine) provided and the regulations for taking them, only the general hygiene and dietary regulations mentioned in the first article of her precautionary texts can be regarded as an effective measure.[65]

The next plague hit Quedlinburg in 1636, when 707 people died in St. Nikolai parish alone.[66] Despite the regular recurrence of plague in a cycle of nine to eleven years, a plague hospital was not built until 1681. Called "zum Lazarener," it was located in front of the Oering city gate at Oeringer Strasse 8.[67] The hospital consisted of "two main buildings and outbuildings. The large building had two floors—still present today—with a cellar, five parlors, three chambers, a kitchen, and adjoining rooms. The small building had five rooms on the ground floor and another four rooms on the upper floor."[68] A garden in front of the New Town was converted into a plague cemetery to bury the dead.[69]

As an intermediate barrier, the plague cemetery set the buildings apart and thus prevented the disease from being carried into the city by strangers. It seems to have fulfilled this function very well, because while 2,197 people died of the plague in neighboring Halberstadt in 1681–82, Quedlinburg was spared that outbreak of the disease.[70] The Quedlinburg barriers were strictly observed, especially against Halberstadt, but this did not mean that the people of Halberstadt were not supplied with food. The Quedlinburgers drove the food five hundred paces across the border to Halberstadt and unloaded it there, and after their retreat the Halberstadters collected it.[71]

The danger of the plague in 1712–13, which had afflicted other towns, passed Quedlinburg by and found expression only in a plague ordinance.[72] After appearing regularly in Europe for almost four centuries, the plague disappeared in the first half of the eighteenth century. In historical research on the plague, this relatively sudden disappearance gives rise to many controversial discussions, which will not be covered here.

On average, in the plague year 1598–99, the proportion of household heads among the victims of the disease was 12 percent, of women 9 percent and of widows 1 percent. The share of maids was comparatively high at 3 percent, compared to 0.7 percent for servants. The maids probably died due to their greater contact with children, because children accounted for the majority of plague deaths with an average of 73 percent.

An attempt to statistically record the effects of the epidemic disease on Quedlinburg and the local tax lists encounters some difficulties. It is possible to obtain information only for the period from 1566 to 1680. Before that, there are no sources suitable for a quantitative evaluation, and after that there were no more (plague) epidemics, due to the establishment of the plague hospital. Although two cholera epidemics in 1850 (431 deaths) and 1866 (1,077 deaths) claimed many lives, tax data was no longer recorded in tax registers.

Conclusion

From the middle of the fourteenth to the end of the seventeenth century, there were at least eleven waves of plague in Quedlinburg. Table 5.6 shows a comparison of the plague mentions found in the chronicles, with data from the different serial registers. This shows the well-known phenomenon that chronicles are often written intentionally and exaggerate information. While in the chronicles the information about the number of victims is partly glossed over, with the help of serial sources such as tax registers, council accounts, death registers, and lists of new citizens, the conditions from the second half of the sixteenth century can be relatively accurately reconstructed.

Within this period, the plague occurred three times. In the years 1566–67, 1577, and 1598–99. These waves demonstrably also affected neighboring towns. Due to the availability of certain special sources of information, topographical data for 1566–67 and 1598–99 can be linked to the death records. This makes it possible to analyze the contagion of individual households, which has been shown here with the example of Schulstrasse 12/Klink 2. Due to the very precise age data in the death register of 1598, demographic aspects of the plague can be shown more precisely. The largest proportion of the dead, over 70 percent, are children. The present study could only take a first look at the possible sources of plague transmission in Quedlinburg during the sixteenth and seventeenth centuries. It turns out that much more information can be obtained from the sources available to us. Although the abbess of the Quedlinburg Damenstift did not have anything like the information available

Table 5.6. Epidemic events from the 14th to the 17th century in chronicle and serial sources.[73]
© Thomas Wozniak

Year	Presumed Disease	Casualties in Chronicles	Casualties in serial Registers	Remarks
1348–51	Plague	4,000	-	750 households
1361/62	Plague	-	-	Only mentioned
1441	Plague	-	-	Only mentioned
1473	Plague	-	-	Only mentioned
1484–86	Epidemic	-	circa 500	
1566/67	Plague	2,500	2,500	
1577	Plague	1,215	843	Chronicles include suburbs
1598/99	Plague / Pox?	3,000–4,000	1,274	
1611	Plague	-	309	Not mentioned in Chronicles
1626	Plague	2,374	2,374	
1636	Plague	707	707	
1681	Plague	0	0	Averted

to today's society, she made decisions that were in the best interests of all the inhabitants of her domain. In doing so, she went against the ruling council and the merchants, placing the common good above the economic interests of individuals. Notably, she did everything she could to contain the number of deaths. The most effective measure seems to have been to shut down public life and to ban the markets, even against the pleas of the city council, until the dangers of the plague were eliminated. The first time this was achieved, however, was in 1680, when the plague was kept away from the city with the help of a plague hospital ("Pesthof") outside the city walls that had been built decades earlier.

Thomas Wozniak was born in Quedlinburg and grew up as an active Catholic under the communist regime of the German Democratic Republic. When the Berlin Wall came down, he did his civilian service instead of joining the army and worked with disabled people in Tabgha, Israel. After returning overland by bike—tracing the route of the crusaders—he studied history. For the analysis of three late medieval taxation lists, which came to light during renovation work in his parents' house, an old half-timbered building, he was awarded his Master of Science. After completing his dissertation, "Quedlinburg in the 14th and 16th Century," at the University of Cologne in 2009, he worked at the University Marburg until 2015 and finished his habilitation (second book) about "Natural Events in Early Middle Ages" in 2017 in Tübingen. This was followed by professorships (*Professurvertretung*) in Tübingen, Munich, and Bamberg, a guest lectureship at Weber State University in Ogden, Utah (USA), and research fellowships at Heidelberg University and the Leibniz Institute for the History and Culture of Eastern Europe (GWZO) Leipzig. He is currently a professor at the Alpen-Adria-University Klagenfurt in Austria.

Notes

1. Ludowici, "Quedlinburg before the Ottonian Kings," 253–60. Ludowici, "Quedlinburg vor den Ottonen," 91–104.
2. Diener-Staeckling, *Himmel über dem Rat*, 132–45; Scheibe, *Studien zur Verfassungsgeschichte*, 66–71.
3. Wozniak, *Quedlinburg im 14. und 16. Jahrhundert*, 66–67.
4. Wozniak and Kanus-Sieber, "Zur Demographie Quedlinburgs," 101–15.
5. *Welterbemanagementplan*, ed. Bittenfeld et al., 90–91.
6. Giese, *Annales Quedlinburgenses*, 381–582.
7. Wozniak, *Quedlinburg im 14. und 16. Jahrhundert*, 26–29.
8. Wozniak, *Abgabenverzeichnisse* (forthcoming).
9. Lorenz, "Die urkundlichen Eintragungen," 194–255; Hobohm, *Der städtische Haushalt*, 102–11.
10. Cf. Bergdolt, *Die Pest*, 119–24; Meier, *Pest*, 377–463; Bergdolt, *Der Schwarze Tod in Europa*, 249–59; Keil, "Seuchenzüge des Mittelalters," 109–28.

11. Fossel, "Geschichte der epidemischen Krankheiten," 736–901.
12. Kahlow, "Pest als Interpretationsproblem," 103.
13. Rodenwaldt, *Pest in Venedig*, 208: *Quando simul eodem tempore plures aegrotant, et aegrotantium maior pars interimitur.*
14. For example, the "pest" in Tyrol in 1611–12 could be identified as an epidemic of typhus. See Schretter, *Pest in Tirol*, 629.
15. Schlotter, *Geschichte der Lepra*, 10.
16. Sieglerschmidt, "Bevölkerungsgeschichte," 249–82.
17. Höhl, *Pest in Hildesheim*, 193–94.
18. Höhl, *Pest in Hildesheim*, 27–29.
19. Rodenwaldt, *Pest in Venedig*, 125. All translations are mine unless noted otherwise.
20. Schretter, *Pest in Tirol*, 629.
21. Ibs, *Pest in Schleswig-Holstein*, 73.
22. Fritsch, *Geschichte*, vol. 2, 14.
23. For the monastery of Wipertikloster, the last Catholic wedding is recorded in 1547. The last provost, Lambert Borse, converted to the Lutheran Church, married Barbara Oelgarte, the widow of mayor Hans Oelgarte, and became the administrator of the monastery estate, see Fritsch, *Geschichte*, vol. 2, 248–49.
24. Höhl, *Pest in Hildesheim*, 172 f.; Schwarz, *Pest in Bremen*, 116–20.
25. Kleemann, *Kulturgeschichtliche Bilder*, 214–15.
26. Lorenz, *Quellen*, 262–64.
27. Storbeck, *Was Sie von Quedlinburg*, 7: "Therefore, the city will have been very desolate and empty during that time."
28. Stadtarchiv Quedlinburg, Schossregister 1567 fol. 127r: *tot Andreas Qûenstedt.*
29. Zapnik, *Pest und Krieg*, 238–53, with maps, 299–330.
30. Vasold, *Die Pest*, 115–16, 122 doubts that the number of plague deaths reached 30 percent and assumes about 10 percent.
31. Stadtarchiv Quedlinburg, Ratsrechnung 1566–1576 fol. 67r–68v: 57; Stadtarchiv Quedlinburg, Ratsrechnung 1566–1576 fol. 98v–99r: 22; Stadtarchiv Quedlinburg, Ratsrechnung 1566–1576 fol. 130v–131r: 21; Stadtrachiv Quedlinburg, Ratsrechnung 1570 fol. 5r–v: 30.
32. Stadtarchiv Quedlinburg, Schossregister 1567 fol. 168r: *Thomas Schotte* [deleted:] † *Jacob Seffert 6 fl.*
33. Winningstedt, "Chronicon Quedlinburgense," 518; Fritsch, *Geschichte*, vol. 2, 17; Kleemann, *Kulturgeschichtliche Bilder*, 214.
34. For Bremen, see Schwarz, *Pest in Bremen*, 120–21; on Venice, see Rodenwaldt, *Pest in Venedig*, 298–328.
35. Kleemann, *Kulturgeschichtliche Bilder*, 214.
36. Evangelisches Kirchen-Archiv Quedlinburg, Sterberegister St. Benedikti 1577.
37. *Illi qui aliis morborum generibus obierunt.*
38. [Anon.], *Opfer der Pest*, 532.
39. Evangelisches Kirchen-Archiv Quedlinburg, Sterberegister St. Benedicti 1570 ff. The designations in the Quedlinburg death registers are identical with those in the Hildesheim plague book, see Höhl, *Pest in Hildesheim*, 106, table 4.
40. The inscription reads: *ANNO DOM*(INI) [15]*77 DEN · 15 SEPTEM*(BR)*IS* [AND] / [REAS LV]*DER IN* [GOTT] *VORSCHEIDEN SA*[M](T) / [SE]*INEN SONEN. MIC*[HAEL] *LVDER IST VORSCHEID*(EN) / [DEN] *25 NOVEMBRIS ANDREAS LVDER DER IVNG*(ERE) / [DEN [2]8 N[OV]*EMBRIS*

GESTORBEN MATTIAS LVDER / [DE]*N 26 IANVAR*(IU)*M VORSCHEIDEN UND ANDRE*[AS] / [LVDER VORSCHEID]*EN DEN 8 NOVEMBRIS* · [WIE CH-]/[RIST] *A*[LL]*EN GNEDICH SEI* [VND...M] / [VN]*SER* [HER LEBEN] *IM SEI* [LOB V]*ND* [EH]*R S*(EI) *M*(IT) / [IR]*BEM* [IM] *SEI LEBEN WIR* [SO] *LEBEN W*(IR) *DEM* / [HER]*REN* [ST]*ERBEN WIR SO STERBEN WIR DEM HERRN* / *DARVM* [WIR L]*EBEN* [OD]*ER STERBEN SO SEIN WIR* / *D*[EM] *HER*[R]*EN.* [DENN DAZU I]*ST* [CH]*RISTVS* [GESTO]*RBE*(N) / [VND] *B*[EGRABEN] *VND WI*[ED]*ER LEBENDIG* [GEWOR]/[DEN DAS ER VBER] *TOD*[TE VND] *LEBENDIGE HERR SEI* [Röm. 14, 8–9.] / [15] *CORIN*(TER) *W*[IE] *IN ADA*[M] *ALLE STERBEN ALSO* / [WERDEN IN CHRI]*STO* [ALLE] *LEBEN NA*[CH] *DE*[M] *TOD* [1. Kor. 15,22].

41. Stadtarchiv Quedlinburg, Schossregister 1570 fol. 16v.
42. Winningstedt, *Chronicon Quedlinburgense,* 521.
43. Fritsch, *Geschichte,* vol. 2, 24.
44. Cf. Höhl, *Pest in Hildesheim,* 182–85; Schwarz, *Pest in Bremen,* 129–34.
45. Voigt, *Geschichte des Stiftes Quedlinburg,* vol. 3, 370.
46. Nagel, "Kindheit einer alten Stadt," 24.
47. Kleemann, *Kulturgeschichtliche Bilder,* 215.
48. The deaths register of St. Nikolai church was recorded by its pastor Johann Arnd, who worked at the church from 1590 to 1599.
49. Evangelisches Kirchen-Archiv Quedlinburg, Sterberegister St. Nikolai 1598, Nr. 52: *Fridag ist der Schefer Erhardt Rodtschmides dochter in der pfarr Benedicti begraben* ("Friday the daughter of the shepherd Erhardt Rodtschmide is buried in the parish of Benedikti"); Nr. 457: *Claus Henenbergs Sohn;* Nr. 517: *Ein Kindt hinder dem Rahthause.* ("A child behind the town hall").
50. Evangelisches Kirchen-Archiv Quedlinburg, Sterberegister St. Nikolai 1598, Nr. 63: *Mittwochen ist Thobias Gerken ein Medlein begraben* ("Wednesday Thobias Gerken is buried a girl"); Nr. 742: *Heinrich Witten Sohnlin* ("From Heinrich Witten a son").
51. Evangelisches Kirchen-Archiv Quedlinburg, Sterberegister St. Benedicti 1598 Nr. 9, 18, 37, 51, 54–56, 73, 74, 84, 104, 117, 120, 138, 158, 172, 181.
52. Evangelisches Kirchen-Archiv Quedlinburg, Sterberegister St. Nikolai 1598 Nr. 102, 106, 143, 149, 168, 173, 175, 347, 433, 443, 528, 567, 624, 721.
53. Specifically Claus Appell, Paul Botticher, Curdt Brincks, Fesel, Peter Karpe, Ziliacus Kegel, Otte Otten, Sattler, Mattias Schröders, Hans Schultzen, Matz Seddeler, Christian Webel, and Willen.
54. Evangelisches Kirchen-Archiv Quedlinburg, Sterberegister St. Nikolai 1598 Nr. 167, 197, 679, 711, 716, 809.
55. Stadtarchiv Quedlinburg, Ratsrechnung 1598 fol. 1v: *Mangeln / Hans Milde obiit 13. Sept. 98 / Joan Steinacker obiit 12 Octob. 98 / Bartholmes Gerhardt obiit 24 May 98 / Christian Webel obiit 13 Sept. 98 / Andreas Kunig obiit 13 Sept. 98 / Claus Apel obiit 17 Sept. 98 / Matz Meisner obiit.*
56. Evangelisches Kirchen-Archiv Quedlinburg, Sterberegister St. Nikolai 1598 Nr. 12.
57. Fritsch, *Geschichte,* vol. 2, 244.
58. Stadtarchiv Quedlinburg, Ratsrechnung 1598 fol. 12v–14v.
59. Inscription in the Kalandkapelle: ... *NVNC PESTIS VIOLENTIA SOLVTVS* ... ; Evangelisches Kirchen-Archiv Quedlinburg, Sterberegister 1598 Nr. 240: *Von 27. August bis den 28. sind gewesen 53 Personen.* ("From 27 to 28 August, there were 53 people [who died].")

60. Stadtarchiv Quedlinburg, Ratsrechnung 1598 fol. 12v.
61. "Dinsedag ist Andreas Mittlach im Gefängnis gerichtet und folgenden Mittwoch auf der Schindergruben mit Feuer verbrannt wegen seiner Zauberei."
62. Lorenz, *Werdegang*, 388.
63. Kleemann, *Kulturgeschichtliche Bilder*, 215.
64. Lorenz, *Quellen*, 308.
65. Lorenz, *Quellen*, 308–10; Lorenz, *Vorkehrungen*, 1366.
66. Kleemann, *Kulturgeschichtliche Bilder*, 215–16.
67. Kleemann, *Kulturgeschichtliche Bilder*, 218–19.
68. Storbeck, *Was Sie von Quedlinburg*, 8.
69. Kleemann, *Kulturgeschichtliche Bilder*, 219.
70. Cf. Kleemann, *Kulturgeschichtliche Bilder*, 217–18; Storbeck, *Was Sie von Quedlinburg*, 8; Voigt, *Geschichte des Stiftes*, 556. Nearby Eisleben suffered 4,000 plague victims during this period, Nordhausen 3,323, and Magdeburg 2,400. In Aschersleben, 670 people died despite its being cordoned off.
71. Cf. Fritsch, *Geschichte*, vol. 2, 39; Kleemann, *Kulturgeschichtliche Bilder*, 216; Gille, "Pesthof zu Quedlinburg," 1197–98.
72. Schwarz, *Pest in Bremen*, 19–88; Lorenz, *Quellen*, 492–97.
73. Voigt, *Geschichte des Stiftes*, vol. 1, 249; Fritsch, *Geschichte*, vol. 1, 173, Fritsch, *Geschichte*, vol. 2, 14; Kleemann, *Kulturgeschichtliche Bilder*, 216.

Bibliography

[Anon.]: "Opfer der Pest." *Am Heimatborn. Beilage zum Quedlinburger Kreisblatt* 128 (12 July 1927): 532.

Bergdolt, Klaus. *Der Schwarze Tod in Europa. Die Große Pest und das Ende des Mittelalters.* Munich: C. H. Beck, 1994.

Bergdolt, Klaus. *Die Pest: Geschichte des Schwarzen Todes.* Munich: C. H. Beck, 2006.

Diener-Staeckling, Antje. *Der Himmel über dem Rat: zur Symbolik der Ratswahl in mitteldeutschen Städten.* Halle/Saale: Mitteldeutscher Verlag, 2008.

Fossel, Victor. "Geschichte der epidemischen Krankheiten," In *Handbuch der Geschichte der Medizin*, edited by Max Neuburger and Julius Pagel, vol. 2, 736–901. Jena: Gustav Fischer, 1903.

Fritsch, Johann Heinrich. *Geschichte des vormaligen Reichsstiftes und der Stadt Quedlinburg* (2 vols.). Quedlinburg: Gottfried Basse, 1828.

Giese, Martina, ed. *Die Annales Quedlinburgenses* (MGH SS rer. Germ. 72). Hanover: Hahnsche Buchhandlung, 2004.

Gille, Willi. "Der Pesthof zu Quedlinburg. Zum 250jährigen Gedächtnis seiner Entstehung dargeboten." *Am Heimatborn* 296 (7.4.1931): 1197–98.

Glaser, Rüdiger. *Klimageschichte Mitteleuropas. 1000 Jahre Wetter, Klima, Katastrophen.* Darmstadt: Wissenschaftliche Buchgesellschaft, 2001.

Hobohm, Walter. *Der städtische Haushalt Quedlinburgs in den Jahren 1459 bis 1509.* Halle/Saale: Gebauer Schwetschke, 1912.

Höhl, Monika. *Die Pest in Hildesheim: Krankheit als Krisenfaktor im städtischen Leben des Mittelalters und der Frühen Neuzeit (1350–1750).* Hildesheim: Stadtarchiv, 2002.

Ibs, Jürgen Hartwig. *Die Pest in Schleswig-Holstein von 1350 bis 1547/48: Eine sozialgeschichtliche Studie über eine wiederkehrende Katastrophe.* Frankfurt/Main: Lang Verlag, 1994.

Kahlow, Simone. "Die Pest als Interpretationsproblem mittelalterlicher und frühneuzeitlicher Massengräber." *Archäologische Informationen* 30, no. 1 (2007): 97–104.
Keil, Gundolf. "Seuchenzüge des Mittelalters," In *Mensch und Umwelt im Mittelalter*, edited by Bernd Hermann, 109–28. Stuttgart: Deutsche Verlags-Anstalt, 1986.
Kleemann, Selmar. *Kulturgeschichtliche Bilder aus Quedlinburgs Vergangenheit.* Quedlinburg: Magistrat der Stadt Quedlinburg, 1922.
Klewitz, Martin. *Geschichtliches aus der Nikolai-Gemeinde zu Quedlinburg.* Quedlinburg, 1925.
Knorre, Alexander von. *Pest im Ruhrgebiet; Seuchen und Krankheiten im 17. Jahrhundert. Ein Beitrag zum Jubiläum "350 Jahre Westfälischer Frieden."* Herne: Emschertal-Museum, 1998.
Lorenz, Hermann. "Die urkundlichen Eintragungen in die Ratsrechnungen der Stadt Quedlinburg von 1454 bis 1509." *Zeitschrift des Harz-Vereins* 39 (1906): 194–255.
Lorenz, Hermann, ed. *Quellen zur städtischen Verwaltungs-, Rechts- und Wirtschaftsgeschichte von Quedlinburg vom 15. Jahrhundert bis zur Zeit Friedrichs des Grossen, 1. Teil: Baurdinge nebst sonstigen obrigkeitlichen Verordnungen und Abmachungen.* Halle/Saale: Hendel, 1916.
Lorenz, Hermann. *Werdegang von Stadt und Stift Quedlinburg.* Quedlinburg: Magistrat der Stadt Quedlinburg, 1922.
Lorenz, Hermann. "Vorkehrungen gegen die drohende Pest vor 300 und 250 Jahren." *Am Heimatborn* 338 (14.12.1933): 1366.
Ludowici, Babette. "Quedlinburg vor den Ottonen: Versuch einer frühen Topographie der Macht." *Frühmittelalterliche Studien* 49 (2015): 91–104.
Ludowici, Babette. "Quedlinburg before the Ottonian Kings. Approaches towards an Early Topography of Power." In *Small Things, Wide Horizons. Studies in Honour of Birgitta Hårdh*, edited by Lars Larsson, Fredrik Ekengren, et al., 253–60. Oxford: Oxford University Press, 2015.
Meier, Mischa, ed. *Pest. Die Geschichte eines Menschheitstraumas.* Stuttgart: Klett-Cotta, 2005.
Nagel, Horst Friedrich. "Die Kindheit einer alten Stadt." In *Festschrift 1000 Jahre Münz-Zoll- und Handelsrecht*, 17–27. Quedlinburg: Stadt Quedlinburg, 1994.
Porzelt, Carolin. *Die Pest in Nürnberg. Leben und Herrschen in Pestzeiten in der Reichsstadt Nürnberg (1562–1713).* St. Ottilien: EOS-Verlag, 2000.
Rodenwaldt, Ernst. *Die Pest in Venedig 1575–1577. Ein Beitrag zur Frage der Infektkette bei den Pestepidemien West-Europas.* Heidelberg: Springer-Verlag, 1953.
Scheibe, Elisabeth. *Studien zur Verfassungsgeschichte des Stifts und der Stadt Quedlinburg.* Borna-Leipzig: Noske, 1938.
Schlotter, Oskar. *Die Geschichte der Lepra und Pocken in Europa.* Munich: Diss. Med. Fak, 1966.
Schretter, Bernhard. *Die Pest in Tirol 1611–1612. Ein Beitrag zur Medizin-, Kultur- und Wirtschaftsgeschichte der Stadt Innsbruck und der übrigen Gerichte Tirols.* Innsbruck: Stadtarchiv, 1982.
Schwarz, Klaus. *Die Pest in Bremen. Epidemien und freier Handel in einer deutschen Hafenstadt 1350–1713.* Bremen: Staatsarchiv, 1996.
Sieglerschmidt, Jörn. "Bevölkerungsgeschichte." In *Sozial- und Wirtschaftsgeschichte. Arbeitsgebiete—Probleme—Perspektiven. 100 Jahre Vierteljahrsschrift für Sozial- und Wirtschaftsgeschichte*, edited by Günther Schulz. 249–82. Stuttgart: VSWG Beihefte, 2004.

Storbeck, Hasso. *Was Sie von Quedlinburg und Umgebung vielleicht noch nicht wussten.* Halberstadt: Kannemann, 2006.
Vasold, Manfred. *Die Pest. Ende eines Mythos.* Stuttgart: Theiss, 2003.
Voigt, Gottfried Christian. *Geschichte des Stiftes Quedlinburg*, vol. 3. Leipzig: Schwickert, 1791.
Welterbemanagementplan, Broschüre 01, edited by Carl Herwarth v. Bittenfeld, Brigitte Holz, et al. Quedlinburg, 2013.
Winningstedt, Johann. "Chronicon Quedlinburgense." In *Sammlung etlicher noch nicht gedruckten alten Chroniken*, edited by Caspar Abel, 479–522. Braunschweig: Verlag Ludolph Schröders, 1732.
Wozniak, Thomas. *Die frühen Abgabenverzeichnisse Quedlinburgs (1310–1600). Edition, Umgang, Topographie* (2 vols.). Marburg: Stiftung Stoye (forthcoming).
Wozniak, Thomas. *Quedlinburg im 14. und 16. Jahrhundert. Ein sozialtopographischer Vergleich.* Berlin: De Gruyter, 2013.
Wozniak, Thomas, and Katrin Kanus-Sieber. "Zur Demographie Quedlinburgs vom 10. bis 21. Jahrhundert." *Quedlinburger Annalen* 15 (2012/13): 101–15.
Zapnik, Jörg. *Pest und Krieg im Ostseeraum. Der "Schwarze Tod" in Stralsund während des Großen Nordischen Krieges (1700–1721).* Hamburg: Kovač Verlag, 2007.

CHAPTER 6

Handling Pestilence during the Thirty Years' War

SIGRUN HAUDE

Introduction

Pandemics in the West seemed a phenomenon of the past, until our experience with COVID-19 changed this sense of relative safety. As one compares measures, behaviors, and circumstances of epidemics over time, one is tempted to look for parallels and differences, some of which can be highly illuminating. The following study examines epidemics during the Thirty Years' War, in particular the plague outbreak of 1634 and 1635. The geographic foci are Munich with its district (*Rentamt*) and Nuremberg with its surrounding countryside, especially the margravate of Brandenburg-Ansbach. These territories—one in the duchy of Bavaria (sometimes called Old Bavaria), the other in Franconia—are now part of modern-day Bavaria.[1] This devastating episode belongs in the long history of plague cycles that ensued after the so-called Black Death in the mid-fourteenth century and continued until the early 1700s. During these cycles, the plague visited most cities in Europe every eleven years on average; thus, by the seventeenth century Europe had a long history of dealing with the epidemic. In the course of its periodic reoccurrences, governments adapted to the reality of pestilence. This involuntary familiarity with the disease makes the early modern period different from the medieval. Many of the scourge's premises during the mid-fourteenth century do not apply to its early modern successors. As scholars have emphasized, old assumptions—that the populace met plague epidemics with panic, that chaos ruled, and that familial relationships broke down—fall short of the overall evidence for the sixteenth and seventeenth centuries.[2] Over time, authorities developed strategies for dealing with these waves of the infectious disease. Rarely did panic set in; instead, ordinances, mandates about proper procedures, and advisory literature directing the populace toward prophylactic measures abounded. The need to control pestilence propelled governments toward a general organization of health management that included epidemics of other diseases as well.[3]

When the Great Plague broke out in the mid-fourteenth century, contemporaries did not know the physical origin of the disease. A persistent explanation located its cause in humanity's sinfulness. According to the Bible, pestilence was one of the four main afflictions God sent to chastise humans for their turning away from him (the others being war, inflation, and hunger). This interpretation endured well into the early modern period, as David Herlicius, one of the most renowned seventeenth-century authors of *Schreibkalender* (recording calendars) and *Prognostica*, illustrates:

> God sends war because he sees that among humans there is no improvement. To the contrary, the world is becoming ever worse and does not care that Mars and brother Veit, that is the terrible war, cannot make us any more pious. Thus *Mors*, that is pestilence, has to creep into our houses and make us more fainthearted, timid, and bendable.[4]

Along with the religious explanation, natural concepts developed—such as the miasma theory—to account for the disease. Since no apparent physical source could be discerned, physicians blamed the bad air, miasma, for the illness. In this view, ill-fated planetary constellations caused earthquakes and eruptions of volcanos, thus setting free poisonous vapors. Natural processes of decay could also produce foul smells, which is why many regulations focused on eliminating the sources of putrefaction in cities and towns.[5] The miasma theory corresponded to the prevalent concept of the four humors in the human body. The impact of the air on a person depended on the mixture and influence of these humors in one's body.[6]

While the miasma theory was quite old, many in the early modern period were swayed by the contagion theory, known since the Great Plague but fully developed only by the Italian physician Girolamo Fracastoro (ca. 1476/78–1553), in his treatise *De Contagione* (1546). As we will see, early modern conceptions and handling of the disease were ever more oriented toward observation and experience with the infection, which confirmed the contagious nature of pestilence. Still, most ordinances and pronouncements of the seventeenth century show an adherence to both theories, as they addressed the cleansing of the air *and* the separation of the infected from the healthy.

During the Thirty Years' War, authorities upheld some of the well-established strategies for dealing with these outbreaks, but the war changed the known parameters in dramatic ways. The military conflict, particularly during the 1630s, transformed the pestilence into an epidemic of vast proportions. During the war, problems of poverty, migration, and disease converged. Inflation, wet summers due to the little ice age, a starved populace, and troops descending on one's region added tremendous potential for sickness and epidemics. Intriguingly, the period before the Thirty Years' War (1614–21) showed low plague activity.[7] During the next cycle (1622–31), however, the course of the plague became intertwined with events and circumstances of the war, especially the increased mobility of the military and of individuals.[8] When in July 1630 the Swedish army landed in Pomerania and the following year marched southward through the plague zones, it set off "Germany's most devastating mortality crisis," the epidemic cycle from 1632 to 1640.[9] The following analysis begins with a comparative appraisal of Bavaria and Franconia as they confronted the epidemic, before focusing more specifically on four areas: (1) administering spiritual care, (2) collecting scientific data, (3) staffing and provisioning health care, and (4) defying restrictions. The study will conclude by considering problems of epidemics then and now.

Bavaria's and Franconia's Respective Situations and Preventive Measures

Bavaria and Franconia entered this grim period from entirely different positions: the former exuded confidence and strength, whereas the latter was in a severely weakened state. In some ways, Bavaria is atypical in the history of pestilence. While most regions in Central Europe experienced high mortality during epidemic cycles, Bavaria continuously showed low epidemic activity, except for the last, most severe cycle (1632–40). This does not mean that there were no cases of pestilence but, rather, that death rates did not approach epidemic proportions, i.e. at least four times the normal death rate. Despite the recurring nature of this resistance to plague, which suggests certain conditions impeding its spread, there is no clear answer as to why Bavaria overall suffered only mildly from the epidemic.[10] Whatever the reasons, Bavaria was not immune to pestilence as the catastrophic losses during the 1630s show. Between September 1634 and April 1635, some seven thousand people died in Munich alone (almost one third of its population).[11]

Until this outbreak, Bavaria had handled the control of pestilence by staying vigilant and publishing ordinances any time it learned of epidemic activity. Even though Bavaria had been spared major mortality crises during the previous century, the authorities had made preparations to meet the challenge, should it actually occur. Munich's ordinances on pestilence from 1532, 1533, and 1596 became progressively more detailed. The 1596 decree of Duke Wilhelm (r. 1579–97; d. 1626) concerning *Sterbeläufe*, released by Munich's burgomaster and council to prepare their subjects for a possible epidemic, has all the signs of a document aimed at the general prevention of misfortune, and none of an acute crisis.[12] Munich's councilors pointed out that these afflictions usually come in cycles every few years and may come upon them again. The following instructions were designed to help people ward off illness and save the God-given "treasure" (*klainot*) of body and life according to his will.[13] It also reflects the perception, shared by many, that the infection could be managed. With God's grace and the physician's skills, the greater part of the sick could be healed, provided they sought medical help at once. Indeed, for such an illness the apothecary held numerous remedies in store.[14] This confidence is intriguing, since, in effect, at the time no medication was available to treat pestilence. The edict's intention was most likely to calm the populace and prevent panic once cases of infection arose. The ordinance then addressed measures to separate the infected (and those who stayed with them) from the healthy, as well as procedures to hire personnel to care for the sick. Finally, clothes and bedding of the plague-ridden were not to be washed nor sold, since they were considered a carrier of the poison. The best thing would be to destroy them, although the government stopped short of forcing people to do so.[15]

When Duke Maximilian of Bavaria (r. 1598–1651, elector from 1623) released a general edict on the fight against pestilence in 1606, the points under discussion were similar to earlier edicts.[16] Once again, he was only preparing for a possible outbreak, not reacting to an epidemic in his territory. A further decree of 1613 instructed the populace (1) to keep their houses clean; (2) to fumigate closed rooms with pleasant-smelling woods in the morning and evening; (3) to practice moderation in food, drink, baths, and dancing, and to stay away from infected persons; and (4) to have some good medicine handy, for which several recipes were provided.[17] All of these constituted customary preventive measures against pestilence.

Besides edicts, authorities released instructions that specified appropriate behavior during an epidemic.[18] In one directed to the common man, Munich's health department (*Gesundheits-Polizei*) addressed the widespread headache and acute fever epidemic, and located the cause in the foul humors of the body, which were triggered by long-standing fright, fear, flights, and hunger. Searching for safer havens, people dwelt in overcrowded places, which led to fetid taste and smell. The wet summer did not help, and, depending on one's disposition of humors, some people were more prone to the illness than others.[19] If not treated properly and quickly, this contagious disease could develop into pestilence. The pamphlet also urged that the poor be provided with food "because what kind of evil and severe illnesses often grow out of such long famine is clearly evident, especially since the physicians are well aware that hunger and the severe lack of victuals count among the foremost causes of pestilence."[20] It then advised the usual measures: cleanliness, moderation in food and liquor consumption, caution when frequenting baths, no mingling with the sick, and fumigation of the sick rooms. The instruction also offered recipes against headache, fever, and sleeplessness. It concluded with the hope that the almighty God might bring such measures to fruition, especially if the poor man with God's help would be aided with more victuals.[21] These guidelines and concerns were in keeping with edicts and measures in other German cities at this time.

Munich's *General Jnstruction* of 1624 provides an intriguing further step in preparation for a possible outbreak of pestilence.[22] The instruction addressed three stages of severity: (1) several locales had contracted pestilence; (2) the pestilence spread to more than four or five places; and (3) the epidemic became rampant. In none of these cases did the council articulate the possibility that the epidemic would actually infiltrate Munich. Indeed, the first priority was to guard against letting the pestilence penetrate the city walls, and thus it was essential to be aware of the areas the elector had placed under a ban (*bannisiert*). To that effect, the burgomaster was to relay such information promptly to the four main gatekeepers, who would examine foreigners accordingly and let no one from the said locales enter the city.[23] In scenario two, i.e. should the pestilence spread to more than four or five places, the city would step up its protection from the outside world. Citizens were warned under threat of punishment not to take anyone in from infected areas. Now only two of the four main gates would admit foreigners after thorough examination, and any traffic between citizens of whatever station and persons from infected places outside the gates was prohibited. In scenario three, the rampant increase of the epidemic, the pigs' market should be moved to the Isar Gate, and one of the council's special deputies for pestilence, the commissioners, would visit the gates daily.[24]

Besides safeguarding against contagion from the outside, the city fathers urged cleansing on the inside so that bad smells were eliminated. Furthermore, the smokehouse would be opened to fumigate letters and small packages.[25] The instruction spelled out precisely how this exchange of items between courier and fumigator was to take place. Larger items of commerce were placed under quarantine.[26] Munich's health department continued to limit traffic into and out of the city.[27] By 1628 the city released an extensive hiring plan, an *Ordnung vnd Anstöllungen*, which specified the personnel to be engaged in preparation for a plague epidemic, "against which God may long protect us."[28]

In short, at the end of the 1620s, even though Munich seemed immune to the contagion, it was well prepared should the worst case indeed occur. The city fathers gave the impression that they had things under control and that the contagion could be mastered. Their instructions sounded as if no harm could come to its citizens as long as they guarded their city carefully against any contagion from the outside and kept the city smelling pleasantly on the inside. Considering that Bavaria had mostly been spared the experience of pest epidemics, this confidence is understandable, although the knowledge of plague epidemics elsewhere must have caused some general concern among the government and populace.

In 1634, finally, after Swedish, Spanish, and other troops had flooded Bavaria, Munich and its countryside faced the kind of plague epidemic that must have surpassed all imagination. While earlier decrees had only envisioned possible scenarios of the pestilence infiltrating the city, now these odds had become a terrifying reality. The first to act, Elector Maximilian issued a *Pestordnung* even before the epidemic escalated.[29] His territory-wide decree was in many respects similar to the one published two months later by Munich's burgomaster and councilors; however, his was more elaborate regarding its religious component. As the plague epidemic increased, both the city and the elector stepped up their efforts. The council sessions for September and October 1634 were preoccupied with reactions to the pestilence. The councilors supervised the gatekeepers more closely and placed them under a special oath. No one coming from infected places was let into the city, and beggars and other common foreign persons as well as sutlers with their wares were not to be allowed inside.[30]

Munich's city government and Maximilian, who were frequently at odds with one another, joined forces, at least temporarily, to combat the by now out-of-control contagion. Munich's *Ratsordnung* of 30 October 1634 laid out principles for encountering the health crisis.[31] Although it built on earlier edicts, it was more detailed and addressed additional aspects. Released at the height of the plague epidemic, its severe tone reflected the seriousness of the situation. With an eye most likely to the elector, who was always critical of what he perceived as Munich's sluggishness, the burgomaster and council underlined that, upon the first news that pestilence was spreading within and outside Bavaria, it had released and distributed instructions on how to protect and save the city from this epidemic.

Similar to the 1596 ordinance, the first article was directed to God and postulated that saving the soul was more important than saving one's life. Thus, the most vital measure to take was to abstain from all sins, since this epidemic was "no doubt" sent by God because of people's wicked, blasphemous life. Humility, repentance, and prayer were called for. Moreover, people needed to beg God to take away the poisonous air and instead grant them a healthy climate.[32] Gone were the admonitions to attend more fervently the weekly processions. The health crisis was such that gatherings of people had to be avoided.

After the foremost directive to correct and improve one's relationship with God, the following twenty-four articles addressed practical measures—among them the cleansing of air, house, and the most important civic places; the best diet; the separation of the sick from the healthy; caution toward foreigners; the curtailing of feasts; and the prevention rather than the subsequent treatment of disease. Here, too, the city fathers displayed a belief in the treatability of the contagion. They admonished every house father to stock up on preventive medicine and pointed to various booklets and pamphlets for advice on the proper medication, which were available from the apothecary for every level of income. However—and this is decidedly different from the 1596 ordinance—the optimism was more muted. Even though no one was to be frightened of the plague and everyone should submit to God's will, the authorities did not intimate, as they had done before, that this should occur "joyfully." Moreover, the city fathers were more cautious about who could be saved, if they sought aid quickly: in this new ordinance, the former "majority" (*dem merern tayl*) shrank to a vague "various" (*mancher*).[33] Intriguingly, in a change from previous stipulations, the ordinance demanded only the cleaning and fumigating of an infected person's clothes and bedding, not their destruction, which may have been an acknowledgment of the populace's dire financial situation.[34] In early 1635 the infection subsided, and Munich's council decided to close the lazaret.[35] The city provisionally hired a chaplain for the lazaret for the next epidemic occurrence and agreed on a salary for that time.[36]

Maximilian ordered vigilance against anything that could lead to another outbreak. He charged the council not to let the Augsburgers with their clothes and bedding into the city.[37] Any foreign or Bavarian subjects trading in bed feathers were to be allowed into the city only if they could furnish a certificate testifying that they came from uninfected, healthy places. He also reminded the council once again to get rid of the filth, whereupon the councilors decided to visit the city quarters.[38] In August 1635, Munich instituted a special council to deal with infections, the *Infektionsrat*, and Maximilian persisted in demanding reports that detailed how the pestilence broke out in the infected houses.[39] During the renewed convergence of troops in 1647, Munich feared another outbreak of the pestilence. Accordingly, it stepped up its personnel and its vigilance at the gates and public places.[40] Fortunately, this time it was spared a similar catastrophe.

Turning from the more unusual case of Munich and Bavaria to Nuremberg and Franconia, one finds both similarities and differences. Franconia experienced the effects of the war on the spread of disease and pestilence much sooner than Old Bavaria because it became a passage way for military troops as early as 1622.[41] While Maximilian and his city council hardly contemplated the possibility of pestilence infiltrating their territory, Franconia was hit with the plague and other epidemics throughout the 1620s and early 1630s, and was thus much weakened when the great epidemic occurred in 1634. The measures and instructions Nuremberg's authorities initiated to prepare for and react to such outbreaks, however, followed the pattern established by authorities in general over the past century and reflected common attitudes toward and perceptions of the plague.

In the 1500s, Nuremberg had experienced bursts of pestilence and other epidemic infections partly linked to food shortages that claimed anywhere from hundreds to thousands of victims, but none as large as those in 1562–63 (9,034 deaths) and 1574–75 (over 6,500 deaths). These developments propelled Nuremberg to get a handle on disease control, and throughout the next decades it was fairly successful in devising measures to contain the contagious disease as much as possible, considering that there was no known medical treatment at the time.[42] The strain of war, however, challenged everyone's ability to control the epidemic.

While the plague of 1634 with its massive death count usually commands the center of attention, Franconia had fought smaller outbreaks of diseases already throughout the 1620s.[43] In 1624, the council released a decree reiterating earlier stipulations against the importing of feathers.[44] As was often the case, mortality rates fluctuated between the summer and fall months (high) and winter (low). In 1627, 115 people died of the epidemic between 4 June and 9 October; the following year 685 succumbed to it.[45]

For the next couple of years, the number of dead dropped considerably, but it then started to rise steeply, which had much to do with the horrendous situation of several large armies settling outside of Nuremberg. The subsequent violence against civilians, the flights into the city, hunger and starvation, and the rise in diseases led to numerous deaths. One chronicle recounts the burden of these years and is particularly sympathetic to the rural population, who had to flee with all their moveable belongings into the city. According to the chronicler, the council feared an infection already in 1632 because of the increased dung and stench due to the influx from the countryside.[46] But, first, the city and suburbs were plagued by hunger and a kind of typhus, the so-called head or Hungarian sickness. A chronicler, who is conservative in his estimates, speaks of 4,263 "registered" dead, but suggests that the real number was double that.[47] Considering the death figures for 1631 (2,100) and 1633 (2,678), this is still a shockingly high mortality. Among the thousands of dead were many young. Every day, six or seven bodies were carried in a procession. Many, however, were collected on carts, carried outside the city, and buried there. The lazaret was so overcrowded, mostly with Swedish soldiers, that their dead were stacked like wood in the courtyard until there was time to dig a pit for them.[48]

When the plague struck the imperial city again in 1634, Nuremberg and its countryside were so weakened and decimated that its mortality assumed unprecedented proportions (Figure 6.1). The chronicler recorded 11,125 deaths for the year 1634, but added that this figure referred only to those who had been buried in the churchyard, implying that the actual number was far higher.[49] This time the pestilence began to spread in late July 1634. Between twenty and sixty infected people were lying in the house of St. Rochus' churchyard, and because the number was rising daily, the hospital in St. Johannis had to be opened. In October the epidemic escalated, with over 1,100 infected people in the hospital and the infection raging in almost all districts. Churches, schools, and the city hall were fumigated, and the council published an edict with instructions on how one ought to behave during this epidemic. In December the mortality rate began to decline, and by 24 January 1635 the hospital could be closed again, while 102 persons were still

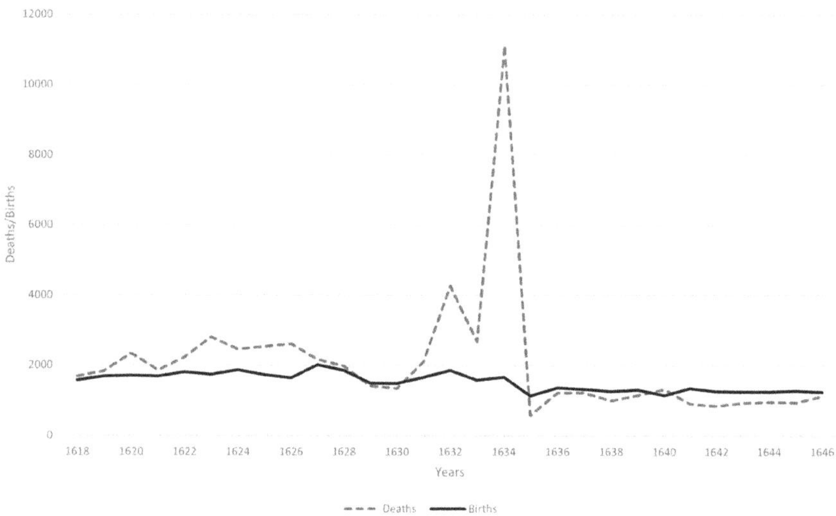

Figure 6.1. Deaths vs. births in Nuremberg, 1618–46. Source: Staatsarchiv Nürnberg, Archivaliensammlung des Historischen Vereins für Mittelfranken, Handschriften 219 (Figure created by Daniel Gladis).

being cared for at St. Rochus.[50] The number of dead for 1635 dropped dramatically, to 582, which reflects the end of the epidemic but also the shrunken number of inhabitants in the city. Baptisms, on the other hand, were twice as high (1,133).[51] Two further waves of pestilence during the war were not demographically severe because of the already decimated population.[52] All in all, during the years 1632 to 1634 Nuremberg suffered about 35,000 deaths, including soldiers and refugees. In contrast to developments in the rest of the Holy Roman Empire, where demographic numbers reached their pre-war status around 1740, the imperial city did not recover from these losses until the middle of the nineteenth century.[53]

From its experience with regularly occurring waves of pestilence and other epidemics, Nuremberg, along with most cities, developed a system of regulations and offices to deal with the predicament, and oriented itself in line with measures taken during similar incidents in previous years. A broad array of publications were designed to help the subjects face this health crisis in the best possible way—from ordinances regarding dying (*Sterbsordnung*), public edicts, and health pamphlets authored by civic physicians, to the so-called *Pestregiment*, with medical advice for the commoner.[54]

The most important difference between Bavaria and Franconia thus concerned the diametrically opposed positions from which they had to fight the catastrophic epidemic of 1634 and 1635. While Franconia had been experiencing epidemic outbreaks and their demographic consequences for years, Bavaria had been spared such trials and losses. However, the territories' preventive measures in response to the plague were very similar and indeed reflected common procedures, although Elector Maximilian's intense resolve may have led to swifter action.

Administering Spiritual Care

Pronouncements from the late sixteenth century through the Thirty Years' War continued to place one's relationship with God ahead of any physical measures one needed to take. A 1596 ordinance for Bavaria began by admonishing everyone to attend more frequently the weekly processions, at which God ought to be entreated to avert his justified wrath, awake them to love God and their neighbor, grant peace and unity throughout Christendom (while bestowing victory over their archenemies, the Protestants), and finally prevent the poisonous pestilence by giving them healthy air.[55] They advised not to be afraid should one get infected but, rather, to submit "joyfully" to God's will and immediately seek help. The ailing had a right to the sacrament, which meant that priests had to visit the infected to administer communion. During the 1634 plague epidemic, Maximilian admonished everyone to turn around their sinful life. The elector showed great concern for the spiritual care of the dying, but the living, too, should make sure to prepare themselves through frequent confession and communion "so that anytime the Lord might come, He finds them awake and not asleep," i.e. ready for death.[56] Secular authorities in every locale should remind the clergy to lead a God-fearing life, and should a priest absent himself from his parishioners because of fear or neglect or should he not be able to visit these houses for any other reason, the secular authorities should inform the clergy's supervisor.

This comment points to the potentially thin presence of ministers on the ground during the epidemic. Bartholomæus Dietwar, a Lutheran minister in Kitzingen near Würzburg, highlights this reality.[57] When several armies converged on their territory and brought disease and then pestilence into the city, the spiritual care of the many sick lay in the hands of only one minister and a chaplain, who quickly fell ill and died. Dietwar, who was asked to assist, recorded the extent of the loss and the progressive deterioration of burial practices. When the plague raged in September and October 1634, not all the 477 dead Dietwar attended to could be buried with a procession.[58]

The consistory of the Principality of Brandenburg-Ansbach in Franconia showed great concern both for the spiritual care of its parishioners and for the physical well-being of its personnel.[59] Already during the 1627 plague epidemic, Feuchtwangen's dean had inquired how the ministers in the parishes ought to conduct themselves toward the sick and the dead. In response, the consistory instructed the pastors to bury each body "with ringing of the bell and hymns" (*mit Klang und Gesang*) and address the survivors with a sermon or lecture of repentance. Should there be no minister in residence and should the next one be far away, the schoolmaster could perform these tasks. No one should be denied communion. Similarly, confession ought to continue, even in abbreviated form. But the minister should take care not to sit too close to the confessing person. In general, ministers were to address the needs of the time in their sermons, especially by encouraging parishioners toward repentance and prayer so that this and other punishments, which they had brought upon themselves because of their many sins, could be averted. The consistory believed that sin was particularly rampant among the common people, who, they charged, did not even recognize their swearing, drinking, overeating, and promiscuity as sins anymore.[60]

The consistory also warned the ministers not to abandon their congregations or raise suspicions that they might leave, since this was the time when the ministers' loyalty and care were needed the most. No one was to be left without physical or spiritual nourishment.[61] Many ministers indeed stayed with their congregation and died performing their office. Their wives and children frequently died as well.[62]

Since the consistory expected its personnel to remain in their parishes and districts, it is only understandable that they released instructions on how their ministers could protect themselves as they cared for the sick. For example, "no one would blame them" if they first sent someone to the houses and rooms where the infected lay, so that the rooms could be cleaned and fumigated. The minister himself should be armed with prayer and some preservative, and certainly he should never go out on an empty stomach. In addition, he needed to have utter confidence that God would keep him safe. Indeed, "[God] was more likely to protect him while in office than if he would not do his duty out of fear, in which case he would be in much greater danger with regard to his body, soul, and conscience and would certainly perish, if the plague caught him after having left his post."[63]

One issue was continuously at the forefront of the consistory's communications: the maintenance of order. The administrators were to act in a way that did not evoke fear and forestalled any kind of confusion and disorder. Those who died of the epidemic should be buried always at a particular hour of the day, and only those who were close to the deceased or whose office required them to be there should come to the burial, because disorder and abhorrence at the sight of the dead often led to greater calamity.[64] Here the consistory most likely referred to the conviction that frightened people were more susceptible to contagions. The infected should stay in their houses, where the clergy would hear their confession separately and give them communion and a comforting lesson. In general, "good order" was to be kept at get-togethers like baptisms and weddings.[65]

When it came to spiritual care, these instructions make clear that the personnel charged with tending to the afflicted souls needed just as much, and maybe even more, support as the parishioners they were to comfort and guide.

Collecting Scientific Data

The fact that the care for one's soul was front and center in many of these pronouncements and in advisory literature did not relegate practical matters to a poor second. As we saw above, in Munich's ordinance of 30 October 1634, one's relationship with God may have been the first and foremost item, but it was followed by twenty-four articles that addressed practical concerns and preventive measures. The practical or "natural" side of plague prevention has always stood alongside spiritual intervention and preparedness, although the emphases between the two tended to change over time. Particularly noteworthy, however, is the increasing focus on gathering reliable data to forestall or diminish the spread of an epidemic.

In Bavaria, a key person in this endeavor was the scribe who was hired during plague epidemics. The city physician was only distantly involved in the care of pest victims, since he prescribed medications but was not obliged to visit the infected in person. With such remote treatment of the disease, Munich's city fathers and the physician needed someone who could furnish them with information about the disease's origin and profile. This was the task of the scribe, who was to document the vital details—e.g. whether the illness stemmed from heat or cold and how long the infected lay sick—and make a daily record of the patients' medical condition available to the city's physician and burgomaster.[66] Additionally, the scribes and the captains (*Hauptleute*) of the city quarters were charged to visit the houses to check on their cleanliness and to report any evidence of filth to the burgomaster so that offenders could be punished.[67]

In Nuremberg, too, the city hired not only the usual assortment of personnel to deal with the pest—barber-surgeons, ministers, gravediggers, carriers of the dead, midwives, wardens, nurses, cooks, etc.—but also someone to be the connecting link between the pest personnel and the council, the *Aufwarter*. His duties were many, including keeping records of the situation, the finances, and the discipline. The chief authority lay with the deputies of epidemics (*Deputierten zu den Sterbsläufften*), a kind of special commission of four to six men which existed only during an epidemic.[68]

The initiatives toward collecting more detailed information on various aspects of the pestilence, especially during the 1634 plague epidemic, were part of a development toward gathering more empirical data on the disease, but in Bavaria it coincided with Maximilian's penchant for meticulous record-keeping. The elector demanded of Munich's city fathers that they send him comprehensive updates every other day. Burgomaster and council were to report who and how many had died of the contagion, how many and which houses were barred, whether the disease had decreased or increased, whether it had been carried in from other places or where it had originated, and whatever other important circumstances might be worth recounting. To Maximilian's dissatisfaction with the city council's incomplete data, Munich's councilors responded with irritation. No doubt, they had their hands full during this epidemic. The councilors pointed out that they had already sent the elector listings and other material, but they now followed up with an assessment of how effective the suggested measures had been.[69]

Munich's report to Maximilian is most enlightening regarding the question whether the contagion had been brought into the city from the outside or where it had originated. The extensive reply, divided into four points, suggests that the city had consulted a physician to answer this point, which was common practice at this time. There was no reference to sin. According to the city authorities, the first reason for the contagion was the lack of victuals, which resulted in the common citizen going hungry.[70] Next came the fright and grief people had experienced, beginning with Munich's occupation, then the quartering of troops, and the concomitant abuse. The council pointed out that, according to the judgment of medical men, fear constituted a "not slight" (*nit geringe*) cause for contagion.[71] A third reason was the lodging of officers and their troops in the city. Some of them fell sick in their houses, but their train and horses also created much uncleanliness that helped spread the contagion. In addition to the soldiers, many foreigners of every social station, whether spiritual or secular, had fled into the city. The heavy influx of refugees and their livestock into Munich led to overcrowded houses, tremendous stench, and squalor. At the same time the poor were begging in the streets and in front of houses and churches, so that the infection spread. These refugees died in the streets either because of their great misery and sadness or because of the lack of victuals, especially warm meals. The most numerous among the victims were the ruined and impoverished peasants.[72]

The fourth and foremost reason for the origin of the contagion, according to the councilors, was the Spanish army. The officers, who had taken up lodging in the citizens' houses all winter and summer, and the many Spanish soldiers in and outside of the city produced an extraordinary amount of refuse and left behind 150 dead, which was where authorities thought the infection originated. As evidence, the report pointed to other places where the Spanish army had left behind similar "relics": the Tyrol, the districts Rosenheim and Griesbach, Aibling, Weilheim, Tölz, Swabia, and other locales.[73] Given the large garrison and the enormous number of foreign people and their livestock in the city, the councilors' efforts to rid the city of its refuse and restore cleanliness had largely been in vain.

Even though early modern political leaders were unaware of the true origin of the plague, they were evidently well informed about how the contagion spread. They knew about the route and centers of contagion and were cognizant of some of the factors that facilitated and exacerbated its proliferation: hunger and crowded living. But we glimpse in these initiatives and reports that governments were eager to go beyond these facts and understand more deeply the profile of this contagion so that they could counteract it more effectively.

Staffing and Provisioning Health Care

As governments were intensely involved in controlling the epidemic, they had to contend with daily challenges and solve problems of a more routine kind, namely, how to provide for all the sick and dying. What did care for the infected look like? How did authorities try to meet the ever-expanding needs created by the epidemic? And how did they pay for the enormous costs of additional personnel and lazarets? Munich offers a good look at these issues.

In terms of staff and in keeping with the earlier noted importance of spiritual care, Munich's city council in 1628 first listed a special priest for the lazaret, whose regular weekly salary of two florins would be raised to six florins, "should God the Almighty indeed strike the city with that sentence."[74] Since the priest had to reside outside the city to prevent bringing the infection inside (the lazaret was also located outside city walls), the Jesuits and Capuchins agreed to care for those infected within the city, who had decided to stay in their houses.[75] Other hires included a nurse, a carrier of the dead, a gravedigger, a midwife, a recordkeeper, and a barber-surgeon. The order stipulated that those who died should be replaced with other qualified personnel, which highlights an awareness that these were hazardous jobs.[76]

In 1634, Munich followed electoral orders to hire a special curate in addition to a fumigator, and to request the assistance of the Jesuits and Capuchins. The curate, however, refused to serve as chaplain during the pestilence unless he was promised the next available benefice belonging to the city. Here one observes some of the deal making for which this crisis provided an occasion. Some took the precarious situation of the pestilence as an opportunity to negotiate a better arrangement for themselves. The chances were that people in contact with the infected would die very soon. If they survived, however, their bargaining for a special bonus to offset the risk they took could place them in a better position than before. In this case, however, the council did not agree to the curate's conditions and hired someone else.[77]

Supplying the infected with all the necessities proved to be an immense task. In late September 1634, H. Schobinger, Munich's *Commissarius* in charge of pestilence, learned that the many poor in the infected and barred houses had no provisions, and he asked the council how they ought to be taken care of. The city fathers settled on a collection for the infected and were willing to pay for the costs until funds had been gathered. For those in the lazaret who were recovering from the pestilence, a separate house with garden was to be opened and equipped so that they could stay there under quarantine.[78]

The epidemic placed great demands on the personnel in charge of caring for the sick, the dying, and the dead. Bernhardt Messenhauser, curate (*Kaplan*) of the lazaret, affords us insight into the grim situation of the health providers and the difficulty of keeping up with the necessity for further hospitals during the epidemic that fall. The lazaret outside the city gate at the Isar River had been opened on 16 September 1634.[79] Soon the Marx House followed as another lazaret, but it was poorly equipped. Patients froze miserably because there was not enough hay to lie on. The cook begged for wood so that she could prepare warm meals. Both nurses and one nurse-in-training lay sick; only the half-ill cook was still of some use. Upon the instruction of the commissioner, the curate hired two new nurses.[80]

Messenhauser was overwhelmed with work in the lazaret and the Marx House, while also overseeing the gravediggers and their labor. His assistant proved to be of no help.[81] Moreover, since both the lazaret at the Isar and the Marx House were entirely filled up, Messenhauser begged the commissioner in charge of the pestilence to repair and open a third house. He requested that this house be well supplied with hay, wood, light, etc. The lazaret's barber-surgeon and his colleague demanded a third master, for otherwise they were unable to take care of the three houses. Luckily, the curate knew of a good candidate.[82] All in all, the council opened three lazarets besides the one at the Isar and a house for recovery from the infection.[83]

The costs during this epidemic rose astronomically, and soon the city had to devise ways to raise extra funds. The council decided to increase the beer tax and use these resources toward their expenses incurred by the epidemic.[84] The next year, in September 1635, Munich requested permission from the elector to add a special tax to meat and, once again, beer so that it could pay for the enormous costs resulting from the infection and other obligations connected with the war. This was to avoid raising taxes in general for the severely impoverished citizenry.[85] The city's billing records illustrate the massive financial burden: the epidemic lasted from September 1634 until April 1635, during which time the council opened, staffed, and equipped five houses altogether. The medication for the infected in the lazarets was paid for out of the city's coffers. In the five houses, more than sixty lazaret attendants continuously cared for over three hundred persons. In order to pay for all these expenses, the administration initiated a collection in the four quarters of the city, which amounted to 1,438 florins and 51 kreutzers.[86] Besides what had been collected from the community, the city treasury paid bills in the amount of 6,425 florins and 20 kreutzers.[87]

Moreover, in 1634 Munich did not collect taxes from its citizenry because of the epidemic, which added to the city's strapped finances.[88] Furthermore, over half of the infected were poor peasants who had fled into the city.[89] In short, the care for the infected consumed vast resources in terms of personnel, supplies, and finances. If a city like Munich, which had entered this catastrophic period on a strong footing, staggered under the massive expenses this health crisis exacted from it, it is easy to understand how much more Nuremberg reeled as it faced this dramatic event, weakened and depleted.

Quarantine and Other Violations

While authorities tried hard to contain the occurrence and spread of pestilence, and expended enormous resources to care for the sick, it is evident that their subjects did not always fall in line with the government agenda. Munich's council complained about people ignoring the separation of the infected from the healthy. This concerned particularly the barring of houses, which people disrespected:

> When the evil pestilence [*böse Sucht*] has penetrated a house or chamber ... and the housefather has been ordered to stay inside together with his household, he nevertheless did not remain in the house but left it or went in and out according to his desire. Other housefathers, who had been ordered to bar their house or chamber, refused to do so and violently resisted the restrictions; or, where the barring had actually been undertaken, the locked-in kept talking with other people on the outside.[90]

Inhabitants also went into infected residences and removed things.[91] People disregarded other orders as well, e.g. citizens housed foreign peasants and other persons, despite directives to the contrary.[92] Moreover, the infected attended church and walked about in the city.[93] Nuremberg's councilmen, too, charged that hardly anyone bothered with their orders. Instead, there were enough "selfish people" (*aigennutzige*), both local and foreign, who smuggled heaps of feathers and bedding into the city to sell them, "through which the general citizenry could easily contract a dangerous infection."[94] The councilors also censured the lack of cleanliness in the streets, since every shop and house emptied their stinking water into the alleys, "which contributed considerably to infections and poisoning."[95] According to district administrators of the rural areas, violations of quarantine were particularly rampant in the countryside.[96] The principal measures in these rural territories involved the quarantining of houses, since no lazaret was available, but such segregation was frequently defied.

Authorities strove to counteract their subjects' lack of compliance in several ways. First, concerned that everyone was aware of the ordinances, Munich's councilors made certain that their ordinances were widely known, as did

Nuremberg's city fathers, who had the text read publicly and sent to the overseers of the quarters so that they could pass it on to every house.[97] The council also sent its pronouncements to the district administrators (*Landpfleger*), who in turn passed instructions to village leaders (*Dorfhauptleute*). Printed edicts were posted at the village entrances and read from the pulpits.[98] Besides ensuring that the information and instructions were available to everyone, these steps also prevented people from feigning ignorance.

Furthermore, in cases of non-compliance, governments threatened severe punishment. These included heavy fines, prison sentences, or shaming by placing the offender in the pillory. Violations of ordinances were nothing new, but, in an epidemic as dramatic as that of 1634, such breaches were particularly harmful. Munich's council threatened to punish transgressions even more severely, but, despite such harsh prospects, people hardly followed the ordinances and indeed acted against them. Accordingly, the council joined forces with Maximilian to put more muscle behind their decree. The elector not only approved the ordinance of 30 October 1634 but made it binding for every level of society, no matter a person's estate or office.[99]

In particular the evidence from the countryside underlines, however, that different levels of government had diverse approaches to dealing with culprits. Maximilian's right-hand man for the district (*Rentamt*) of Munich chastised the burgomaster and council of the market town of Altmannstein for not punishing quarantine offenders severely enough. During the pestilence in 1634, Wolf Mänhardt Crammer had been placed in the tower with bread and water for just one day for having gone to Riedenburg, where the infection raged. Not only should he have been punished more harshly; since he could have brought back the contagion, he should have been placed under quarantine outside of the market town at his own cost. The town should have used Crammer to make an example of quarantine violators.[100] Another case comes from the district (*Pfleggericht*) of Vohburg, where Maximilian's administrator reprimanded the local official for insufficient punishment. Because of the military turmoil, Simon Präutl of Gaimersheim had brought his bedding to Ingolstadt and came to fetch it as the pestilence was raging in that city. When he arrived at the gate of Gaimersheim and the bailiff (*Amtmann*) refused to let him pass because he came from an infected locale, Präutle forced his way past the gate, hit the officer, and took his bedding home. Since Präutl was poor, he was placed in chains for fourteen days. The elector's right-hand man sternly reproached the bailiff that the offender should never have been tolerated in the market town but should have been chased outside of its gates and placed under quarantine. Only after having spent the appropriate time in quarantine and after having cleaned his bedding should he have been let back inside the gates. Moreover, this case should have been reported to the electoral court, which would have decided on the proper punishment.[101]

These two cases reveal a rather moderate approach to quarantine by the local authorities. One can only guess at the possible reasons for the administrators' reaction. It is doubtful that they lacked an understanding of the principles of quarantine. More likely they placed other local interests, such as social and economic considerations, above containing the infection. As soon as the epidemic declined, rural administrators begged the electoral council to relax the quarantine so that their subjects could pursue their business, which suggests that economic considerations played a significant role in their decisions.[102] Maximilian, however, had no patience with such light handling of the culprits during this health crisis. Breakers of quarantine were a major threat to his territory and subjects, and exemplary sentencing was needed to keep people from following their own—faulty—advice.

An example from Nuremberg corroborates the weight of economic concerns. According to a chronicler, the deaths from the 1625 epidemic caused fear, but did so because they disrupted commerce, since passes were blocked and neither people nor goods could get through.[103] This report helps one understand why people might break the quarantine: anxiety about the plague's impact on business could be more pronounced than about its effect on one's health.

Even Munich's city council dealt leniently with Brigitta Millerin in January 1635, when the infection had begun to subside. After her father had died of the plague, Brigitta had moved him into a different room and had sold some of his clothes. At this point, the city had been opened again, and, rather than punishing her harshly, the council pardoned her and merely reprimanded her severely for her crime.[104]

Conclusion

To conclude, in the seventeenth century, strategies were in place to deal with plague epidemics, and governments were adamant about the practical side of checking the contagion. While they continued to be concerned about humanity's role in bringing about pestilence and placed a "call-to-spiritual-order" at the top of their directives, the concrete handling of the epidemic gained ever more ground. Still, the war, with its uneven geographic effect, positioned Franconia and Bavaria very differently as they confronted the pestilence of 1634. During this outbreak that broke all boundaries and showed up the inadequacy of well-established strategies, both territories suffered severely, but Franconia was critically ruined, since it had already been decimated by troops, disease, and hunger during the 1620s.

Turning our gaze toward our own time, how do the experiences of the 1600s compare with those of the twenty-first century? Continuities and discontinuities are particularly discernible when looking at the four aspects examined: spiritual care, scientific data, adequate health care, and quarantine violations. During the Thirty Years' War, we noted an increasing attention to recordkeeping and scientific data in order to determine the origin and characteristics of the contagion so that governments could curtail its spread. It is thus evident that the usefulness of scientific information in fighting epidemics is not only a mantra of the modern age but resided at the forefront of how governments approached disease control in the seventeenth century. The purpose of arriving at a better understanding of the epidemic's spread and profile was its more successful containment. Controlling the epidemic through developing vaccines, however, belonged in the era of modern times.

Continuities also abound when it comes to the complex and daunting task of staffing and supplying health care for the afflicted, as well as the enormous resources these efforts take. The urgent pleas of Munich's curate, Bernhardt Messenhauser, for further personnel and supplies bring to mind more recent realities of hospital physicians' desperate calls for equipment—from basic facemasks to ventilators. Reports and images of doctors and nurses exhausted beyond measure as they care for an endless stream of COVID victims are still fresh in our minds.

Another common refrain concerns violations of the restrictions placed upon one's life that are meant to help fight the epidemic. Then as now, the dread of economic repercussions or social isolation was often greater than the fear of disease, and critics of limitations on commerce point to the economic fallout of such stipulations. The political contexts are, of course, not the same. Efforts today are not complicated by a horrendous war, and current governments work in many ways that are different from those in the seventeenth century. Also, the global response to COVID-19 demonstrated a broad spectrum of political leadership. The early modern period distinguishes itself also in that governments continued to invoke God in fighting the pandemic, whereas such reliance on religion is largely absent in political pronouncements today. In our multicultural society, communities and individuals may place their faith first and foremost in God, but public policy decisions concerning health issues rest on scientific insights.

Beyond comparing methods and behaviors then and now, the most comforting message from looking at the past may be the fact that the epidemic did end. Measures eventually did help to contain the contagion and save lives.

Sigrun Haude is the Walter C. Langsam Professor of European History at the University of Cincinnati. She is the author of *Coping with Life during the Thirty Years' War* (Brill, 2021) and *In the Shadow of "Savage Wolves": Anabaptist Münster and the German Reformation during the 1530s* (Humanities Press, 2000), and has published on Anabaptism and gender. She is the co-editor of *Challenging Orthodoxies: The Social and Cultural Worlds of Early Modern*

Women (Ashgate, 2014) and *Rethinking Europe. War and Peace in the Early Modern German Lands* (Brill/CHLOE, 2019).

Notes

1. In the following, I will frequently refer to the duchy or Old Bavaria simply as Bavaria. For a brief discussion of the governmental handling of epidemics during the war, see my study *Coping with Life during the Thirty Years' War*.
2. These insights are underlined by Eckert, *Structure of Plagues*; Ulbricht, ed., *Die leidige Seuche*; and Feuerstein-Herz, ed., *Gotts verhengnis und seine straffe*.
3. For example, Nuremberg's ordinance concerning pestilence (*Pestordnung*) evolved by 1562 into the more general regulation concerning deadly diseases (*Sterbsordnung*). Porzelt, *Pest in Nürnberg*, 69. Documents only gradually became more explicit about the kind of infection with which they were dealing, whether it was a form of pestilence, typhus, dysentery, or smallpox.
4. Hauptstaatsarchiv München, Manuskriptensammlung, Nr. 522, Schreibkalender 1636, 9. Kap. Von Kranckheiten des Leibes dieses 1636. Jahrs, D[r]. All translations are mine.
5. For a discussion of the powers of smell and the plague, see Le Guérer, *Scent*, 39–62.
6. Porzelt, *Pest in Nürnberg*, 29–30.
7. Eckert, *Structure of Plagues*, 78–132.
8. Edward Eckert also underlines the influence of seasonal factors on plague activity. The peak usually occurred during the fall months (September until November), whereas February to July showed limited activity. In addition, he stresses the great variations in mortality between individual communities within clusters. *Structure of Plagues*, 143–44.
9. Eckert, *Structure of Plagues*, 134, 136.
10. See Eckert's fascinating epidemiological research on Bavaria (*Structure of Plagues*, 98, 112, 142, 145–46). Bavarian Swabia, especially Augsburg, however, suffered high mortality in 1627–31. Eckert suggests a few possibilities to explain this anomaly: the type of settlement, which in Bavaria was more dispersed and thus did not reflect the interactive village and town life of many other areas; a different linkage of these settlements; biological factors, such as concentration and types of rodents; and modes of building construction. As I submit in my study *Coping with Life*, Elector Maximilian's vigilance regarding the epidemic likely contributed as well to Bavaria's fortunate situation.
11. Heimers, *Krieg, Hunger, Pest und Glaubenszwist*, 42. Munich's normal population was roughly 23,000, but this number does not include the refugees and military.
12. At this time, Wilhelm's son, Maximilian (r. 1598–1651), was already heavily involved in the governing of the dukedom, even though he did not officially become duke of Bavaria until 1598.
13. Stadtarchiv München, Gesundheitswesen 3, Sterbeläufe, Mandat Herzog Wilhelms "die Sterbeläufe betreffend" (1 Nov. 1996).
14. Stadtarchiv München, Gesundheitswesen 3.
15. Stadtarchiv München, Gesundheitswesen 3.
16. Stadtarchiv München, Bürgermeister und Rat, 60 A 1, Landesherrliche Generalmandate und Verordnungen Bayerischer Herzöge und Kurfürst Maximilian I (1514–1651), Pestbekämpfung (9 Sept. 1606).

17. Stadtarchiv München, Bürgermeister und Rat, 60 B 3, Sammlung von landesherrlichen Erlassen, fol. 10v–11r: Pest, Vorbeugungs- und Verhaltensmaßnahmen (5 Sept. 1613). A princely edict of 1625 contained positions similar to the earlier decrees. See Stadtarchiv München, Bürgermeister und Rat 60 B 9, Sätze und Ordnungen des Landesherrn, 1613–1674, fol. 1r: Gedrucktes Mandat über Pestbekämpfungsmaßnahmen (1625).
18. See, e.g., Stadtarchiv München, Gesundheitswesen 43, Seuchenverhaltensmaßregeln. Polizei-Verfassung. Gesundheits-Polizei. Betreff: Bericht, wie sich der gemaine Mann in jetzt grassierendem Kopfweh vnd hitzigem Fieber zu verhalten habe. Aus dem 17. Jahrhundert.
19. Stadtarchiv München, Gesundheitswesen 43.
20. Stadtarchiv München, Gesundheitswesen 43.
21. Stadtarchiv München, Gesundheitswesen 43.
22. Stadtarchiv München, Gesundheitswesen 52. Polizeiverfassung. Gesundheitspolizei. Sterbeläufe Pest vnd Contagien vnd die dagegen getroffenen Anstalten betreffend. 1592–1632. *General Jstruction* [sic] 1624. Wie es alhie gehalten würdt, wann ihm Lanndt oder auch ausser Landt die laidige Sucht der Pest Einreist.
23. Stadtarchiv München, Gesundheitswesen 52, fol. 1r–v.
24. Stadtarchiv München, Gesundheitswesen 52, fol. 2r–v.
25. For an instruction how letters and small packages were to be fumigated, see Stadtarchiv München, Gesundheitswesen 52, *Instruction* für den brief Raucher ihm Rauch hauß.
26. Stadtarchiv München, Gesundheitswesen 52.
27. Stadtarchiv München, Gesundheitswesen 52, Wegen der Sterbläuf (1625).
28. Stadtarchiv München, Gesundheitswesen 52, Ordnung vnd Anstöllungen (1628). Wie es alhie wan die Laidige sucht der Pesst (darvor vnß Gott lang behietten wölle) einreissen wurde, gehalten würdet, fol. 1r.
29. Stadtarchiv München, Bürgermeister und Rat 60 B 14, Sammlung landesherrlicher Mandate in Justiz- und Polizeisachen, 1562–1698, Nr. 26, Pestordnung (19 Aug. 1634). Maximilian (who had become elector in 1623 after his victory for the emperor at the Battle of the White Mountain in 1620) had left Munich before the Swedes arrived in 1632 and did not return to the city until 1635.
30. Stadtarchiv München, Ratssitzungsprotokolle (Unterrichterserie) 249, fol. 308v (7 Sept. 1634).
31. Stadtarchiv München, Gesundheitswesen 5, Ratsordnung, die Pestilenz betreffend.
32. Stadtarchiv München, Gesundheitswesen 5.
33. Stadtarchiv München, Gesundheitswesen 3.
34. Stadtarchiv München, Gesundheitswesen 5.
35. Stadtarchiv München, Ratssitzungsprotokolle (Unterrichterserie) 250/1, fol. 71r (12 Feb. 1635).
36. Stadtarchiv München, Gesundheitswesen 34, Peuers von H: Georgs Mosman besteltem Lazaret Caplan (21 April 1535), fol. 433r–v.
37. Stadtarchiv München, Ratssitzungsprotokolle (Unterrichterserie) 250/2, 2v (1 June 1635).
38. Stadtarchiv München, Ratssitzungsprotokolle (Unterrichterserie) 250/2, fol. 3v–4r (4 June 1635).
39. Stadtarchiv München, Ratssitzungsprotokolle (Unterrichterserie) 250/2, fol. 98v (31 Aug. 1635) and fol. 139r (5 Oct. 1635).
40. Stadtarchiv München, Stadtverteidigung 251/b, fol. 2r–v.

41. Staatsarchiv Nürnberg, Archivaliensammlung des Historischen Vereins für Mittelfranken, Handschriften 219, Nürnberger Chronik bis 1687 (no author or date of publication), fol. 190r. The chronicle speaks of 6,000 Cossacks who quartered by Führt and demanded to be fed by the city. From then on, there occurred an almost continuous stream of companies through their territory.
42. Porzelt, *Pest in Nürnberg*, 40–42, 176–77. Like Eckert, Carolin Porzelt (291) underlines the lack of pest activity from 1614–1623.
43. Chronicles testify to a series of epidemics beginning in August 1624, when fifty children alone succumbed within eight days. In October "pestilence" began to spread. The city council undertook measures to forestall any increase of the disease, but it still took a while for it to subside completely. Staatsarchiv Nürnberg, Archivaliensammlung des Historischen Vereins für Mittelfranken, Handschriften 219; fol. 202r. As mentioned earlier, the sources are not always reliable on the kind of epidemic. Porzelt (*Pest in Nürnberg*, 42) speaks of dysentery that came down on the city in October 1624.
44. Staatsarchiv Nürnberg, Rep. 63/2, Reichsstadt Nürnberg, Mandate, lose, III, Nr. 448 (3 Dec. 1624).
45. Staatsarchiv Nürnberg, Archivaliensammlung des Historischen Vereins für Mittelfranken, Handschriften 219, fol. 212v and 215r.
46. Staatsarchiv Nürnberg, Reichsstadt Nürnberg Handschriften Nr. 472; 632.
47. Staatsarchiv Nürnberg, Archivaliensammlung des Historischen Vereins für Mittelfranken, Handschriften 219, fol. 230r. Another chronicle speaks of 5,785 buried bodies, including the Swedes. Staatsarchiv Nürnberg, Archivaliensammlung des Historischen Vereins für Mittelfranken, Handschriften 473, Nürnberger Chronik bis 1678, *von anderer Hand fortgesetzt bis 1689*, fol. 285r.
48. Staatsbibliothek München, Cgm 5642, Cronica von Nürnberg bis 1679, 389. This chronicler's count of a total of 29,406 is too high as well.
49. Staatsarchiv Nürnberg, Archivaliensammlung des Historischen Vereins für Mittelfranken, Handschriften 219, fol. 236v. The author contends that travelers had brought the infection into the city. Regarding the 11,125 buried in the churchyard, historian Ernst Mummenhoff judged that the real number was more than twice as high, between 18,000 and 22,000, which would mean a loss of one half to two-thirds of the city population. Mummenhoff, *Altnürnberg*, vol. 2, 72–73; Porzelt, *Pest in Nürnberg*, 43.
50. Staatsarchiv Nürnberg, Archivaliensammlung des Historischen Vereins für Mittelfranken, Handschriften 219, fol. 235v–36r.
51. Staatsarchiv Nürnberg, Archivaliensammlung des Historischen Vereins für Mittelfranken, Handschriften 219, fol. 241v. In 1640 small pox (*Kindts Blattern*) erupted and took the lives of several hundred children (fol. 255r).
52. Porzelt, *Pest in Nürnberg*, 43.
53. Porzelt, *Pest in Nürnberg*, 35. A census taken in Nuremberg in 1806 counted only 25,176 inhabitants.
54. Porzelt, *Pest in Nürnberg*, 55–57. Curiously, a general edict on contagion for the entire Frankish Circle was not published until 1708, when an infection was spreading from Poland, but European cities and territories usually cooperated to fight epidemics (Ibid., 140–44).
55. Stadtarchiv München, Gesundheitswesen 3. As we saw in the previous section, at the height of the 1634 epidemic, attendance of processions was discouraged.
56. Stadtarchiv München, Bürgermeister und Rat 60 B 14, Nr. 26, Pestordnung (19 Aug. 1634).

57. Landeskirchliches Archiv der Evangelisch-Lutherischen Kirche in Bayern, Markgräfliches Dekanat Uffenheim, Akt. 95, Chronick Bartholomæus Dietwar. Kitzingen lay in the margravate Brandenburg-Ansbach to the west of Nuremberg in Franconia.
58. Landeskirchliches Archiv der Evangelisch-Lutherischen Kirche in Bayern, Markgräfliches Dekanat Uffenheim, Akt. 95:67, 70, 77, 80, 84.
59. The consistory was the central ecclesiastical institution in Brandenburg-Ansbach's Lutheran church, followed by the deans (middle authorities) and then the parish ministers.
60. Landeskirchliches Archiv der Evangelisch-Lutherischen Kirche in Bayern, Markgräfliches Dekanat Feuchtwangen, Miscellanea 153a, Kirchliche Verhältnisse während des 30 jähr. Krieges, 1. Verhalten bei Pest (1627), fol. 1r–v.
61. Landeskirchliches Archiv der Evangelisch-Lutherischen Kirche in Bayern, Markgräfliches Dekanat Feuchtwangen, Miscellanea 153a, fol. 3r–v.
62. Landeskirchliches Archiv der Evangelisch-Lutherischen Kirche in Bayern, Markgräfliches Dekanat Konsistorium Ansbach C, Spez. 14, Alfershausen, vol. 1, 1497–1653. Bittschrift des Pfarrers Gottfried Feist, von Alfershausen, an den Grafen Friedrich von Solm und Räte (2 July 1633); ibid., Spez. 883, Uffenheim Dekanat, Vol. I, 1491–1743, Copia Schreibens An Decanum zue Vffenheim, Bericht vndt Bedencken. Der aniezo Verordneten *Consistorialium* alhier zu Onolzbach [Ansbach], an den fürstl. Landhoffmeister des Dekanats Uffenheim (17 March 1635).
63. Landeskirchliches Archiv der Evangelisch-Lutherischen Kirche in Bayern, Markgräfliches Dekanat Feuchtwangen, Miscellanea 153a, fol. 2v–3r.
64. Landeskirchliches Archiv der Evangelisch-Lutherischen Kirche in Bayern, Markgräfliches Dekanat Feuchtwangen, Miscellanea 153a, fol. 2r.
65. Landeskirchliches Archiv der Evangelisch-Lutherischen Kirche in Bayern, Markgräfliches Dekanat Feuchtwangen, Miscellanea 153a.
66. Stadtarchiv München, Gesundheitswesen 52, Lazarethschreibers Instruction (zwischen 1622–1644 [added in pencil]).
67. Stadtarchiv München, Ratssitzungsprotokolle (Unterrichterserie) 249, fol. 347v (14 Oct. 1634).
68. Porzelt, *Pest in Nürnberg*, 62–63.
69. Stadtarchiv München, Gesundheitswesen 34, Seuchen—Vorbeugemaßnahmen, Antwort Bürgermeister und Rat der Stadt München an den Kurfürsten (25 Sept. 1634), fol. 59v–60r. The earlier report had been sent on 5 Sept. 1634.
70. Stadtarchiv München, Gesundheitswesen 34, fol. 60v–61r.
71. Stadtarchiv München, Gesundheitswesen 34, fol. 61r.
72. Stadtarchiv München, Gesundheitswesen 34, fol. 61r–v.
73. Stadtarchiv München, Gesundheitswesen 34, fol. 62v–63r.
74. Stadtarchiv München, Gesundheitswesen 52, Ordnung vnd Anstöllungen (1628). Wie es alhie wan die Laidige sucht der Pesst (darvor vnß Gott lang behietten wölle) einreissen wurde, gehalten würdet, fol. 1r.
75. These dwellings were subsequently barred so that no one could leave the house or receive visitors, and the healthy were separated from the infected within the house. The *patres* and *fratres* willing to care for the sick had to separate from the rest of their convent as well. Stadtarchiv München, Ratssitzungsprotokolle (Unterrichterserie) 249, fol. 319r (13 Sept. 1634).

76. Stadtarchiv München, Gesundheitswesen 52, Ordnung vnd Anstöllungen (1628), fol. 1r–3r.
77. Stadtarchiv München, Ratssitzungsprotokolle (Unterrichterserie) 249, fol. 310r (7 Sept. 1634).
78. Stadtarchiv München, Ratssitzungsprotokolle (Unterrichterserie) 249, fol. 333r –v (28 Sept. 1634).
79. Stadtarchiv München, Kämmerei 1/241, fol. 158r: Vncosten So dits 1634 Jars über die Lazaret Heüser, auch derselben diener, zutrager, vnd warther von .16, Septbris . anno. 1634. bis auf den 10. Febr: Anno .35. in die .22. wochen lang aufgeloffen.
80. Stadtarchiv München, Gesundheitswesen 34, Memoriale an die herrn *Commissarios de dato* den 19 *Octobris* (1634), fol. 177v.
81. Stadtarchiv München, Gesundheitswesen 34, fol. 178r.
82. Stadtarchiv München, Gesundheitswesen 34, An die Herrn *Commissarios* der *infection* von dem 20 *Octobris* (1634). Von Bernhardt Messenhauser; fol. 180r–v.
83. Stadtarchiv München, Kämmerei 1/241, fol. 158r.
84. Stadtarchiv München, Ratssitzungsprotokolle (Unterrichterserie) 249, fol. 344r (11 Oct. 1634).
85. Stadtarchiv München, Ratssitzungsprotokolle (Unterrichterserie) 250/2, fol. 123v (22 Sept. 1635).
86. Stadtarchiv München, Kämmerei 1/241, Kammerrechnungen 1634, fol. 158r–v.
87. Stadtarchiv München, Stadtverteidigung 251/b, Verzaichnuß. Etlich vnderschidlicher *Extra ordinari* Außgaben, so der Statt München von Anno .32. biß auf Anno .35. aufgeloffen, vnd waß der Statt noch vf dato für Purdten obligen. Verfaßt: 15. Sept. 1635. Infections Vncosten, fol. 5v. The treasury also kept records, according to which the entire costs for the lazaret houses and the personnel from 16 September 1634 until 10 February 1635 came to 5,282 fl. 25 kr. 2 dl.
88. The city, however, did go after taxes that were still outstanding for 1633. Stadtarchiv München, Kämmerei 1/241, Kammerrechnungen 1634, fol. 54r.
89. Stadtarchiv München, Stadtverteidigung 251/b, Memorial. Ettlicher vnderschüdlicher extraordinari ausgaben, vnd anderer beschwerlicheiten So der Statt München Camer von Anno 1632 seider der feindts einfahl, bis vf Anno 41. zugetragen: vnd waß der Statt noch in vielen dingen abligt, 1832–1641 (25 March 1641), fol. 2r.
90. Stadtarchiv München, Gesundheitswesen 5.
91. Stadtarchiv München, Ratssitzungsprotokolle (Unterrichterserie) 249, fol. 355r–v (18 Oct. 1634).
92. Stadtarchiv München, Ratssitzungsprotokolle (Unterrichterserie) 249, fol. 321v (19 Sept. 1634) and 344r (11 Oct. 1634).
93. Stadtarchiv München, Ratssitzungsprotokolle (Unterrichterserie) 249, fol. 346r (13 Oct. 1634).
94. Staatsarchiv Nürnberg, Rep. 63/2, Reichsstadt Nürnberg, Mandate, lose, III, Nr. 448 (3 Dec. 1624).
95. Staatsarchiv Nürnberg, Rep. 63/2, Reichsstadt Nürnberg, Mandate, lose, III, Nr. 448.
96. Staatsarchiv München, Kirchen in der Herrschaft Hohenaschau, A 2608, esp. letter of 6 Sept. 1634 to the judge of Wildenwart.
97. Stadtarchiv München, Gesundheitswesen 5; Staatsarchiv Nürnberg, Archivaliensammlung des Historischen Vereins für Mittelfranken, Handschriften 219; fol. 202v.
98. Porzelt, *Pest in Nürnberg*, 146.
99. Stadtarchiv München, Gesundheitswesen 5.

100. Staatsarchiv München, Rentmeister—Literalien, fasc. 33, 124, Umbriths-Prothocoll gegen der Thonau, Rentambts Minchen, 1636. Marckht Altmanstain, fol. 159v.
101. Staatsarchiv München, Rentmeister—Literalien, fasc. 33, 124, Umbriths-Prothocoll gegen der Thonau, Rentambts Minchen, 1636. Marckht Altmanstain, fol. 225v–26r.
102. Staatsarchiv München, Kirchen in der Herrschaft Hohenaschau A 2608, letter of the judge of Wildenwart to the electoral council (6 Feb. 1635).
103. Staatsarchiv Nürnberg, Archivaliensammlung des Historischen Vereins für Mittelfranken, Handschriften 219; fol. 206r.
104. Stadtarchiv München, Ratssitzungsprotokolle (Unterrichterserie) 250/1, fol. 22r (10 Jan. 1635).

Bibliography

Archival Sources

Hauptstaatsarchiv München

Manuskriptensammlung, Nr. 522
Landeskirchliches Archiv der Evangelisch-Lutherischen Kirche in Bayern [Nuremberg]
Markgräfliches Dekanat Feuchtwangen, Miscellanea 153a
Markgräfliches Dekanat Uffenheim, Akten 95
Markgräfliches Konsistorium Ansbach C, Spez. 14
Markgräfliches Konsistorium Ansbach C, Spez. 883, Dekanat Uffenheim, vol. I

Staatsarchiv München

Hohenaschauer Archiv, vol. 2: Akten 348
Kirchen in der Herrschaft Hohenaschau, A 2608
Rentmeister—Literalien, fasc. 33, 124

Staatsarchiv Nürnberg

Archivaliensammlung des Historischen Vereins für Mittelfranken, Handschriften 219
Archivaliensammlung des Historischen Vereins für Mittelfranken, Handschriften 473
Reichsstadt Nürnberg, Handschriften, Nr. 472
Reichsstadt Nürnberg, Mandate, lose, III, Nr. 448

Staatsbibliothek München, Handschriftensammlung

Cgm 5642

Stadtarchiv München

Bürgermeister und Rat, 60 A 1
Bürgermeister und Rat, 60 B 3
Bürgermeister und Rat, 60 B 9

Bürgermeister und Rat, 60 B 14, Nr. 26
Gesundheitswesen 3
Gesundheitswesen 5
Gesundheitswesen 34
Gesundheitswesen 43
Gesundheitswesen 52
Kämmerei 1/241
Ratssitzungsprotokolle (Unterrichterserie) 249
Ratssitzungsprotokolle (Unterrichterserie) 250/1
Ratssitzungsprotokolle (Unterrichterserie) 250/2
Stadtverteidigung 251/b

Primary Sources

Fracastoro, Girolamo. *De contagione et contagiosis morbis et eorum curatione*, vol. 3. Venice, 1546.

Secondary Sources

Eckert, Edward A. *The Structure of Plagues and Pestilences in Early Modern Europe: Central Europe, 1560–1640*. Basel: Karger, 1996.

Feuerstein-Herz, Petra, ed. *Gotts verhengnis und seine straffe—Zur Geschichte der Seuchen in der Frühen Neuzeit*. Ausstellungskatalog der Herzog August Bibliothek. Braunschweig: Schönberg, 2005.

Guérer, Annick Le. *Scent: The Mysterious and Essential Powers of Smell*, translated by Richard Miller. New York: Turtle Bay Books/Random House, 1992 [1988].

Haude, Sigrun. *Coping with Life during the Thirty Years' War (1618–1648)*. Leiden: Brill, 2021.

Heimers, Manfred P. *Krieg, Hunger, Pest und Glaubenszwist: München im Dreißigjährigen Krieg*. Munich: Buchendorf, 1998.

Mummenhoff, Ernst. *Altnürnberg in Krieg und Kriegsnot*, vol. 2. Nuremberg: Schrag, 1916.

Porzelt, Carolin. *Die Pest in Nürnberg: Leben und Herrschen in Pestzeiten in der Reichsstadt Nürnberg (1562–1713)*. St. Ottilien: Eos, 2000.

Ulbricht, Otto, ed. *Die leidige Seuche: Pest-Fälle in der Frühen Neuzeit*. Cologne: Böhlau Verlag, 2004.

CHAPTER 7

Plague Control in the Absolutist Territorial State

Ideal and Reality in Electoral Hanover, 1709–16

ULF WENDLER

Introduction

In 1720, the plague in Marseille caused great anxiety and fear all over Europe. In response, the eminent physician Richard Mead (1673–1754) published a *Short Discourse Concerning Pestilential Contagion* in England with advice on how to combat the epidemic. While he was partly critical of the measures taken in France, he praised the arrangements made a decade earlier in the Electorate of Hanover. They had achieved the desired success and stopped the spread of the plague, so that only a small number of towns and villages were affected.[1]

Yet Mead did not consider the Electorate of Hanover to be a model state for disease control because new procedures had been devised in the territory while old familiar measures[2] had been consistently applied. Besides quarantine, these were either cordoning off, which blocked movement in and out of the entire territory and of individual locations, or isolation measures, which blocked movement from inside to the outside. When the Black Death had led to mass deaths in the mid-fourteenth century, people developed measures to protect themselves and prevent the spread of the disease. The pathogens could not be controlled directly, so for actual or perceived carriers (people and goods), access to certain areas was restricted and regulated. Quarantine was the best-known measure against an epidemic and had been used to contain plague since the fourteenth century.[3] It involved isolating travelers in a special place for a certain period before allowing them to enter a city or area. Residents could also be isolated at a specific quarantine point if necessary. Quarantine implies regulation of access to a place, so it is somewhat related to cordons.

Blocking access at gates was already reported in connection with the plague of 1348 in Milan and Parma, but also in Gloucester.[4] While access points to walled cities were comparatively easy to close off from the inside, this was more difficult in the case of entire territories. In the Duchy of Milan, for example, this was attempted unsuccessfully in 1576, in Spain in 1589, in Russia in 1551, 1571, and 1602, in the Papal States in 1656, and in the Prince-Bishopric of Westphalia in 1664–68.[5] Territorial states north of the Alps propagated cordoning off in some cases, but often only for their key cities. More far-reaching measures were beyond their possibilities. Early modern states did not have the means to devise effective measures to combat epidemics until the development of absolutism, i.e. for Central Europe during the last plague epidemics in the second half of the seventeenth century and the early eighteenth century. Now territorial states were at least somewhat able to protect their extensive borders with a health cordon: "A cordon sanitaire was a vigorous, physical protective barrier against foreign areas with epidemics established by military troops."[6] It came comparatively late in history that a place or territory did not seal itself off but was isolated from the outside.[7] Only absolutist states were able to effectively isolate individual places from the outside world after an outbreak of the disease in order to prevent the spread of the epidemic.

Comprehensive measures could be successfully implemented only in a larger territory with the power resources of an absolutist state. The newly acquired possibilities for action can be well traced in the example of the Electorate of Hanover, ruled by a line of the Guelphs. The Principality of Calenberg, with its capital Hanover, experienced a great increase in power around 1700. In 1692 Calenberg attained the status of an Electorate of the Holy Roman Empire, and in 1705 it was united with the Principality of Lüneburg, the associated Duchy of Lauenburg, and the County of Hoya. During the Second Northern War (1700–20) the Electorate of Hanover occupied parts of the Duchies of Bremen and Verden in 1712, which it was able to acquire permanently in 1719 (Map 7.1). Finally, in 1714, Elector Georg Ludwig became King George I of England (Figure 7.1). The politically successful Electorate of Hanover was an absolutist-dominated territory with a strong army and a well-organized administration. It was confronted with the last great plague in Central Europe in the early eighteenth century.

In the early eighteenth century, the plague appeared in Istanbul and Transylvania (1701–2) and spread over Ukraine (1703–4), Poland and Silesia (1706–9), Pomerania (1709–10), East Prussia (1708–10), and the Baltic States to Sweden and Denmark (1710–11), finally reaching Hamburg (1712) and threatening the Electorate of Hanover. The disease also occurred in southwestern Central Europe, where Hungary, Bohemia, Austria, as well

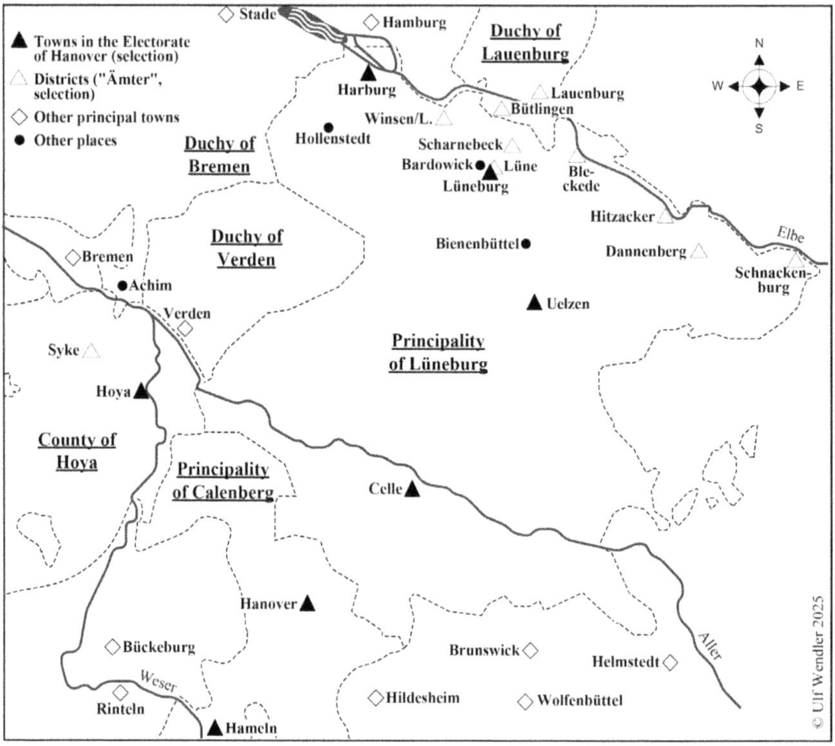

Map 7.1. The North of the Electorate of Hanover in 1705 and the acquisitions in 1719 (simplified). © Ulf Wendler

as Regensburg were affected (1713–14). This plague epidemic ended in early 1714 in most areas of Central Europe,[8] although there were still suspected cases of the disease in the Electorate of Hanover until 1716.[9]

The medical police orders of this territory during the epidemic corresponded to the demands of the time. This chapter will investigate the guiding principles of the Electorate of Hanover's government on which their orders were based. Two goals can be distinguished here. (1) The invasion of the plague had to be stopped at the borders of the territory and the spread of the plague in the country had to be prevented, respectively. (2) If there were cases of plague in one place, every effort was to be made to confine the outbreak to that village or town. The measures were staggered over time in three phases of initially low, then high, and finally diminishing threat from the epidemic.

While the possibilities for enforcing orders had grown under absolutism, they remained limited. Many orders issued by absolutist princes or their governments in reality were not or only partially implemented, or were adapted,

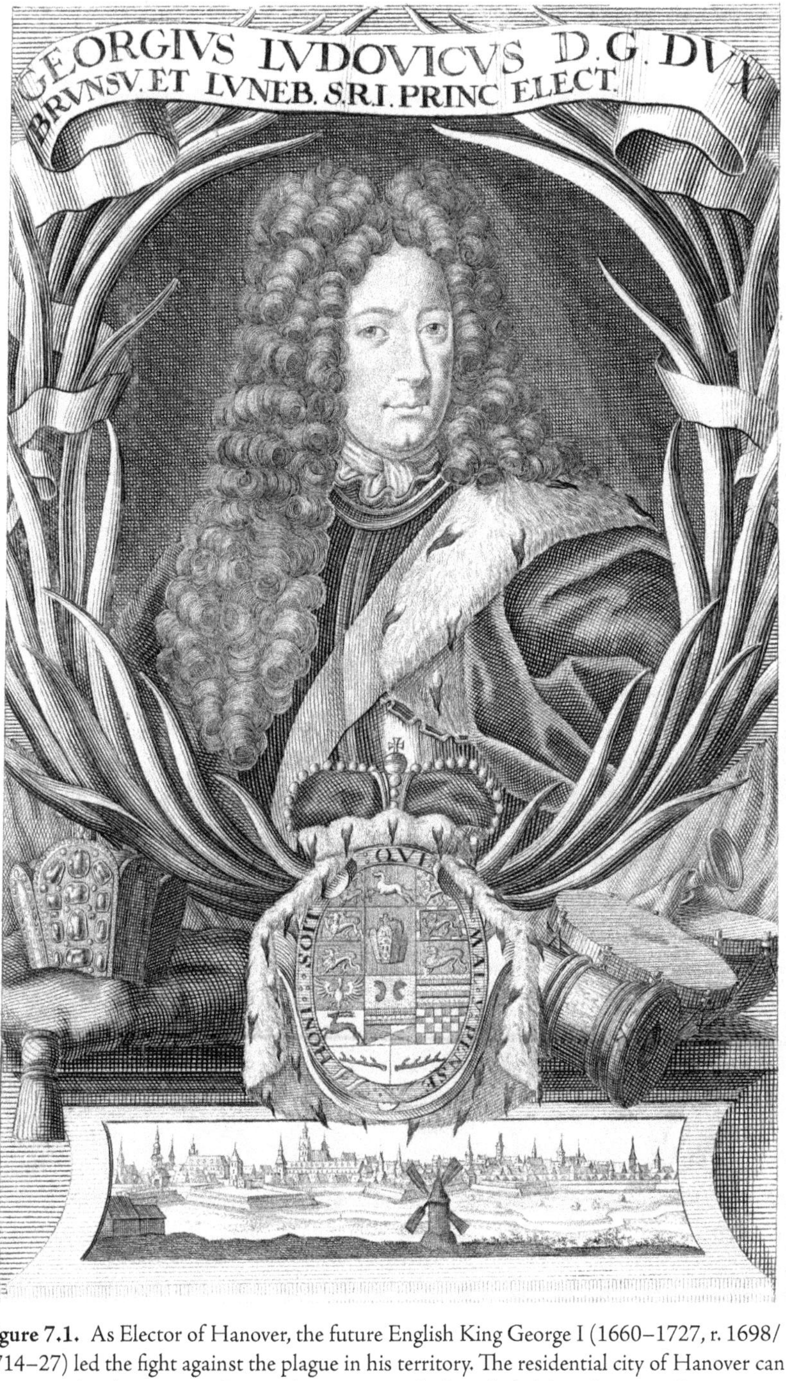

Figure 7.1. As Elector of Hanover, the future English King George I (1660–1727, r. 1698/1714–27) led the fight against the plague in his territory. The residential city of Hanover can be seen under the portrait. Copperplate engraving by Joseph de Montalegre, 1712, private collection. © Ulf Wendler

circumvented, or ignored by officials and subjects according to local circumstances and ideas. This can also be seen in relation to the containment of the plague. For this reason, the importance of disease control by absolutist states is assessed differently in the literature. While some authors attribute a decisive role to early modern state measures (especially cordons sanitaires) in the disappearance of plague epidemics from Europe at the end of the seventeenth century and in the course of the eighteenth century,[10] others consider them to be of secondary importance.[11]

Phase 1: Low Danger and the Exclusion of Vagrants, 1709–10

The Electorate of Hanover was in no way prepared for a health crisis in the early eighteenth century. For example, there was no central *Collegium Sanitatis*. Although one was suggested around 1685 and a proposal was formulated in 1710, it did not come to fruition.[12] The most important source for the government's ideas about fighting the plague were decrees, some of which were promulgated separately for the two principalities of Calenberg and Lüneburg. Between 1709 and 1716, the government issued at least 47 dated edicts related to plague. Their large number and distribution over the years reflects the sense of threat. While only one decree, or none at all, were issued in 1709, 1715, and 1716, there were many in 1710 and 1712 (Table 7.1). The government reacted on short notice to current threat situations. As a result, most edicts were promulgated during the warm, late summer and early fall months of August through October, when plague was particularly likely to spread (Table 7.2).

The government of the Electorate began to fight the plague before the disease reached the borders of the territory.[13] In Phase 1 of the disease control, trade was only slightly restricted. There was a perception that the plague could attach itself to objects with rough surfaces as well as textiles and the like. Consequently, a decree of January 1710 prohibited the importation of old clothes, bedding, hair, furs, wool, flax, hemp, feathers, etc. into the Electorate of Hanover.[14] However, goods were only a marginal concern during this stage.

Under the pretext of prevention, the government intensified its persecution of marginal groups.[15] Vagrant lower classes, whose members temporarily or permanently had no fixed place of residence where they could be controlled, were excluded from the territory (Figure 7.2).[16] They were under general suspicion for being itinerant, poor, and allegedly living in unsanitary conditions. These marginalized groups were believed to spread the disease easily. The government also feared that they would produce disorder through lack of discipline and their stay could cause food prices to rise.[17] Although other measures were later enacted, the association of vagrant marginal groups and members of the lower classes with the epidemic continued to be emphasized

Table 7.1. The distribution of plague edicts by year, 1709–16*

YEAR	NUMBER
1709	1
1710	15
1711	6
1712	15
1713	5
1714	4
1715	0
1716	1
Total	**47**

* *Landes-Ordnungen Lüneburg*, part 3, vol. 1, 1030–32, 1041–47; part 3, vol. 2, 1528–1656; *Landes-Ordnungen Calenberg, part* 3, 637–772.

© Ulf Wendler

Table 7.2. The distribution of plague edicts by month, 1709–16*

MONTH	NUMBER
January	3
February	1
March	0
April	2
May	1
June	1
July	2
August	13
September	9
October	6
November	3
December	3
Total	**44**

* *Landes-Ordnungen Lüneburg*, part 3, vol. 1, 1030–32, 1041–47; part 3, vol. 2, 1528–1656; *Landes-Ordnungen Calenberg*, part 3, 637–772. For three decrees, the year can be determined but not the month.

© Ulf Wendler

Table 7.3. Decrees against vagrant marginal groups, 1709–14*

Year	Number	Beggars, Vagrants, etc.	(Beggar) Jews	Roma	Deserters	Reference to the Plague
1709	2		1	1		1
1710	8	6	5	5		6
1711	6	4	5	1	2	4
1712	6	2	2	1	3	4
1713	1	1	1			1
1714	1	1	1			1
Total	24	14	15	8	5	17

* *Landes-Ordnungen Lüneburg*, part 3, vol. 1, 1021–47; part 3, vol. 2, 1528–1656; *Landes-Ordnungen Calenberg*, part 3, 148–64, particularly 154; 637–772, particularly 689–90.
© Ulf Wendler

throughout Phases 2 and 3 and served as a pretext for their exclusion. A total of twenty-four relevant decrees date from 1709 to 1714, seventeen of which make direct reference to the epidemic (Table 7.3). Persecution was particularly intense from 1710 to 1712.

In September 1709 the pastors of the Electorate read from the pulpits a decree expelling all Jews without a residence permit from the territory. The reason given was that plague was rampant in Pomerania, Prussia, and Poland, and could be further spread by Jews, and especially by the poor beggar Jews (*Bettel-Juden*) from these areas.[18] The decree was confirmed in January and August 1710.[19] At the end of August, foreign beggars, vagrants, and dissolute servants were forbidden to enter and stay in the Electorate of Hanover.[20] In an epidemic decree of September 1710, the government banned not only all beggars, Jewish and Christian, but also masterless servants and vagrants, discharged soldiers, dissolute craftsmen, vagrant students, sick people, and Roma (*Zigeuner*) from the Electoral Hanoverian territory.[21] Members of these itinerant and hardly controllable social groups were also forbidden to enter or stay in the territory in the following years (see Table 7.3).

Of these groups, the Jews were the most strongly opposed by the government and the most extensively dealt with in the decrees. There were differences among the Jews. The privileged ones were the protected Jews (*vergeleitete Juden* or *Schutzjuden*), who were placed under the protection of the absolutist sovereigns after providing evidence of sufficient assets or paying a sum of money. Most people of the Jewish faith did not belong to this group and did not enjoy as secure a status as the recognized members or servants of the Jewish

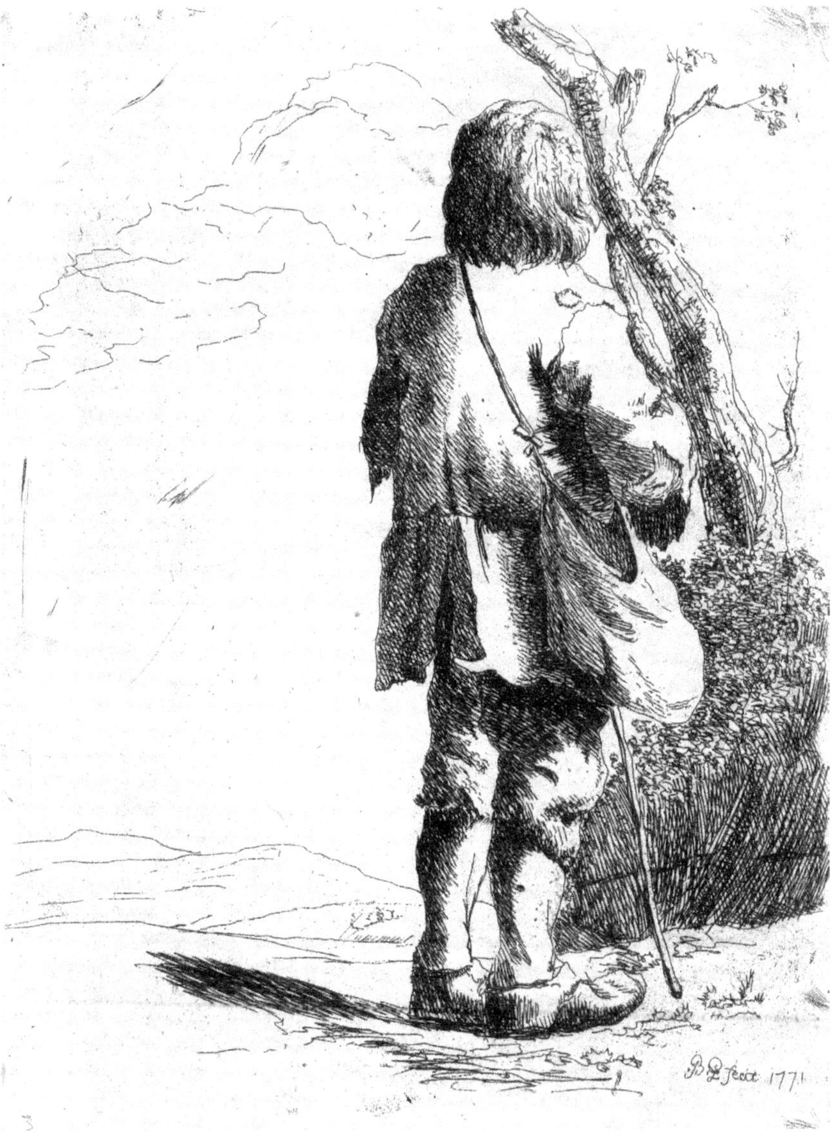

Figure 7.2. Vagrants, like this poor man, were defamed by the absolutist governments as spreaders of the plague. Etching by monogrammist B. G., 1771, private collection. © Ulf Wendler

community. This majority, without any rights of residence and legal livelihood, were sweepingly defamed as beggar Jews (*Bettel-Juden*), although in fact they had various professions and activities.[22]

A particularly hostile image was held of the allegedly impure, mostly Polish beggar Jews, who often traded in goods in which the plague could take root.[23] On the whole, foreign Jews were under general suspicion, especially if they came from distant regions. On the other hand, the protected Jews of northern and southern German territories and towns (Hamburg, Brunswick and the entire Guelph territories, Hildesheim, Halberstadt, Hesse-Kassel, Frankfurt, and Upper Germany) were allowed, at least initially, to stay in the Electorate of Hanover for necessary business and with official certificates.[24] However, they had to wait until the government allowed them to enter by means of a passport.[25] They often were suspected of giving their attestations to Jews from other regions.[26] The local protected Jews remained largely exempt from restrictions but were not allowed to bring the goods of foreign Jews into the country in their place.[27] Moreover, when they returned to their hometown from a trip, the elder of the local Jewish community had to confirm their identity.[28]

In 1711 and 1712, beggar Jews (as well as beggars, vagrants, and dissolute servants) were further prohibited from staying in the Electorate of Hanover. But in the decrees any reference to the spread of plague was absent because the danger of epidemic had decreased. In 1712, the government expressly forbade protected Jews from giving alms to or harboring beggar Jews. Instead, they were to report them to the authorities.[29]

When the plague raged in parts of South Germany and Austria in 1713, the anti-Jewish regulations were not only reinstated but also tightened. The government in Hanover feared that other territories would expel population groups such as beggars and beggar Jews as a first measure, just as it had done. Especially in Vienna and Prague, there were allegedly not only many beggar Jews but also numerous Jews who traded in used goods. According to the government's ideas, these people knew that they were not allowed to cross the established border checkpoints into other territories or into the Electorate of Hanover. Therefore, they tried to bypass the official routes to get to places where they could live. In this way, the epidemic could be imported into the Guelph territory. While its own protected Jews were tolerated in the Electorate of Hanover, other Jews wishing to pass through or reside in the area had to apply to the government for permission beforehand. All other people of the Jewish faith, with or without health passes from foreign authorities, had to leave the territory within eight days.[30] When the danger of epidemics in the Electorate of Hanover came to an end in 1714, the government nevertheless emphasized that the exclusion of beggar Jews as well as beggars and vagrants had not been canceled but should be continued.[31]

Under the threat of the epidemic, the government intensified the exclusion of marginalized groups, even if they were not linked to the spread of the disease. This is particularly striking in the case of the Roma, who were mentioned only in passing in connection with the plague threat. They, too, were forbidden to stay in the Electorate. At the end of November 1709 another pertinent edict was issued, this time about alleged criminal activities of the Sinti and Roma. The potential spread of epidemics did not play a role, which was assumed to be the case with the beggar Jews.[32] At all borders, posts bearing an inscription were to warn Roma against entering the Electorate of Hanover on pain of drastic penalties.[33]

Border regions that were particularly vulnerable but easy to control were already more closely monitored in Phase 1. The Electorate of Hanover had militias from the rural population, known as *Ausschuss*, that supported the regular army. In the Principality of Lüneburg, for example, for every nine peasants in each village one man between twenty and thirty-two years of age had to be drafted. Draftees had to remain militiamen (*Ausschussknechte*) for six years and were called up a few times a year for drills.[34] Similar institutions existed in the other Guelph territories.[35] After the Duchy of Lüneburg was united with the Electorate of Calenberg, four companies were formed. Long-serving soldiers, some of them retired, served as officers and sergeants.[36] In November 1709, militiamen from four districts (*Ämter*) close to the Elbe River[37] had to control and turn away strangers at various crossings over the river in the Principality of Lüneburg and in the Duchy of Lauenburg (Map 7.2).[38] They were supervised by the chairman of the Estates of the Principality of Lüneburg, Ernst Wilhelm von Spörcken (1665–1726, Figure 7.3). This capable man was repeatedly appointed by the government for special tasks. He supervised the actions of the responsible higher local officials, inspected the crossings, and reported to the government in Hanover.[39] Von Spörcken remained an important personality in the fight against the plague in the particularly endangered Principality of Lüneburg until the end of the plague. Some of the selected border checkpoints continued to be important crossing points for the next years but some were soon to be closed. This proves that the local knowledge of the government in Hanover was sometimes poor. This is also shown by the circumstances of the decree of September 1710, which will be discussed below.

Phase 2: Great Dangers and Decisive Action, 1710–14

In Phase 1, the Electorate of Hanover mainly issued decrees and used largely existing infrastructure to keep marginal social groups and some goods out of the territory. Because the situation had become more threatening in the second half of 1710, Phase 2 intensified measures. The Elector issued stricter edicts

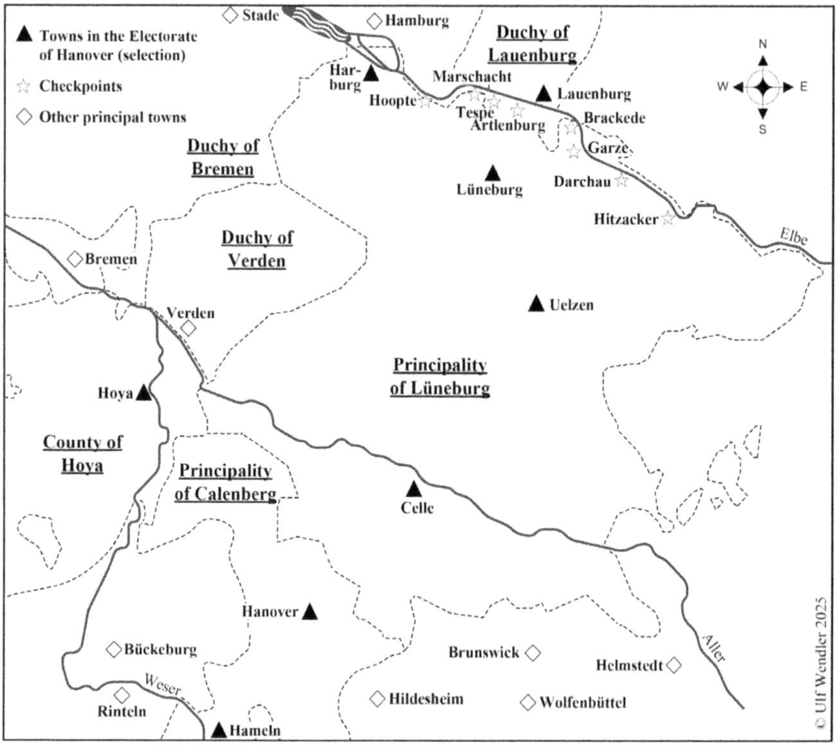

Map 7.2. Checkpoints along the Elbe River in November 1709. This border region was already monitored in Phase 1 (see Wendler, "Zirkulation," 82). © Ulf Wendler

that regulated access to the territory for almost all classes of the population and tightened the control of goods. Most importantly, an organization was established to enforce the measures, which did not exist in normal times. Plague secretaries and, later, plague inspectors were appointed to monitor the drastically reduced number of border crossings, and soldiers and militias manned the boundaries.

As the danger in the Electorate of Hanover grew in the late summer and fall of 1710, restrictions were placed both on the areas directly affected by plague, Western and Eastern Pomerania, Prussia, Poland, and Silesia, as well as on the neighboring territories of Mecklenburg, the Mark Brandenburg, and Saxony. No persons were allowed to enter from the infected areas, nor were goods that potentially carried the plague allowed to be brought in. The importation of these goods from neighboring territories was also prohibited. A little later, the government stipulated that travelers from infected areas had to prove by

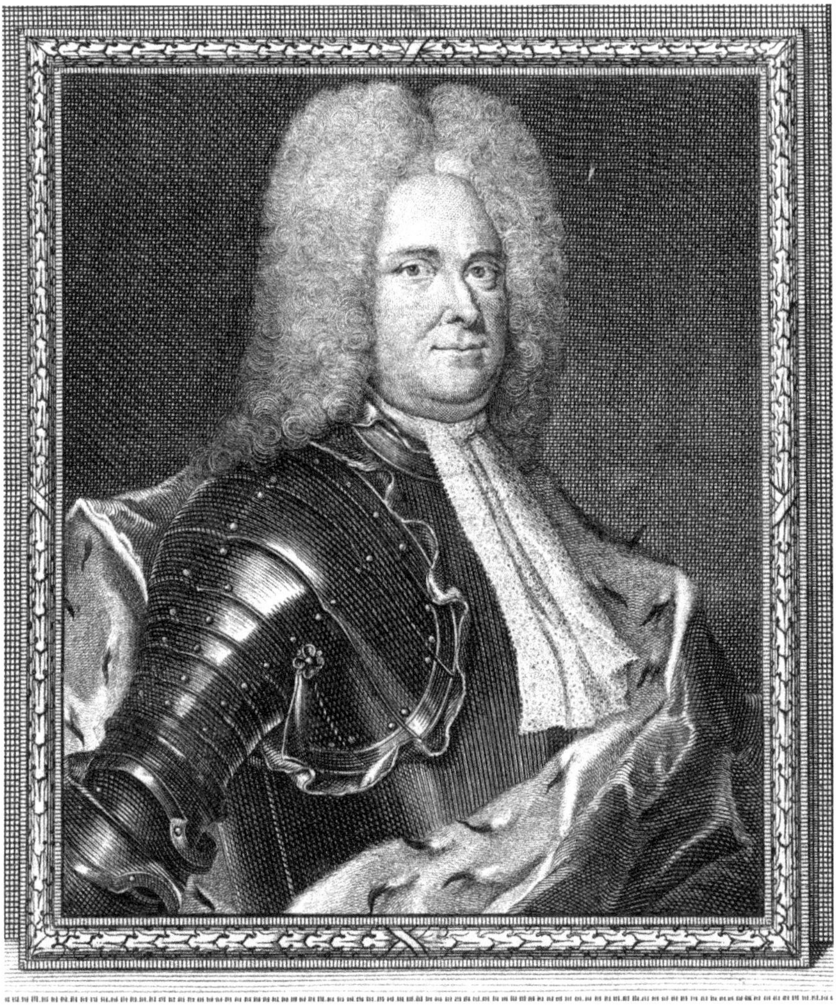

Figure 7.3. Ernst Wilhelm von Spörcken (1665–1726) led the fight against the plague along the Elbe River in 1712. Copperplate engraving by J. G. Fritsch, 1726, private collection. © Ulf Wendler

means of an official health certificate that during the last forty days they had not stayed in plague-infected places. They had to confirm their declarations by taking an oath at the borders of the Electorate. Comparable proof was mandatory for goods. Hanover also required certificates, or at least sworn affidavits, for persons and goods from non-suspicious places that they had not been in contaminated places for the previous forty days.[40]

The government not only issued decrees but also wanted to see them implemented. To do this, an organization had to be established to protect the borders that did not exist in this form in normal times. This was especially necessary for the Principality of Lüneburg, which was particularly threatened by the epidemic due to its geographical location, first in the east, then in the north, and finally in the west. The Elector did not get serious about epidemic defense until September 1710, when border checkpoints were established that all travelers and freight carriers had to use (Map 7.3). At the designated points, plague secretaries controlled the entry, especially checking health passes. Such checks were to take place not only at the designated border sites but also at the gates of individual towns. Innkeepers were forbidden to accommodate travelers without health certificates.[41] The goal was to control travelers several times at three levels: at the external border, at the city gates, and at inns.

Plague secretaries were required to check travelers or transported goods at the borders and at important inland stations. They had to turn away potentially dangerous people and goods. In September 1710 these were appointed,

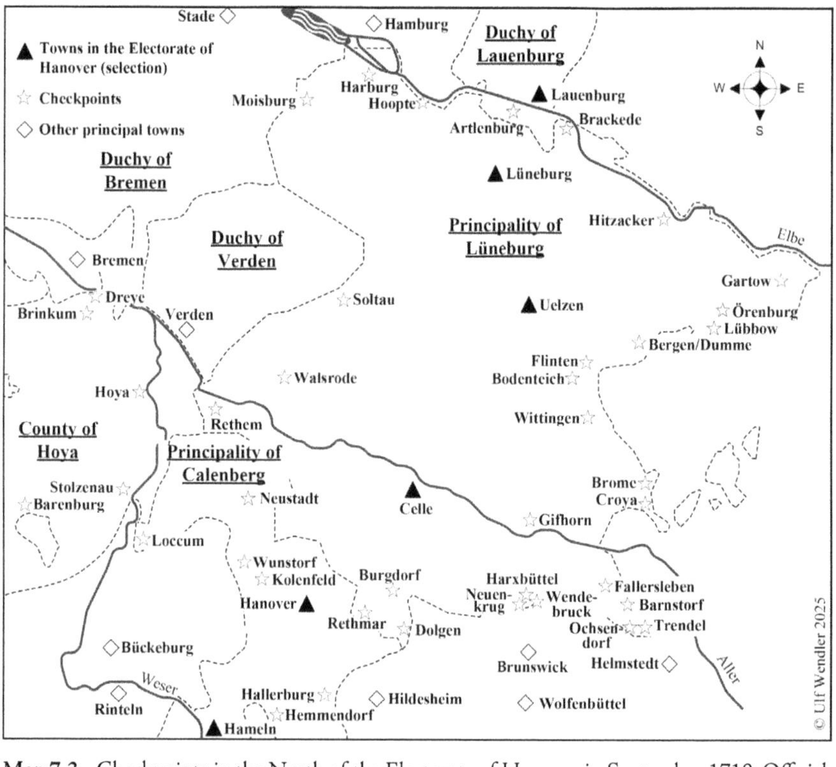

Map 7.3. Checkpoints in the North of the Electorate of Hanover in September 1710. Official crossings were established along all borders (see Wendler, "Zirkulation," 84). © Ulf Wendler

or gate and border scribes were made plague secretaries.[42] They were instructed by a comprehensive decree in November.[43] Officials were to keep a sharp watch on all travelers not only at the external borders but also inside the territory.[44] Health passes and certificates were to be issued and sealed only by state institutions. First, officials had to verify that there was no contagious disease at the place of issue. Then the full name, occupation, and appearance of the passport holder had to be listed, also where he came from, where he had stayed for how long, and where he intended to travel. In the case of goods, the place of manufacture, sale, and packing, as well as the route of transportation, were to be specified.[45]

Due to the government's lack of local knowledge the September decree listed only a few border checkpoints, which affected travel disproportionately. But not all small roads could or needed to be guarded, because at that point the danger was not so great. The government realized that the measures could not be enforced in this way. Still, it wanted all those who did not enter through the official border checkpoints to be severely punished. The problem could be alleviated only by opening more checkpoints. Therefore, officials had to report which important border crossings had been left unmentioned in the edict.[46] A new decree in November listed significantly more checkpoints where health passes could be presented (Map 7.4).[47] Due to the objections of the government of the Duchy of Lauenburg, the subjects there received a few additional privileges with regard to traffic routes.[48] These processes show the interplay between the government and local officials, in the course of which the official border crossings were determined.

The various instructions against the plague were repeated, summarized, and supplemented by additional regulations in a decree at the beginning of November 1710. Courland and Livonia were now also considered infected areas. The following month, the government confirmed this edict. All innkeepers and village leaders were to be informed of it, so that the regulations could be disseminated as widely as possible.[49] In another edict, the duke informed his subjects that they had to present their health passes at certain places when entering the duchies of Bremen and Verden.[50]

In the spring of 1711, the threat of plague temporarily subsided. For this reason, goods from Mecklenburg (except Friedland), the Mark Brandenburg west of Berlin, all of Saxony, and Silesia west of the Oder River were now permitted to be transported through the Electorate of Hanover once again, under certain conditions. In the Guelph territories, these goods were not allowed to be opened under any circumstances. The restrictions on the movement of people and goods with the duchies of Bremen and Verden were removed, and the corresponding plague secretaries withdrawn.[51] At the end of May 1711, the border passes were maintained only against the Mark Brandenburg and along the Elbe River. The others were abolished.[52]

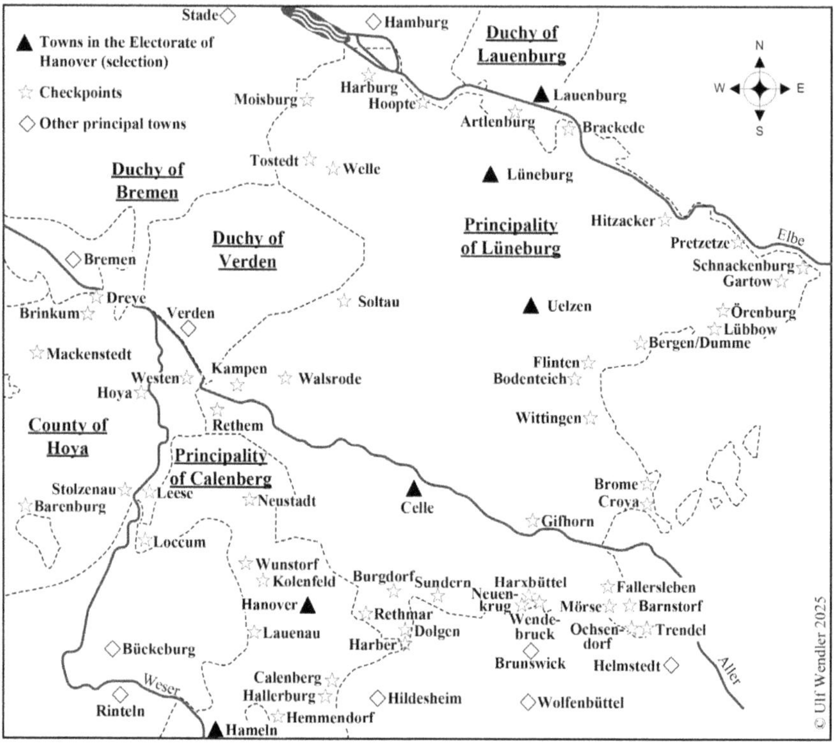

Map 7.4. Checkpoints in the North of the Electorate of Hanover in November 1710. A larger number of official crossings were established along all borders (see Wendler, "Zirkulation," 85). © Ulf Wendler

While conditions in Eastern Europe began to improve in 1711, the danger in the north increased. After the Netherlands restricted trade with the Electorate of Hanover, decisive action was taken again in the early autumn. To protect this trade and the inhabitants altogether, no more travelers were allowed to land from the Danish islands and from Scania, and no more goods were allowed to be brought into the country. The importation of any goods from Hamburg, Altona, Lübeck, Holstein, Lauenburg, Mecklenburg, and Pomerania to which the plague might potentially be attached was prohibited. All other goods could be imported with an official certificate that provided information about their origin and transport route. Persons were allowed to enter if they proved by health passes that they had not been in an infected place for six weeks.[53]

The outbreak and spread of the plague were promoted by the Great or Second Northern War of 1700–20, in which Sweden fought Russia, Denmark, Saxe-Poland, Prussia, and the Electorate of Hanover (from 1713) for power in northern and northeastern Europe. In 1709, the Swedes suffered a decisive defeat in Russia. In the years that followed, the opposing alliance (including, above all, Denmark) attempted to neutralize or conquer the Swedish possessions in the Baltic region and northern Germany. A key role was played by Schleswig-Holstein, which was ruled partly by the Danish king and partly by the duke of Gottorp, who was allied with Sweden. The armies of the time were frequently plagued by epidemics. For example, after an unsuccessful campaign by the Danes against Sweden in 1710, the plague spread from Scania via Denmark to Schleswig-Holstein, where numerous cases of the disease occurred in 1711–12.[54] Therefore, in the summer of 1711 the Electorate of Hanover harbored fears regarding deserters from the Danish army who could possibly come across the Elbe River from Schleswig-Holstein (see Table 7.3). No one was allowed to cross the river without permission, and boats had to be tied up at night.[55]

The threat in the north was joined by that in the west. The duchies of Bremen and Verden belonged to Sweden since 1645/48. Denmark tried to take the duchies, but the Guelphs also wanted to expand their territory by annexing this area.[56] On 31 July 1712 the invasion by the Danish army began from Holstein. Stade, the heavily fortified capital and administrative center of the duchies, fell on 7 September; the territory of Bremen was now in Danish hands.[57] In a manifesto of 27 July, shortly before the invasion, the Swedish governor pointed out that the Danish army had spread the plague in Holstein and would do the same in the duchies of Bremen and Verden in case of war.[58] In reality, however, plague was already rampant in Stade beginning on 18 July and continued to claim victims until the beginning of 1713.[59]

The Electorate of Hanover had secured part of the booty even before the Danish attack. Hanoverian troops moved into the Duchy of Verden at the end of July. This occupation and the establishment of a chain of guards on the Este and Wümme rivers in the Duchy of Bremen were intended to prevent the plague from spreading to the Electorate from the west. In the posting, in the interest of expedience, no consideration was to be given to the official border between the principalities of Lüneburg and Bremen.[60] The area occupied by the Danes, including Stade, had to be rigorously cordoned off.[61]

In 1712, the danger of epidemics increased for the Electorate of Hanover. The plague was rampant in Holstein, which belonged to Denmark, so since July 1712 the entry and import of goods from the area were prohibited.[62] On 23 July members of the Danish army were generally forbidden from entering the country, and all boats on the Elbe and Weser rivers were to be carefully tied up to prevent any illegal river crossing.[63]

Now plague decrees were issued at short intervals in an attempt to avert the danger once again.[64] On 4 August the government issued a comprehensive edict. It stated that there were probably cases of plague among the Danish troops who had invaded the Duchy of Bremen. The border, especially with Holstein, not only had to be marked by posts and straw as before, but additionally black boards had to be attached to the poles. They warned that anyone trying to enter from infected or suspicious places would be shot.[65]

Entry from the Duchy of Bremen and from Holstein was prohibited. From Hamburg, Lübeck, and Mecklenburg, travelers were allowed to enter the Electorate of Hanover via only five border crossings, with health passes and after taking an oath.[66] Controls were now not only carried out at the border crossing points and town gates but also in the interior of the territory along the Aller River. Locals could cross the river on seven bridges, but foreigners were allowed to use only the four bridges in the west of the Principality of Lüneburg (Map 7.5).[67]

In addition to the manning of the borders by militiamen and soldiers, the plague secretaries were crucial for the control of traffic flows. Every fifteen to twenty kilometers an official crossing point was created where the plague

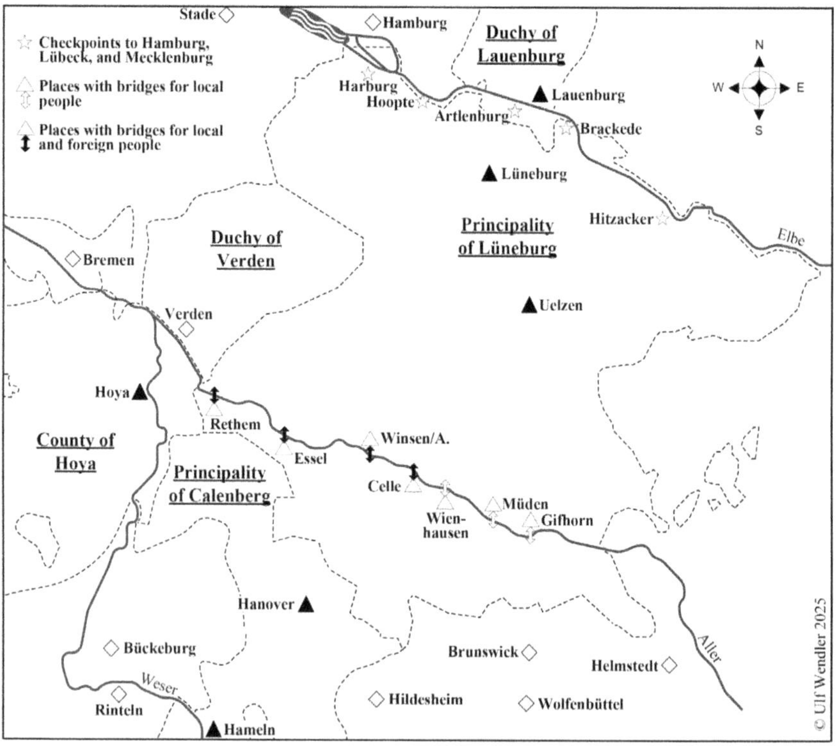

Map 7.5. Checkpoints to Hamburg, Lübeck, and Mecklenburg as well as bridges in the Principality of Lüneburg in November 1712 (see Wendler, "Zirkulation," 88). © Ulf Wendler

secretaries were posted together with guards. The secretaries had to check travelers and turn them away if necessary. If unauthorized persons tried to break through, they were first to be warned and then shot if unresponsive.[68] The plague secretaries were subordinate to the districts. In the summer of 1712 plague inspectors were appointed, who had to inform the plague secretaries about all official regulations, as well as supervise them day and at night.[69]

In four decrees of 11, 12, and 20 August and of 5 September 1712, the earlier prohibitions were partially reconfirmed. In particular, beggar Jews and Danish deserters were repeatedly forbidden to stay (see Table 7.3). Entry from the Duchy of Bremen and, especially, from plague-stricken Stade was prohibited.[70] The government tried to enforce the strict regulations.[71]

In November, the Elector and the Privy Council entrusted Ernst Wilhelm von Spörcken with the overall supervision of all epidemic matters for the particularly threatened northern part of the Principality of Lüneburg and southern part of the Duchy of Lauenburg. In the affected districts[72] along the Elbe River officials had to follow his instructions.[73]

The year 1713 initially brought an apparent easing of the situation. However, the plague was not yet over, as became apparent in the summer. In August 1713 a decree stated that the plague was rampant in Austria, Bohemia, Regensburg, and the Principality of Oels in Silesia. From these territories, as well as from Moravia and Silesia east of Wroclaw, no one was allowed to enter the Electorate of Hanover, nor were goods to be imported from there. The stay of non-protected (*nicht vergeleiteten*) Jews and beggars in the territory was forbidden once again.[74]

However, the threat of the epidemic spreading was not from the south but from the north. In 1713 the plague raged in the most important neighboring trading city. In Hamburg, the disease broke out for the first time in September 1712 but died down in the following winter months. It occurred a second time in midsummer 1713 and lasted until spring 1714. In 1713 alone, an estimated six thousand to seven thousand Hamburg residents died from the plague.[75] On 22 March 1714 the city celebrated its deliverance from the disease with thanksgiving services and by firing small cannons.[76]

The government in the Electorate kept a close eye on the situation in the Hanseatic city. It not only received reports from its diplomats in Hamburg but also sent a surgeon[77] there in early 1713 to make unobtrusive inquiries. When it became clear in 1713 that the plague was rampant, Danish and Hanoverian troops sealed off the city. Traffic with the important trading center was completely interrupted. This was intended not only to prevent the spread of the plague but also at the same time to divert as much of Hamburg's trade traffic as possible to Altona in Danish territory or to Harburg in the Electorate of Hanover.

From October 1713 on, people from Hamburg could enter the Electorate only after a quarantine of thirty days. Apart from wine, brandy, wine vinegar, herrings, metals, and minerals, no goods were allowed to be imported from the city. There was a designated district, Grasbrook, for the transfer of trade goods, where traders from Hamburg had to deposit their goods according to certain rules. In addition, new docks were built there for seagoing vessels. Electoral Hanoverian bargemen unloaded the goods from the seagoing ships and handed them over to the Hamburg traders in accordance with a specified procedure. The loading of the seagoing vessels with trade goods from the city was just as complicated. The mediation of Hanoverian skippers prevented English and Dutch seamen from coming into direct contact with people from Hamburg who might have fallen ill.[78]

These strict measures were intended not only to prevent the disease from entering the city but also to ensure that no other states issued bans against the Electorate of Hanover. The magistracy of Hamburg gave assurances at the end of December that the epidemic had abated in the city, which further news confirmed. Nevertheless, the central government in Hanover admonished its officials in Harburg not to deviate under any circumstances from the existing regulations. Although such diseases subsided in the winter, they could increase again in the spring.[79] Despite these concerns, facilitation of trade in certain goods was allowed under specific conditions.[80] Distrust remained high because merchants of Hamburg were accused of disregarding protective regulations in the greedy quest for profits.[81]

In Phase 2, the activities of the Electorate of Hanover to combat the epidemic represented a major effort, not only organizationally but also financially. For five years, from 1709 to 1714, around 1,400 Reichsthaler were reportedly needed monthly just to pay plague officials in the Electorate of Hanover. In addition, there were costs for the localities isolated from the outside, some of which had to be fed for eight months, the replacement payments for burned-down houses with the furniture in them, etc.[82] The government tried to keep the costs low or to pass them on to the local level or to find new sources of money. Thus, the towns themselves had to provide quarantine houses if they did not already exist. In the villages, these were not to be newly built but a suitable existing building was to be designated for this purpose. If possible, the quarantines had to be financed from local revenues. On the other hand, the government paid for the construction of guardhouses at the Aller River bridges and for the firewood for the guards. The militia received no pay when they were deployed within their districts. However, with the onset of winter in 1712 the necessary firewood appeared too expensive to the government, so the militiamen were to be sent home. Nevertheless, the officers had to impose controls to prevent suspicious persons from staying in their areas.[83]

The government tried to find additional sources of money. In July 1713 a collection was announced to replace the objects and houses burned because of the plague. Fundraisers had to go from house to house in the villages and towns, collecting money from the inhabitants and recording the amounts in a book.[84] However, the costs of fighting the plague were covered mainly by taxes. In the Principality of Lüneburg the estates approved and collected these levies. They raised over 14,000 Reichsthaler from 1 October 1713 to 31 July 1714 alone (of which over 1,600 Reichsthaler came from the collection mentioned above). This money was not enough, because the Lüneburg share of the expenditures during this period amounted to about 18,000 Reichsthaler. The central government in Hanover therefore demanded an additional payment.[85]

Phase 3: Diminishing Danger and the Return to Normality 1714–16

After the danger of epidemic had subsided, the restrictions were partially withdrawn and finally abolished in Phase 3. The organization was slowly dismantled, i.e. the border guards were abandoned and the plague secretaries dismissed. The implementation of the measures took place through many individual commands over a longer period of time. While the important decrees of Phases 1 and 2 were carefully preserved and later printed in law collections, this did not happen for the edicts of Phase 3. This makes the source situation for this period more difficult than for the first two phases.

The measures against Hamburg were gradually lifted in 1714. In February the Hanoverian Elector significantly expanded the scope of goods that could be imported, with a bill of lading now sufficing for importation. Two months later, the quarantine for noble people and merchants was reduced to five days. Vagrants, beggars, Jews, craftsmen, and discharged soldiers from Hamburg and the areas beyond the Elbe River remained prohibited from entering the country. Goods to which the plague could adhere were still not allowed to be brought in. All other goods could be imported if they came from a merchant whose house had been spared from the plague and who had employed only healthy people for packing.[86]

In Electoral Hanover, the measures to contain the plague were officially lifted on 30 May 1714. Thanksgiving services for deliverance from the plague were held in July.[87] The celebrations were a bit premature. In the following year, the outbreak of the plague was again feared in certain locations in the south of the Duchy of Lauenburg and in the Principality of Lüneburg.[88] There was also still a danger of epidemics in neighboring foreign territories.[89]

The longer the measures were in place, the more of a burden they became. Yet, it took quite some time before the restrictive orders on the Electorate of Hanover's borders were gradually revoked. For example, the men stationed against Hamburg on the Elbe River and in the Duchy of Lauenburg were not allowed to leave their posts until the end of June. Nevertheless, even though trade and commerce were permitted without sworn passes, dangerous goods (feather beds, rags) as well as beggars, beggar Jews, or other vagrants still were not let in.[90]

By the end of July 1714 all measures to combat the plague were finally discontinued. The plague secretaries in Harburg, Lüneburg, and at the border crossings along the Elbe River were informed accordingly.[91] But it was not until March 1716 that the last plague secretaries in Lüneburg and along the Elbe River could be dismissed.[92] Now the danger was finally over.

Fighting Individual Outbreaks of Plague

When Richard Mead praised the measures of the Electorate of Hanover in 1722, he was not primarily referring to the shut-off measures against foreign countries. The action at the country borders had been effective but had little relevance to the situation in the British Isles. For Mead, the primary focus was on how plague outbreaks were controlled locally in the Electorate.

In the Hanoverian territory, disease control measures were similar everywhere because they were implemented and coordinated at the highest level. The early modern state used all its resources of power to effectively contain the epidemic even in small villages and prevent it from spreading further. Beginning with the 1722 edition, Mead's *Short Discourse* quoted in its introduction a revealing report, dated 10 February 1722, sent to him by Secretary Backmeister, an employee of the Hanoverian government chancellery. The account, an extraordinary and unique primary source for the Electorate, described in detail the principles and procedures for combating the plague in 1712 and 1713. Backmeister, "who was the Person, that issued out the Orders that were given," reported in a somewhat idealized way on the measures taken after an outbreak of the plague.[93] In retrospect, these seemed very successful.[94]

According to the description, the sick and the healthy had to be separated from each other. The government isolated an infected village so that the inhabitants could not communicate with others. Those trapped in the village were reportedly immediately provided with all the necessities of life. The physical and spiritual needs of the villagers were taken care of by medical personnel, like a doctor and surgeons, and a plague pastor. Nurses and gravediggers were also employed.

The sick came to a specially built lazaretto. Their unaffected housemates had to undress at night, burn their clothes, and move into quarantine in a separate building in new clothes they were given. The changing of clothes and burning of the old textiles were repeated whenever it was necessary. For example, this happened when someone recovered and left the lazaretto to go into quarantine. Or if a sick person died, his nurse, the gravedigger, and the surgeons had to change clothes before isolating themselves. In summer, the quarantine places were huts that were set on fire after use.

The houses abandoned by their inhabitants were to be boarded up and guards placed in front of them. In the countryside, buildings were burned down if they were of low value, as long as this could be done without endangering neighboring farms. Public funds compensated the owners. In towns, burning down was not possible without endangering them. Therefore, men were hired to clear the houses of all goods potentially bearing the contagion. They burned them in the yards or in front of the buildings. If neighbors felt that this endangered them too much, the goods were taken outside the town on funeral carts and destroyed there. Initially the suspicious objects had only been buried—but they were sometimes dug up again, whereupon the infection continued.

Until those affected had been compensated for the loss of their homes and goods, they hid individual items, thus spreading the disease. However, when they received adequate compensation for their losses from the public funds, they consented to burning without hiding anything.

The authorities left the cattle outside the farms in summer. The inhabitants of non-contaminated farms were obliged to take care of the animals of those who were quarantined. In winter, before leaving an infected property to go into quarantine, healthy people were required to kill the livestock and bury them ten feet deep.[95]

Backmeister's descriptions are not later ideas that were projected back but, rather, present as a unique contemporaneous source. The account was essentially in line with the government's intentions and policies during the epidemic that are also found in the edicts of the time. For example, in 1712 cleanliness was generally decreed inside and outside the houses, and individual towns had to select buildings to quarantine plague sufferers. All residents had to purchase food and fuel for a year within six weeks so that there would be no famine if infected places were isolated by guards and ditches. Pharmacists as well as brewers and merchants had to stock up on the necessary medicines and supplies for this period. Towns had to build up their own stocks. Fairs as well as trade in old clothes were prohibited.

If the plague broke out in a town, the government was to be notified immediately. The village had to be isolated, for which purpose palisades were to be erected or deep ditches dug on occasion. Guards were to man the entrances. No one was allowed to leave and communication with the outside was cut off. If anyone tried to leave the place, he could be shot. In the villages, plague hospitals and quarantine houses were to be selected and the government was to be informed. The local administrations had to provide food and medicine for those who were trapped. During deliveries, a safety distance of forty paces was to be maintained. Preachers, physicians, and surgeons were allowed to enter infected places.[96]

Regulations were issued, probably in 1712, for plague physicians and plague surgeons. Physicians had to perform their duties faithfully and obediently and had to stay in a place where they could be easily found when needed. The physicians had to send a report about the sick to the government every two weeks. Surgeons were additionally admonished to obey their superior physicians and keep them informed of everything. Mainly, both decrees consisted of brief instructions on how to treat the sick.[97]

How the government attempted to implement the principles formulated in these decrees on the local level is shown by an order dated 11 September 1712. This was issued for the village of Brinkum, south of Bremen (see Maps 7.3 and 7.4) in the County of Hoya, that belonged to the Electorate of Hanover.[98] Officials from the district[99] had to isolate the village and specifically seal off infected houses with militiamen. A sergeant and four ordinary soldiers were also sent from Verden. Anyone who tried to leave Brinkum or the infected houses had to be shot.

In front of the village, huts were to be erected for the sick. The healthy people from the infected houses had to bring the sick to the huts and board up the residential buildings. Nothing was to be taken from the farms. The healthy ones should then quarantine in other huts. The guards had to watch everything, but without coming closer than forty paces. A bench was erected in an open field, and what the isolated needed in medicine and food was to be put on it. When the bearer had left, the isolated were allowed to fetch the goods.

The doctor was to stay outside Brinkum and get reports from the two surgeons in the village. He could be spoken to only from forty paces away, and only in the open and against the blowing wind. The doctor and the surgeons should receive well-waxed overgarments for visiting the sick. The existing surgeon was to be prevented from leaving so that he could be called upon in case of emergency.

On occasion, the cattle were to be driven through the water to another pasture. Fowl as well as dogs and cats had to be shot immediately. In addition, a plan of the village had to be made to decide whether the infected houses could be set on fire without danger to the other buildings. The district should lay out all costs and make an account of it.[100]

In 1713 the Elector of Hanover personally described similar measures to the Saxon Privy Councils in Dresden regarding the plague-infected village of Bienenbüttel (south of Lüneburg, see Map 7.1). He had ordered the place to be isolated on all sides. Thus, no one could leave the village and communication with the outside world was no longer possible. The inhabitants had to leave their infected houses, with the sick moving into plague huts and the healthy into quarantine huts. The healthy should first burn all objects from the infected houses that could transmit the plague. The Elector asserted that the measures were successful. He also intended to have the infected buildings burned down.[101]

Implementation Problems in Reality

The Electoral Hanoverian government made determined attempts to prevent the advance of the plague. But it remains doubtful whether the early modern state had the necessary resources of authority, personnel, and money to implement its measures. The central government sent officials and soldiers to the borders and to infected localities. It provided money and other resources. Above all, based on its ideas, the government ordered drastic measures through decrees and numerous letters. But what was the likelihood that these were actually implemented? Research in recent decades has demonstrated that absolutist states often achieved little with their edicts. For governments of territorial states of the time, it was particularly difficult to influence local conditions directly and to impose their will on individual subjects. Orders from the superiors were modified, mitigated, or overridden by local officials and subjects considering current conditions.[102] In addition, cities such as Bremen sometimes succeeded in obtaining special relief by bribing leading members of the Hanoverian government or the officials they sent to gather information.[103]

In the Electorate of Hanover the main measures were to control external borders and to isolate places affected by the plague. But the implementation was necessarily incomplete. It is easy to find cases of non-compliance.[104] For example, in July 1713 a woman traveled to Hamburg and returned to her home village of Hollenstedt (south of Hamburg, see Map 7.1) with rags from the city. There she infected a farm before she died of the disease herself. Not only the illicit passing but also the strictly forbidden trade in old clothes and rags could not be stopped.[105] Backmeister's 1722 report that was printed by Richard Mead tells the story of three men who came from Hamburg to Achim (east of Bremen, see Map 7.1) without permission. There they spent the night in a barn, where they were found dead the next day with signs of plague. The barn was burned down, supposedly stopping the spread of the plague.[106] This allegation was not true, because in this village of about three hundred inhabitants more than fifty people fell victim to the plague.[107] Backmeister's account thus is not only idealized but false.

The most controversial measure taken by the central government was the burning down of buildings, which it considered to be the safest means. Yet there was strong opposition to this, even from local electoral officials designated to carry out appropriate orders. This was the case, for example, in the above-mentioned village of Bienenbüttel.[108] Therefore only the insignificant shepherd's house was burned down there, while the other infected houses were cleaned.[109] The villagers received no monetary compensation for the value of the building but got a commitment for the timber for the reconstruction and the assumption of craftsmen's expenditures. But the residents had to do the actual work and ultimately also had to procure some of the wood themselves. Despite the difficulties, the house was rebuilt in 1714–15.[110] Backmeister's description of the unproblematic burning down and financing of the destroyed houses corresponded to reality only to a limited extent.

There is an interesting eyewitness account from Bienenbüttel by the local pastor Philipp Julius Toppius (1649–1727). He described the measures taken to protect the borders of the Electorate of Hanover against the plague. The inhabitants of the village felt safe because they lived roughly in the middle of the Principality of Lüneburg. However, in the summer of 1713 travelers brought the epidemic to the village. As a result, Bienenbüttel was isolated from the outside world by militiamen and regular soldiers. The pastor criticized the measures taken in detail and sharply condemned the behavior of the authorities' plague officials as well as the plans to burn down buildings. For example, he did not kill his two dogs as ordered as a preventive measure but chained them up for five months. When the epidemic was over in the village at Easter 1714, but public worship was still prohibited, the pastor and many but not all parishioners defied this. Yet, despite the criticisms and the individual transgressions, Toppius was essentially in agreement with the measures taken.[111]

Further examples could be provided to show that central government regulations were not or only partially implemented at the local level or that absolutist power was limited in reality. Frequently, broad assumptions about the power of absolutist states do not hold. One particular document provides information about the possibilities and limits of the absolutist state: the health pass of Margaretha Raehnen. The twenty-seven-year-old woman had this passport issued to her at her residence in Lüneburg on 24 May 1712. The town was not infected with the plague, as affirmed in the document. Margaretha Raehnen was of medium build, had a narrow face, and wore a blue jacket (*Kamisol*) with red flowers, but no wig, as the description says. In an arm basket she carried spigots (*Bier Haan*), spoons, and ribbons for sale, with which she wanted to go to "Bron" (perhaps Brome) and Uelzen

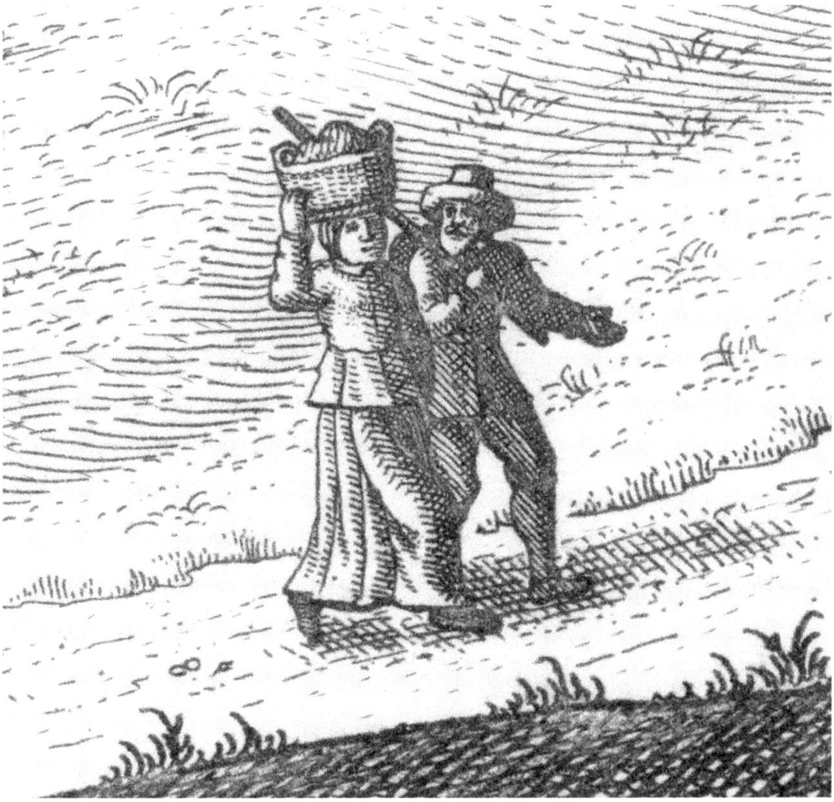

Figure 7.4. This woman in the Lüneburg area, like Margaretha Raehnen, wears a "Kamisol" and carries a basket of goods. Etching, city view of Lüneburg (detail) by Merian, 1654, private collection. © Ulf Wendler

(Figure 7.4). With the goods and the health pass, she traveled to the extreme south of the Principality of Lüneburg before arriving back in her hometown on 3 July. On the way, she was checked at seven places and finally in Lüneburg (Table 7.4, Map 7.6).

Although the passport was limited to twenty days and had long since expired, Margaretha Raehnen undertook a second journey with it shortly thereafter. She again went to the east and south of the Principality of Lüneburg before returning at the end of August or beginning of September. This time Margaretha Raehnen was checked in nine locations (Table 7.4, Map 7.7). But there is no proof of where she had stayed for more than a month. Either she remained in one place for this time or she crossed the border to a different state. In general, she stayed in many border places without it being known whether she had left the Electorate of Hanover. Her health pass has no foreign entries.

Table 7.4. The journeys of Margaretha Raehnen, 1712*

Places	Date
[Journey 1]	**24 May to 3 July**
Lüneburg (today Kreisfreie Stadt)	24 May
Bad Bodenteich (today Landkreis Uelzen)	28 May
Brome (today Landkreis Gifhorn)	30 May
Ahnebeck (today part of the municipality Parsau (Landkreis Gifhorn))	1 June
Tiddische (today Landkreis Gifhorn)	2 June
Trendel (today estate in the municipality of Rennau, joint municipality of Grasleben (Landkreis Helmstedt))	9 June
[Expiration of the health pass]	**12 or 13 June**
Brome (today Landkreis Gifhorn)	17 June
Wittingen (today Landkreis Gifhorn)	19 June
Lüneburg (today Kreisfreie Stadt)	3 July
[Journey 2]	**6 July to 31 August**
Hitzacker (today Landkreis Lüchow-Dannenberg)	6 July
Pretzetze (today part of the municipality Langendorf/Elbe (Landkreis Lüchow-Dannenberg))	9 July
Schnackenburg (today Landkreis Lüchow-Dannenberg)	14 July
Brome (today Landkreis Gifhorn)	20 July
Croya (today part of the municipality Parsau (Landkreis Gifhorn))	22 July
Ahnebeck (today part of the municipality of Parsau (Landkreis Gifhorn))	22 July
Fallersleben (today part of Wolfsburg (Kreisfreie Stadt))	23 July
Stederdorf (today part of the municipality of Wrestedt (Landkreis Uelzen))	29 August
Bad Bevensen (today Landkreis Uelzen)	31 August

* StadtA LG, St. Mich., Rep. B 22, Nr. 11, Health pass Margaretha Raehnen, Lüneburg May 24, 1712.
© Ulf Wendler

At the end of the journey, her passport, which had been expired for months, was confiscated in Lüneburg.[112]

Not only was Margaretha Raehnen checked frequently but this happened even in places that were not designated as checkpoints in the official decrees. Yet she was able to use her health pass even though it had expired. It can be noted that control was comprehensive by early modern standards but by no

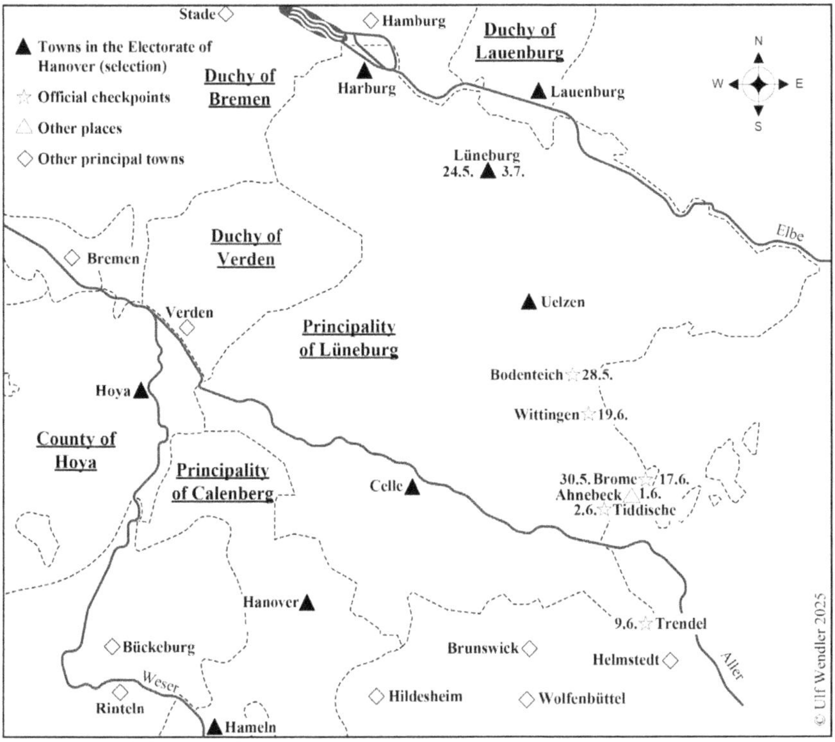

Map 7.6. The first journey of Margaretha Raehnen, from 24 May to 3 July 1712. © Ulf Wendler

means complete. Such a conclusion can also be drawn for the Electorate of Hanover's efforts as a whole: they were intensive for the time but not perfect.

Conclusion

When the plague reached Northern Germany in the early eighteenth century, the government in Hanover gained a reputation among neighboring states for its resolute fight against the epidemic.[113] The territory's medical police arrangements during the 1709–16 plague epidemic met the demands of the time in an almost ideal way. Quarantine, cordoning off, and isolation were the most important measures to prevent the invasion and spread of epidemics. They were suitable for fighting a contagious epidemic.

The procedure in Electoral Hanover followed a specific scheme. Phase 1 (1709–10) largely used the existing infrastructure to exclude and control

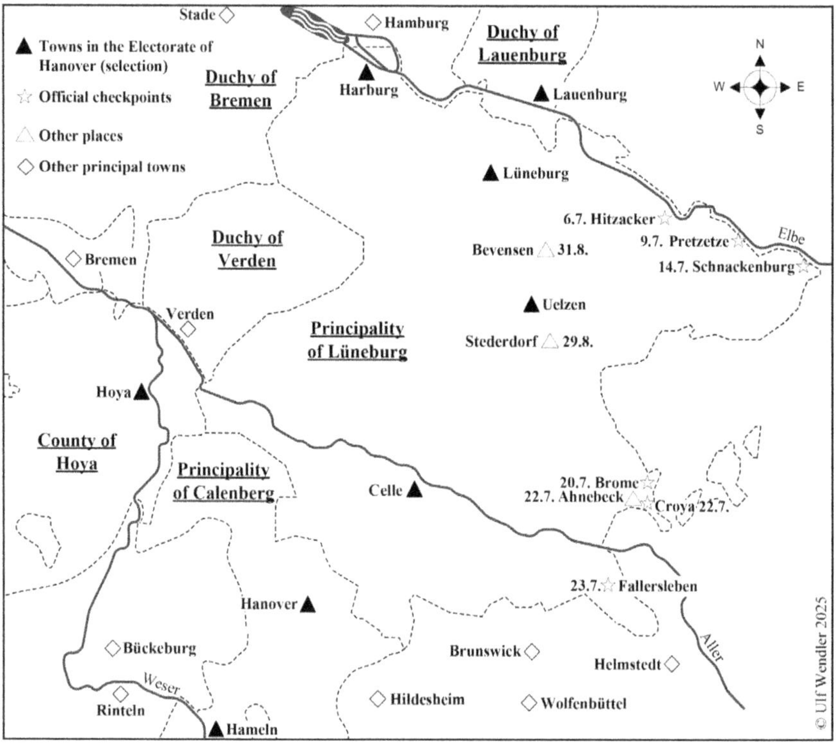

Map 7.7. The second journey of Margaretha Raehnen, from 6 July to 31 August 1712. © Ulf Wendler

marginal social groups and some goods. These were no longer allowed to enter or be imported into the territory. It is already clear from the first decrees that the absolutist state combined disease prevention with the fight against disliked social groups, which were also excluded and persecuted in normal times. While in the beginning it was mainly then the non-protected beggar Jews, the circle was quickly expanded to include all vagrant population groups. Vagrants were blamed for possibly unintentionally or negligently spreading the epidemic. However, they were not held responsible as scapegoats for the epidemic itself.

As the threat situation intensified, the government stepped up measures. In Phase 2 (1710–14) the aim was to combat the plague with determination. Not only were more edicts promulgated but also, above all, great organizational and financial efforts were made. It was a matter of cordoning off the territory so that the movement of people and goods could be regulated. Militiamen and regular soldiers manned the borders, which could be crossed only at certain points, with plague secretaries and plague inspectors controlling travelers and goods. In the interior, traffic was also monitored at town gates and bridges. For coordination and supervision in a particularly threatened region, a high and capable nobleman was given special powers. Hanoverian troops even moved into the neighboring duchies of Bremen and Verden to establish a health cordon. Depending on the threat situation, the measures were relaxed or tightened again.

In Phase 2 the plague appeared sporadically in the territory. There were clear rules for the procedure in the contaminated villages and towns. The settlement was isolated and within the village the (still) healthy were separated from the sick. The patients had to be treated in a kind of lazaretto. Medical and spiritual personnel took care of the physical and spiritual needs of the sick. All potentially infected objects were to be burned, including, in the countryside, even buildings of little value.

As the threat of epidemic decreased, normalization began in Phase 3 (1714–16). Restrictions and controls had been gradually introduced and were only reluctantly lifted. The epidemic regime lasted significantly longer than the real threat situation would have actually required. Gradually, the militiamen and regular soldiers, and finally also the plague secretaries, were withdrawn from the border. In 1714 the population in the territory celebrated the liberation from the plague, but there was disturbing news about plague cases until 1716.

The sporadic outbreaks of plague in the Electorate of Hanover remained isolated events; a widespread epidemic did not occur. Accordingly, government officials later proudly and confidently described the measures taken in a report sent to the famous English physician Richard Mead, who published it in his *Plague Treatise*. The officials exaggerated the effect of the measures and idealized the government's approach.

The success of the Electorate of Hanover stood in marked contrast to earlier conditions and to other early modern states. Referring to the conditions of the seventeenth century, one historian wrote about a neighboring territory: "My research from Braunschweig-Wolfenbüttel demonstrates the unevenness of plague legislation and its limited enforcement and efficacy. It shows that the financial limitations on the central government hampered its effectiveness, and it suggests a lack of centralized sovereignty in matters relating to the health of the territory's subjects and to threats from outside the boundaries of the territory."[114] In view of this conclusion, it is not surprising that historians formulated fundamental doubts about the abilities of absolutist states to control epidemics. In the Electorate of Hanover, too, numerous cases can be identified in which central government measures failed, were circumvented, or were inadequately implemented. This would seem to confirm the view that it was fundamentally impossible for an absolutist central state to implement its directives and thus achieve its ambitious goals in disease control. But this conclusion falls short and is too general. An early modern territorial state could achieve considerable success in the eighteenth century under certain circumstances. Two conditions were required for this.

First, the central government had to be determined to respond decisively and consistently.[115] This presupposed the conviction that the absolutist state was capable of successful disease control. The Electorate of Hanover did not have a disaster plan for combating an epidemic in advance, but it could draw on experience from previous epidemics.[116] Above all, the promising methods (quarantine, cordoning off, isolation) had been known for centuries. The decisive innovation was that they were now applied with great effort to an entire territory. The government obviously had a clear vision of what to do but reacted ad hoc to each threat situation. The great resources of the early modern state were mobilized for fighting the epidemic. Within a comparatively short time, an organization for the control of and defense against suspicious people and goods at the borders and town gates could be established and maintained for several years. The government was also able to enforce drastic measures in individual infected places and effectively isolate villages from the outside world. In the process, early modern state power took hold of a village and its inhabitants in a way that would not have been possible in normal times for organizational and financial reasons. Fortunate circumstances contributed to the success of the Electorate of Hanover. The plague did not get out of control in the territory at any time. For the most part, only individual villages were infected at different times, which could be isolated and supplied with everything necessary one after the other with manageable resources.[117] The Electorate of Hanover would probably not have been able to contain a large-scale outbreak of the disease.

Second, the central government needed the cooperation of local officials and the population to ensure the effectiveness of the measures ordered. The sources examined provide only rudimentary evidence of their support. For example, when the government excessively restricted the number of border crossings in the fall of 1710, complaints about this quickly led to a correction. Research has found that when an epidemic threatened, there was an increased willingness at the local level to obey orders from the central government.[118] Evidence for the Electorate of Hanover also shows that orders from above were implemented and largely followed. It is clear that in combating the plague in the early eighteenth century there was not only an unusual determination on the part of the central government, but also a new acceptance of the prescribed measures on the part of the subjects. This points to new attitudes. In the face of the epidemic, the government felt obligated, responsible, and able to care for the health of the population. This was also expected by the subjects, who in return more or less supported the measures taken by the authorities, or at least accepted them to a certain extent.

Thus, for all the imperfections of implementation, the fundamental effectiveness of the great efforts of the Electorate of Hanover cannot be denied. The determined action of the government between 1709 and 1716 was a major factor in ensuring that the last plague outbreak in the region did not have worse consequences.

In the introduction, the controversial question among researchers whether the measures of the absolutist states contributed significantly to the disappearance of the plague in the eighteenth century was mentioned. Absolutist states like the Electorate of Hanover were basically able to use the means at their disposal to ensure that the epidemic did not spread as quickly and widely as in previous centuries. However, other territories were partially unwilling or unable to take such measures. The actions implemented to combat epidemics by the absolutist states differed. The regulations and procedures of the early modern territories contributed to the disappearance of the plague in Western and Central Europe but cannot fully explain it; for a full answer a range of other factors will have to be examined as well.

Ulf Wendler served as City Archivist of Chur, Grisons, Switzerland, from 2006 to 2024. He has been working as a freelance historian since 2024. Ulf Wendler studied history and European ethnology in Hamburg and Zurich. He received his MA (1991) and PhD (1997) degrees from the University of Hamburg. His primary research field is German early modern historical demography and plague history, and his secondary field is Swiss social history. His best-known publications about the plague include *Nicht nur Pest und Pocken. Zur Bevölkerungsgeschichte des Fürstentums Lüneburg 1550–1850* (Hanover 2008), *Pestilentz im Norden. Seuchen in der nördlichen Lüneburger Heide und im Süden Hamburgs 1657–1716* (Ehestorf 2012), and *Pest, Fleckfieber, Ruhr und Typhus. Epidemien auf dem Land und ihre Deutung im Fürstentum Lüneburg 1565–1666* (Göttingen 2024).

Notes

Some of this material was previously published in German in Wendler, "Zirkulation," 77–101. See for the Principality of Lüneburg Wendler, *Pestilentz*, 99–143.

1. Mead, *Short Discourse*, XXXI. See Slack, *Impact*, 327–34.
2. See the overview at Rödel, "Obrigkeiten," 192–204.
3. Sticker, *Abhandlungen*, vol. 1/II, 295–96.
4. Sticker, *Abhandlungen*, vol. 1/I, 51–52, 55–56; vol. 1/II, 222, 264, 294.
5. Sticker, *Abhandlungen*, vol. 1/I, 109–10, 123, 182–83; vol. 1/II, 319; Dinges, "Pest," 305–6.
6. Christensen, *Politics*, 136.
7. Sticker, *Abhandlungen*, vol. 1/I, 135–36 (Digne 1629).
8. Eckert, "Retreat," 17–21; Friemann, "Diarium," 137; Wohlwill, *Hamburg*, 57; Haeser, *Lehrbuch*, vol. 3, 454–59; Sticker, *Abhandlungen*, vol. 1/I, 213–21; about East Prussia see Sahm, *Geschichte*, 35–175.

9. Wendler, *Pestilentz*, 198–211.
10. Mattmüller, *Bevölkerungsgeschichte*, vol. 1, 239–44; Rödel, "Obrigkeiten," 204–5.
11. Dinges, "Pest," 83–85; see the differentiated judgement of Schlenkrich, *Gevatter Tod*, 380.
12. Deichert, *Geschichte*, 15–18. Hamburg established its "Collegium" in 1710. Wohlwill, *Hamburg*, 44.
13. The Electorate of Hanover apparently reacted as early as 1707 to the plague that was spreading in Eastern Europe, but little is known about the measures taken. See Wendler, *Pestilentz*, 99–101.
14. *Landes-Ordnungen Lüneburg*, part 3, vol. 2, 1530–32.
15. Bulst, "Krankheit," 34–35.
16. See Küther, *Menschen*.
17. *Landes-Ordnungen Lüneburg*, part 3, vol. 1, 1030, 1041–42.
18. *Landes-Ordnungen Lüneburg*, part 3, vol. 2, 1528–32.
19. *Landes-Ordnungen Lüneburg*, part 3, vol. 2, 1530–35.
20. *Landes-Ordnungen Lüneburg*, part 3, vol. 1, 1030–32.
21. *Landes-Ordnungen Lüneburg*, part 3, vol. 2, 1544; see Schnath, *Geschichte*, vol. 3, 274; Schwarz, *Pest*, 21, note 6.
22. Breuer, "Frühe Neuzeit," 132–40; Lowenstein, "Anfänge," 174–76; Marx, *Geschichte*, 59–66, 92–95.
23. *Landes-Ordnungen Lüneburg*, part 3, vol. 2, 1528. Hamburg thought and acted similarly. Wohlwill, *Hamburg*, 43–44.
24. *Landes-Ordnungen Lüneburg*, part 3, vol. 2, 1534, 1544.
25. *Landes-Ordnungen Lüneburg*, part 3, vol. 2, 1539; 1567–68.
26. *Landes-Ordnungen Lüneburg*, part 3, vol. 2, 1536, 1539.
27. *Landes-Ordnungen Lüneburg*, part 3, vol. 2, 1531.
28. *Landes-Ordnungen Lüneburg*, part 3, vol. 2, 1568.
29. *Landes-Ordnungen Lüneburg*, part 3, vol. 1, 1032–41.
30. *Landes-Ordnungen Lüneburg*, part 3, vol. 2, 1633–41.
31. *Landes-Ordnungen Lüneburg*, part 3, vol. 1, 1043–47.
32. *Landes-Ordnungen Lüneburg*, part 3, vol. 1, 1021–25.
33. *Landes-Ordnungen Lüneburg*, part 3, vol. 1, 1026.
34. *Landes-Ordnungen Lüneburg*, part 2, 212–15.
35. For Calenberg see *Landes-Ordnungen Calenberg*, part 3, 193–203.
36. Sichart, *Geschichte*, vol. 1, 278–81; vol. 2, 115–17.
37. Districts (Ämter) of Winsen/Luhe, Lüne, Bleckede and Dannenberg (see Map 7.1).
38. Hoopte, Marschacht, Brackede, Garze, Darchau, and Hitzacker in the Principality of Lüneburg and Tespe and Artlenburg in the Duchy of Lauenburg (see Map 7.2). Stadtarchiv Lüneburg (hereafter: StadtA LG), St. Mich., B 22, Nr. 8/I, Elector Georg Ludwig to Landschaftsdirektor von Spörcken, Görde 14 November 1709.
39. StadtA LG, St. Mich., B 22, Nr. 8/I, Elector Georg Ludwig to Landschaftsdirektor von Spörcken, Görde 14 November 1709. See also Gebhardi, *Kurze Geschichte*, 108–10; Weyhe-Eimke, *Aebte*, 340–54.
40. *Landes-Ordnungen Lüneburg*, part 3, vol. 2, 1532–35; 1543–44.
41. *Landes-Ordnungen Lüneburg*, part 3, vol. 2, 1535–39.
42. *Landes-Ordnungen Lüneburg*, part 3, vol. 2, 1541–51; see Schnath, *Geschichte*, vol. 3, 274.

43. *Landes-Ordnungen Lüneburg,* part 3, vol. 2, 1561. The questionnaire on persons and goods is quoted in Wendler, *Pestilentz,* 106–7.
44. *Landes-Ordnungen Lüneburg,* part 3, vol. 2, 1567, 1583.
45. *Landes-Ordnungen Lüneburg,* part 3, vol. 2, 1535–51.
46. *Landes-Ordnungen Lüneburg,* part 3, vol. 2, 1555–57.
47. *Landes-Ordnungen Lüneburg,* part 3, vol. 2, 1565–66; see Schnath, *Geschichte,* vol. 3, 274.
48. Due to objections of the Lauenburg government, a little later Lauenburg subjects with valid health passes were allowed additionally to use the Darchau ferry across the Elbe River. StadtA LG, St. Mich., B 22, Nr. 10/I, "Extract der nach und nach von Hhr. Churfürstl. Durchl. Gdst. ergangenen Verordnungen," 1712–13, Nr. 88 (6 September 1712). The duties of a plague secretary were taken over by the local customs officer Rautenkranz. Ibid., Nr. 121 (9 September 1712). See ibid., Nr. 115 (13 September 1712?), that the inhabitants of the Neuhaus district were allowed to cross the Elbe River with permits but were not allowed to transport passengers.
49. *Landes-Ordnungen Lüneburg,* part 3, vol. 2, 1557–75, 1593–98.
50. At the Burger Schanze and in Hastedt, Achim, Verden, Langwedel, Scheßel, and Altenkloster. StadtA LG, AA, V 3, Nr. 12, Regulation of Elector Georg Ludwig, Göhrde 30 November 1710.
51. *Landes-Ordnungen Lüneburg,* part 3, vol. 2, 1598–1600; Schnath, *Geschichte,* vol. 3, 274; Schwarz, *Pest,* 24.
52. *Landes-Ordnungen Calenberg,* part 3, 689–90.
53. *Landes-Ordnungen Lüneburg,* part 3, vol. 2, 1604–08. On the approach of the Netherlands see Schwarz, *Pest,* 24–25.
54. Persson, "Boy," 175–85; Frandsen, "Krieg," 206–15; Frandsen, *Last Plague,* 467–79; Gaul, *Möglichkeiten,* 19–28; Hansen, *Geschichte,* 98–109.
55. *Landes-Ordnungen Lüneburg,* part 3, vol. 2, 1600–02.
56. Krüger, *Erwerb,* 16–20; Schnath, *Geschichte,* vol. 3, 653–61.
57. Krüger, *Erwerb,* 33–42, 53–55; Schnath, *Geschichte,* vol. 3, 672–73; *Stade,* 196–97.
58. Krüger, *Erwerb,* 45. According to Gaul, the first appearance of the plague in Schleswig-Holstein cannot be precisely dated but the epidemic can be traced to various places as late as September and October 1712. Gaul, *Möglichkeiten,* 25–28.
59. Kroll, "Pest," 47–48; *Stade,* 207–8.
60. Krüger, *Erwerb,* 48–51; Schnath, *Geschichte,* vol. 3, 668–72; StadtA LG, St. Mich., B 22, Nr. 11, Privy Council to Oberhauptmann von Spörcken in Harburg, Hanover 1 August 1712.
61. StadtA LG, St. Mich., B 22, Nr. 10/I, "Extract der nach und nach von Hhr. Churfürstl. Durchl. Gdst. ergangenen Verordnungen," 1712–13, Nr. 18 (14 August 1712), 19 (15 August 1712), 23 (9 August 1712), 59 (25 August 1712), 67 (29 August 1712), 70 (29 August 1712), 86 (6 September 1712), 129 (22 September 1712). Generalmajor von Klinckowström's mission was recorded in an instruction that gives a good overview of his duties and the measures taken to regulate traffic. It is quoted in Wendler, *Pestilentz,* 123–25.
62. *Landes-Ordnungen Lüneburg,* part 3, vol. 2, 1608–9.
63. *Landes-Ordnungen Lüneburg,* part 3, vol. 2, 1610–12; StadtA LG, St. Mich., B 22, Nr. 11, Privy Council to Oberhauptmann von Spörcken in Harburg, Hanover 1 August 1712.

64. See also the edict of 4 August 1712, Schnath, *Geschichte*, vol. 3, 274–76.
65. "Diejenigen, welche sich von inficirten oder der Pest halber verdächtigen Orten einschleichen werden, sollen ohne Gnade am Leben gestrafet und erschossen werden." *Landes-Ordnungen Lüneburg*, part 3, vol. 2, 1576–77.
66. The border crossings were Harburg and Hoopte for Hamburg, Artlenburg for Lübeck, and Brackede and Hitzacker for Mecklenburg. About the conditions in Hoopte see Puffahrt, "Maßregeln," 53–58.
67. The bridges at Wienhausen, Müden, and Gifhorn were passable only for locals; at Rethem, Essel, Winsen, and Celle, foreigners were also allowed to cross the river. *Landes-Ordnungen Lüneburg*, part 3, vol. 2, 1576–77, 1579, 1581–82.
68. StadtA LG, St. Mich., B 22, Nr. 11, Instruction for the plague inspector Niepot, Hanover 1 August 1712.
69. StadtA LG, St. Mich., B 22, Nr. 11, Instruction for the plague inspector Niepot, Hanover 1 August 1712.
70. See the summary of the regulation in StadtA LG, St. Mich., B 22, Nr. 10/I, "Extract der nach und nach von Hhr. Churfürstl. Durchl. Gdst. ergangenen Verordnungen," 1712–13, Nr. 1 (11 August 1712); *Landes-Ordnungen Lüneburg*, part 3, vol. 2, 1614–18, 1624–28, 1637–40; see Krüger, *Erwerb*, 54, note 255, that many Danish soldiers did not desert, only because, as potential plague infected persons, they had nowhere to go.
71. See the examples in Wendler, *Pestilentz*, 130–34.
72. Districts (Ämter) of Harburg, Winsen/Luhe, Bütlingen, Scharnebeck, Lüne, Bleckede, Hitzacker, Dannenberg, and Schnackenburg as well as Lauenburg (see Map 7.1).
73. StadtA LG, St. Mich., B 22, Nr. 11, Privy Council to the Districts of Harburg, Winsen/Luhe, Bütlingen, Scharnebeck, Lüne, Bleckede, Hitzacker, Dannenberg, Schnackenburg, and Lauenburg, Hanover 13 November 1712.
74. *Landes-Ordnungen Lüneburg*, part 3, vol. 2, 1633–41.
75. Friemann, "Diarium," 131–40; Wohlwill, *Hamburg*, 50–70; Boyens, "Krise," 295.
76. Lieboldt, "Dankfest," 159–60.
77. Wohlwill, *Hamburg*, 57.
78. Wohlwill, *Hamburg*, 56–60, 70–77; *Landes-Ordnungen Lüneburg*, part 3, vol. 2, 1641–43; Puffahrt, "Maßregeln," 54–55; Boyens, "Krise," 310–11.
79. StadtA LG, St. Mich., B 22, Nr. 10/II, Privy Council to Oberhauptmann von Spörcken, Hanover 24.12.1713.
80. StadtA LG, St. Mich., B 22, Nr. 10/II, Privy Council to Oberhauptmann von Spörcken, Hanover 24 December 1713; ibid., Elector Georg Ludwig to Landschaftsdirektor von Spörcken, Hanover 9 January 1714; see ibid.: Instruction for the plague secretary Bergmann in Hoopte by Landschaftsdirektor von Spörcken, Lüneburg 10 January 1714.
81. StadtA LG, St. Mich., B 22, Nr. 10/II, Elector Georg Ludwig to the City of Hamburg, Hanover 4 January 1714.
82. StadtA LG, St. Mich., B 22, Nr. 10/II, Elector Georg Ludwig to Landschaftsdirektor von Spörcken, Hanover 3 August 1713 (recte 1714).
83. *Landes-Ordnungen Lüneburg*, part 3, vol. 2, 1628–31.
84. *Landes-Ordnungen Lüneburg*, part 3, vol. 2, 1632–33.
85. StadtA LG, St. Mich., B 22, Nr. 10/II, Elector Georg Ludwig to Landschaftsdirektor von Spörcken, Hanover 3 August 1713 (recte 1714).
86. *Landes-Ordnungen Lüneburg*, part 3, vol. 2, 1644–49.

87. Wendler, *Pestilentz,* 32–34; Schnath, *Geschichte,* vol. 3, 276.
88. 1714–15 in Tespe and Artlenburg (see Map 7.2), 1715 in Bardowick (north of Lüneburg, see Map 7.1), and 1715–16 in Celle. Wendler, *Pestilentz,* 198–208; Pagel, "1715/16," 106–22; *Landes-Ordnungen Lüneburg,* part 3, vol. 2, 1653–56; Spangenberg, *Beschreibung,* 54–55; Cassel, *Geschichte,* vol. 1, 484.
89. For example, in Boizenburg/Elbe in Mecklenburg. StadtA LG, St. Mich., B 22, Nr. 8/IV, Privy Council to Landschaftsdirektor von Spörcken, Hanover 13 September 1715; ibid., Surgeon Feder to Landschaftsdirektor von Spörcken, Lüneburg 13 September 1715; ibid., Surgeon Feder to Landschaftsdirektor von Spörcken, Lüneburg 14 September 1715; ibid., Landschaftsdirektor von Spörcken to the District of Bleckede, Lüneburg 15 September 1715; ibid., Duchy of Lauenburg to Landschaftsdirektor von Spörcken, Ratzeburg 16 September 1715.
90. StadtA LG, St. Mich., B 22, Nr. 10/II, Elector Georg Ludwig to Landschaftsdirektor von Spörcken, Hanover 29 June 1714; ibid., Elector Georg Ludwig to Generalmajor von Gauvain, Pyrmont 29 June 1714.
91. In Hoopte, Artlenburg, Brackede, Hitzacker, Schnackenburg, and at the dam of Pretzetze (see Map 7.4). StadtA LG, St. Mich., B 22, Nr. 10/II, Elector Georg Ludwig to Landschaftsdirektor von Spörcken, Hanover 14 July 1714; ibid., Letter by Landschaftsdirektor von Spörcken, Lüneburg 19 July 1714. For the dam of Pretzetze see Wendler, *Pestilentz,* 112–13.
92. In Lüneburg at the Bardowicker Gate and in Hoopte, Artlenburg, and Brackede (see Map 7.4). StadtA LG, St. Mich., B 22, Nr. 8/II, Regulation of King Georg, Hanover 18 March 1716; Puffahrt, "Maßregeln," 58.
93. Mead, *Short Discourse,* 1722, XXX–XXXVI.
94. Mead, *Short Discourse,* XXX.
95. Mead, *Short Discourse,* XXXI–XXXVI.
96. *Landes-Ordnungen Lüneburg,* part 3, vol. 2, 1575–93; see Schnath, *Geschichte,* vol. 3, 274–75.
97. *Landes-Ordnungen Lüneburg,* part 3, vol. 2, 1618–24; similar StadtA LG, AA, C 3, Nr. 7, "Instruction vor dem H. Pestmedico e. e. hochweis. Rath übergeben von denen beyden Herren Physicis 1712" (quoted in Wendler, *Pestilentz,* 243–51); ibid., "Instruction vor die beyden Pest-Chirurgos auff e. e. hochweisen Raths Verlangen entworffen und überreichet von denen beyden Herren Physicis," Lüneburg 24 October 1712 (quoted in Wendler, *Pestilentz,* 252–54).
98. See Schwarz, *Pest,* 50, 56–57.
99. District (Amt) Syke (see Map 7.1).
100. StadtA LG, St. Mich., B 22, Nr. 10/I, "Extract der nach und nach von Hhr. Churfürstl. Durchl. Gdst. ergangenen Verordnungen," 1712–13, Nr. 108 (11 September 1712). See the measures in Welle at Deichert, *Geschichte,* 238–39.
101. StadtA LG, AA, C 3, Nr. 8, Elector Georg Ludwig to the Privy Council in Dresden, Hanover 9 September 1713.
102. Brakensiek, "Akzeptanzorientierte Herrschaft," 395–97, 404; Tammen, *Staatlichkeit,* 346–62.
103. Schwarz, *Pest,* 32–34, 53–55, 67, 78, 80, 82, 87; see Wohlwill, *Hamburg,* 60.
104. Examples among others in Wendler, *Pest und Pocken,* 93.
105. Wendler, *Pestilentz,* 99–101, 131–32, 165–66.
106. Mead, *Short Discourse,* XXXI–XXXII.

107. Gerhold, "Narren," 156.
108. Wendler, *Philipp Julius Toppius*, 150.
109. StadtA LG, St. Mich., Rep. B 22, Nr. 10/II, District of St. Michaelis to Privy Council, Lüneburg 14 January 1714.
110. StadtA LG, St. Mich., Rep. B 22, Nr. 19, Municipality of Bienenbüttel to Landschaftsdirektor von Spörcken, Bienenbüttel 9 October 1714 (with decision of Landschaftsdirektor von Spörcken, Lüneburg 11 October 1714); ibid., Nr. 8/II, "Anno 1714 Waß zu Bienenbüttel an der Hirten Kohte … ."
111. Wendler, *Toppius*, 147–70, 399–405.
112. StadtA LG, St. Mich., Rep. B 22, Nr. 11, Health pass Margaretha Raehnen, Lüneburg 24.5.1712.
113. See for example Wohlwill, *Hamburg*, 57, note 1.
114. Christensen, *Politics*, 89.
115. In particular the neighboring large trading cities of Bremen and Hamburg lacked such a will, so that they sometimes perceived the Electorate of Hanover's measures as harassment. Schwarz, *Pest*, 44–47, 53–62, 65–68, 73–74, 78–83, 86–87; Wohlwill, *Hamburg*, 48–50, 56–63, 68–70, 76–79, 90–102, 104–7, particularly 98–102, 105–6.
116. See Wendler, *Pestilentz*, 71–98.
117. Wendler, *Pestilentz*, 147–211.
118. Christensen, *Politics*, 206–7, 218.

Bibliography

Archival Sources

Stadtarchiv Lüneburg (StadtA LG)

AA, C 3, Nr. 7: "Actorum betr. die eingelangten Churfürstl. Verordnungen und Rescripta wegen der Contagion, auch desfalls gemachte ordnungsmäßige Vorkehrung de 1709–14."

AA, C 3, Nr. 8: "Actorum betr. die eingelangten Churfürstl. Verordnungen und Rescripta wegen der Contagion, auch desfalls gemachte ordnungsmäßige Vorkehrung de 1709–14."

AA, V 3, Nr. 12: "Verordnungen," 7 January 1710–28 December 1719.

St. Mich., B 22, Nr. 8 (new: St. Mich., Nr. 689/1–5): "Acta betr. Contagionssachen," 1709–19.

St. Mich., B 22, Nr. 10 (new: St. Mich., Nr. 691, 692/1–2): "Acta betr. Kontagionssachen in specie die Veranstaltung gegen die Stadt Hamburg wegen der dort herrschenden Seuche," 1712–14.

St. Mich., B 22, Nr. 11 (new: St. Mich. Nr. 693/1–3): "Acta betr. varia in Kontagionssachen," 1712–15.

St. Mich., Rep. B 22, Nr. 19 (new: St. Mich., Nr. 701): "Ashausische und Bienenbüttelsche Kontagionssachen item Geldausgaben für die Pestbedienten," 1713–14.

St. Mich., Rep. B 22, Nr. 24 (new: St. Mich., Nr. 707): "Die Geldausgaben wegen des mit der Viehseuche infizierten Dorfes Bienenbüttel," 1714.

Primary Sources

Chur-Braunschweig-Lüneburgische Landes-Ordnungen und Gesetze, Dritter Theil worinnen enthalten CAPVT TERTIUM vom MILITAR-Wesen und CAPVT QVARTVM von POLICEY-Sachen, Zum Gebrauch der Fürstenthümer, Graf- und Herrschafften Calenbergischen Theils. Göttingen: Universitäts Buchhandlung, 1740.

Chur-Braunschweig-Lüneburgische Landes-Ordnungen und Gesetze, Zweyter Theil, worin enthalten CAPUT SECUNDUM, von Administration der Justiz in Civil- und Criminal-Fällen auch andern das Justiz-Wesen angehenden Punkten und CAPUT TERTIUM, welches alle das Militair-Wesen angehenden Verordnungen in sich begreiffet. Zum Gebrauch des Fürstenthums Lüneburg, auch angehöriger Graf- und Herrschaften Zellischen Theils. Lüneburg: Sternische Buchdruckerey, 1742.

Chur-Braunschweig-Lüneburgische Landes-Ordnungen und Gesetze, Dritter Theil, worin enthalten CAPUT QVARTUM, von Policey-Sachen. Erster Band, Mit den zwölf erstern Sectionen desselbigen. Zum Gebrauch des Fürstenthums Lüneburg, auch angehöriger Graf- und Herrschaften Zellischen Theils. Lüneburg: Sternische Buchdruckerey, 1743.

Chur-Braunschweig-Lüneburgische Landes-Ordnungen und Gesetze, Dritter Theil, worin enthalten CAPUT QVARTUM, von Policey-Sachen. Zweiter Band, Mit den zehn letztern Sectionen desselbigen. Zum Gebrauch des Fürstenthums Lüneburg, auch angehöriger Graf- und Herrschaften Zellischen Theils. Lüneburg: Sternische Buchdruckerey, 1743.

Mead, Richard. *A SHORT DISCOURSE CONCERNING Pestilential Contagion, AND THE METHODS To be used to Prevent it*. 8th edition, London: Sam. Buckley, 1722.

Secondary Sources

Boyens, Kathrin. "Die Krise in der Krise. Die Maßnahmen Hamburgs während der letzten Pest 1712–1714." In *Die leidige Seuche. Pest-Fälle in der Frühen Neuzeit*, edited by Otto Ulbricht, 295–325. Cologne-Weimar-Vienna: Böhlau Verlag, 2004.

Brakensiek, Stefan. "Akzeptanzorientierte Herrschaft. Überlegungen zur politischen Kultur der Frühen Neuzeit." In *Die Frühe Neuzeit als Epoche*, edited by Helmut Neuhaus, 395–406. Munich: Oldenbourg, 2009.

Breuer, Mordechai. "Frühe Neuzeit und Beginn der Moderne." In *Deutsch-jüdische Geschichte in der Neuzeit, vol. 1: 1600–1780*, edited by Mordechai Breuer and Michael Graetz, 83–247. Munich: C. H. Beck, 2000.

Bulst, Neithard. "Krankheit und Gesellschaft in der Vormoderne. Das Beispiel der Pest." In *Maladies et société (XIIe–XVIIIe siècles). Actes du colloque de Bielefeld*, edited by Neithard Bulst and Robert Delort, 17–47. Paris: Éditions du centre national de la recherche scientifique, 1989.

Cassel, Clemens. *Geschichte der Stadt Celle mit besonderer Berücksichtigung des Geistes- und Kulturlebens der Bewohner*. 2 vols. Celle: W. Ströher, 1930–34.

Christensen, Daniel. *Politics and the Plague in Early Modern Germany. Political Efforts to Combat Epidemics in the Duchy of Braunschweig-Wolfenbüttel during the Seventeenth Century*. Saarbrücken: VDM Verlag Dr. Müller, 2008.

Deichert, H. *Geschichte des Medizinalwesens im Gebiet des ehemaligen Königreichs Hannover*. Hanover-Leipzig: Hahnsche Buchhandlung, 1908.

Dinges, Martin. "Pest und Politik in der europäischen Neuzeit." In *Pest. Die Geschichte eines Menschheitstraumas*, edited by Mischa Meier, 283–313. Stuttgart: Klett-Cotta, 2005.

Dinges, Martin. "Neue Wege in der Seuchengeschichte?" In *Neue Wege in der Seuchengeschichte*, edited by Martin Dinges and Thomas Schlich, 7–24. Stuttgart: Franz Steiner Verlag, 1995.

Eckert, Edward A. "The Retreat of Plague from Central Europe, 1640–1720: A Geomedical Approach." *Bulletin of the History of Medicine* 74 (2000): 1–28.

Frandsen, Karl-Erik. "Das konnte nützen. Krieg, Pest, Hunger und Not in Helsingør im Jahr 1711." In *Städtesystem und Urbanisierung im Ostseeraum in der Frühen Neuzeit. Urbane Lebensräume und Historische Informationssysteme. Beiträge des wissenschaftlichen Kolloquiums in Rostock vom 15. und 16. November 2004*, edited by Stefan Kroll and Kersten Krüger, 205–25. Berlin: LIT Verlag, 2006.

Frandsen, Karl-Erik. *The Last Plague in the Baltic Region 1709–1713*. Kopenhagen: Museum Tusculanum Press, 2010.

Friemann, Martin. "Das Diarium als Quelle Hamburger Familienforschung." *Zeitschrift für Niedersächsische Familienkunde* 22 (1940): 131–40.

Gaul, Volker. *Möglichkeiten und Grenzen absolutistischer Herrschaft. Landesherrliche Kommunikationsstrategien und städtische Interessen während der Pest in den Herzogtümern Schleswig-Holstein-Gottorf (1709–1713)*. Tönning-Lübeck-Marburg: Der andere Verlag, 2005.

Gebhardi, Ludwig Albrecht. *Kurze Geschichte des Klosters St. Michaelis in Lüneburg*. Celle: Capaun-Karlowa'sche Buchhandlung, 1857.

Gerhold, Karlheinz. "Seht den Narren mal, er will sich vorm lieben Gott verstecken!—Die Pest in Achim im Jahre 1712." *Heimatkalender für den Landkreis Verden 2003*: 135–61.

Haeser, Heinrich. *Lehrbuch der Geschichte der Medicin und der epidemischen Krankheiten, Bd. 3: Geschichte der epidemischen Krankheiten*. Jena: Gustav Fischer, 1882.

Hansen, Peter. *Geschichte der Epidemien bei Menschen und Tieren im Norden. Nach Untersuchungen ausgehend von Schleswig-Holstein*. Glückstadt: J. J. Augustin, 1925.

Kroll, Stefan. "Die Pest in Stade 1712 und ihre Opfer." *Stader Jahrbuch N.F.* 80 (1990): 47–67.

Krüger, Lutz Erich. *Der Erwerb Bremen-Verdens durch Hannover. Ein Beitrag zur Geschichte des großen Nordischen Krieges in den Jahren 1709–1719*. Hamburg: Niederelbe-Druck Otterndorfer Verlagsdruckerei, 1974.

Küther, Carsten. *Menschen auf der Straße. Vagierende Unterschichten in Bayern, Franken und Schwaben in der zweiten Hälfte des 18. Jahrhunderts*. Göttingen: Vandenhoeck & Ruprecht, 1983.

Lieboldt, J. "Dankfest in Hamburg vom 22. März 1714." *Mittheilungen des Vereins für Hamburgische Geschichte* 5 (1882): 159–60.

Lowenstein, Steven M. "Anfänge der Integration 1780–1871." In *Geschichte des jüdischen Alltags in Deutschland*, edited by Marion Kaplan, 123–224. München: C. H. Beck, 2003.

Marx, Albert. *Geschichte der Juden in Niedersachsen*. Hanover: Fackelträger-Verlag, 1995.

Mattmüller, Markus. *Bevölkerungsgeschichte der Schweiz, part I*, 2 vols. Basel, Frankfurt am Main: Helbing & Lichtenhahn, 1987.

Pagel, Marianne. "1715/16—Die Pest in Bardowick." In *Damals. Viertes Heimatbuch für den Landkreis Lüneburg*, 101–22. Lüneburg: Landkreis Lüneburg, 2001.

Persson, Bodil E. B. "The Boy with the Rake and the Girl with the Broom. Pestilences in Early Eighteenth Century Southern Sweden." In *Städtesystem und Urbanisierung im Ostseeraum in der Frühen Neuzeit. Urbane Lebensräume und Historische Informationssysteme. Beiträge des wissenschaftlichen Kolloquiums in Rostock vom 15. und 16. November 2004*, edited by Stefan Kroll and Kersten Krüger, 172–204. Berlin: LIT Verlag, 2006.

Puffahrt, Otto. "Maßregeln zur Pestabwehr im Kreis Harburg—Bemerkungen zur Pestepidemie 1712/13." *Harburger Kreiskalender 1986*: 53–58.

Rödel, Walter G. "Die Obrigkeiten und die Pest. Abwehrmassnahmen in der frühen Neuzeit—dargestellt an Beispielen aus dem süddeutschen und Schweizer Raum." In *Maladies et société (XIIe-XVIIIe siècles). Actes du colloque de Bielefeld*, edited by Neithard Bulst and Robert Delort, 187–205. Paris: Éditions du centre national de la recherche scientifique, 1989.

Sahm, Wilhelm. *Geschichte der Pest in Ostpreußen*. Leipzig: Duncker & Humblot, 1905.

Schlenkrich, Elke. *Gevatter Tod. Pestzeiten im 17. und 18. Jahrhundert im sächsisch-schlesisch-böhmischen Vergleich*. Stuttgart: Franz Steiner Verlag, 2013.

Schnath, Georg. *Geschichte Hannovers im Zeitalter der neunten Kur und der englischen Sukzession 1674–1714, vol. 3: 1698–1714*. Hildesheim: Lax, 1978.

Schwarz, Klaus. *Die Pest in Bremen. Epidemie und freier Handel in einer deutschen Hafenstadt 1350–1713*. Bremen: Selbstverlag des Staatsarchivs, 1996.

Sichart, Louis von. *Geschichte der Königlich-Hannoverschen Armee*. 5 vols. Hanover-Leipzig: Hahn'sche Buchhandlung, 1866–98.

Slack, Paul. *The Impact of Plague in Tudor and Stuart England*. Oxford: Clarendon Press 2003.

Spangenberg, Ernst. *Historisch-topographisch-statistische Beschreibung der Stadt Celle im Königreiche Hannover*. Celle: G. E. F. Schulze'sche Buchhandlung, 1826.

Stade. Von den Siedlungsanfängen bis zur Gegenwart. Stade: Krause Druck, 1994.

Sticker, Georg. *Abhandlungen aus der Seuchengeschichte und Seuchenlehre*. 2 vols. Gießen: Alfred Töpelmann, 1908–12.

Tammen, Annika. *Frühmoderne Staatlichkeit und lokale Herrschaftsvermittlung. Normgebung und Herrschaftspraxis im Herzogtum Holstein des 17. und 18. Jahrhunderts*. Bielefeld: Verlag für Regionalgeschichte, 2017.

Wendler, Ulf. "Die 'Pest' in den Dörfern: Das Hamburger Umland 1663/64." *Kreiskalender 2009. Jahrbuch für den Landkreis Harburg*: 83–96.

Wendler, Ulf. *Pest, Fleckfieber, Ruhr und Typhus. Epidemien auf dem Land und ihre Deutung im Fürstentum Lüneburg 1565–1666*. Göttingen: Wallstein Verlag, 2024.

Wendler, Ulf. *Nicht nur Pest und Pocken—Zur Bevölkerungsgeschichte der Lüneburger Heide, des Wendlandes und der Marschen des Fürstentums Lüneburg 1550–1850*. Hanover: Hahnsche Buchhandlung, 2008.

Wendler, Ulf. *Pestilentz im Norden. Seuchen in der nördlichen Lüneburger Heide und im Süden Hamburgs 1657–1716*. Ehestorf: Förderverein Freilichtmuseum am Kiekeberg, 2011.

Wendler, Ulf. "Der letzte Pestzug in Kurhannover." *Heimatkalender für Stadt und Kreis Uelzen* 1995: 115–22.

Wendler, Ulf. *Philipp Julius Toppius (1649–1727). Selbstzeugnisse eines Pastors und die Disziplinierung der ländlichen Gesellschaft*. Uelzen: Initia Medien und Verlag UG, 2017.

Wendler, Ulf. "Zirkulation und Kontrolle im frühmodernen Flächenstaat. Die Pestbekämpfung des Kurfürstentums Hannover 1709–1716." In *Zirkulation und Kontrolle. Dynamiken des 18. Jahrhunderts*, edited by Marian Füssel, 77–101. Berlin: Schwabe Verlag, 2025.

Weyhe-Eimke, Arnold von. *Die Aebte des Klosters St. Michaelis zu Lüneburg. Mit besonderer Beziehung auf die Geschichte des Klosters und der Ritterakademie*. Celle: Schulze'sche Buchhandlung, 1862.

Wohlwill, Adolf. *Hamburg während der Pestjahre 1712–1714*. Hamburg: Lucas Gräfe & Sillem, 1893.

PART III

Broader Academic and Social Responses to Plague

CHAPTER 8

About What Is Right in Times of Plague

Contagious Debates in Natural Philosophy, Medicine, Law, and Theology at the University of Helmstedt, 1681–83

BENJAMIN WALLURA

In memory of Holger Hübbe (1968–2024)

Introduction and Scope: The University of Helmstedt and the Threat of Plague in the Seventeenth Century

The question of what is "right" in times of plague—or, more broadly speaking, in times of epidemics[1]—was a constant challenge in early modern societies. Since the onset of the global COVID-19 pandemic in early 2020, modern researchers have rightly intensified their interest in the history of epidemics.[2] However, caution should be taken not to take a one-size-fits-all approach in considering historical pandemics.[3] Historically, Central Europe was among the hot spots of severe epidemics, both during the late medieval Black Death and during subsequent recurring outbreaks of plague, the so-called Second Pandemic.[4] The answer to the question of what was considered "right" (in the sense of "what is right to do," "correct," "valid," "reasonable," or "advisable") in such historical times of epidemic was (and *mutatis mutandis* still is) complex. How should we address historical concepts of "right" with regard to epidemics or plague and how can we identify them? What in early modern European intellectual thought was considered to be "right" in times of epidemic, and why?

Based on different historical and social contexts, the terms "right," "correct," or even "true," and so forth could cover a variety of often conflicting meanings.

"Knowledge" on the hand, and "validity," "authority," or "reason" on the other, combine to form a most dynamic relationship and depend heavily on the epistemic assumptions of certain groups within a society. In particular, what academic communities in history regarded as "valid," "legitimate," or "reasonable" was based on their specific cultural knowledge, their perspective on authority and how they—in their early modern academic contexts—evaluated various proposed arguments given for a specific subject matter.[5]

Early modern European natural philosophy and medicine, for instance, naturally focused on other aspects of epidemic diseases than did law and theology. Even natural philosophy (*philosophia naturalis* or *physica*) and medicine did not necessarily share the same opinions on how epidemic diseases should be explained, treated, and fought against.[6] And even within these university disciplines themselves, we find many differing and conflicting assumptions and arguments. European natural philosophers in the seventeenth century, for instance, were arguing over the existence and behavior of the smallest particles, so-called corpuscles, and their possible role in the spread of diseases and the process of contagion or infection.[7] University-trained physicians, on the other hand, broadly acknowledged the ancient Hippocratic miasma theory that explained contagion through bad air. At the same time, they were arguing over the exact fermentation processes taking place within the human body during a contagion. From the point of view of historical epistemology and methodology, the discursive field opens up here into a very diffuse and heterogenic phenomenon. Moreover, the exact origin of epidemic diseases, such as plague, was fiercely disputed.[8] As a consequence, necessary precautions to prevent contagion, and the possible remedies and measures which might help prevent and cure the disease, were also widely discussed among fellow physicians, doctors, and various kinds of medical practitioners.[9]

While the natural philosophical and medical arguments were mainly concerned with the question of how to "rightly" classify, prevent, or medically cure the disease, the very notion of "right" applied also very directly to law and moral philosophy in the strict sense of which specific legal and moral issues had to be addressed in times of epidemic. When death rates were high, legal experts were highly sought after by authorities in order to draft officially binding plague ordinances and implement them. In the seventeenth century, all the fields of knowledge mentioned here were governed by theology and Christian beliefs as they were taught at the higher schools. No philosophy, no medicine, no law, no moral teachings, and no political measures could be implemented without God and theology. Likewise, physics, medicine, law, moral philosophy, and theology displayed connections and intersections in seventeenth-century European discourses of plague.[10]

Due to the comprehensiveness of the argument followed in this chapter, it seems necessary to narrow down the scope. The main interest will focus on mere academic debates in a Lutheran scholarly and university context. In spite of the extensive devastation resulting from the Thirty Years' War (1618–48), the Holy Roman Empire possessed a variety of confessionalized universities in the second half of the seventeenth century. One of the most important universities founded after the Reformation in the center of the empire was the Academia Julia at Helmstedt (1576–1810), founded by Duke Julius of Braunschweig-Lüneburg (1528–89). More than a century later the university of Helmstedt was still counted among the important and well-frequented educational institutions of the empire. Around 1680, many universities, including Helmstedt, underwent noticeable curricular changes. The paradigm of academic education mostly driven by contemporary Aristotelianism and late Renaissance scholasticism, an academic phenomenon that built the core of the established *Schulphilosophie* at the majority of European universities at that time, was under attack. By the second half of the seventeenth century, academics and university professors all over Europe, regardless of confession, found themselves facing a tremendous variety of new currents in philosophy that initiated several controversies about scientific methodology and philosophical reasoning about natural phenomena. Philosophers such as Francis Bacon, René Descartes, Pierre Gassandi, or later somewhat less radical reformers, such as Kenelm Digby, Robert Boyle, or Gottfried Wilhelm Leibniz, challenged in their respective ways the established *Schulphilosophie* traditionally driven by locally and historically diverse kinds of Aristotelian, peripatetic, or scholastic conceptions of philosophy and academic teaching, leading to a *philosophia reformata,* a restituted or even reformed and renewed philosophy.[11]

In this climate of gradual philosophical and academic reforms the threat of plague hit the city of Helmstedt roughly from 1681 to 1683. The threat immediately called for an academic response, and the topic of plague, in one form or another, underwent a thorough re-examination in all the academic faculties at Helmstedt, i.e. philosophy, medicine, law, and theology.[12] This chapter aims to provide a case study on the historical discussions on what is "right" in times of plague and how scholars in four different faculties addressed the issue at the Academia Julia in Helmstedt.

Helmstedt, and more broadly the whole ducal territory of Braunschweig-Lüneburg and the free cities situated within it, were threatened by the plague several times in the seventeenth century (1625–26, 1657–58, and 1681).[13] As the archival records and the academic productions in Helmstedt, in particular between 1681 and 1683, show, the plague was seen as an imminent threat to the university and the town and was taken very seriously by scholars and authorities.[14]

In what follows I will highlight some of the measures implemented or proposed against the plague as they were discussed by the local academic scholarship. In four miniatures dedicated to each faculty and field (i.e. philosophy, medicine, law, and theology), I will analyze the particular constellation of debates centered on the imminent threat of plague in Helmstedt from 1681 to 1683. I will do this by referring to a balanced selection from extant printed academic works (especially academic dissertations) and archival materials. We will see how the different academic faculties in Helmstedt issued recommendations, warnings, interjections, and reflections, echoing important local voices concerning a serious epidemic threat at a well-defined place within a short period of time.[15] The academic dissertations and disputations discussed here will provide an impression of how differently a specific academic community of university professors as well as practicing doctors and ministers with a university affiliation addressed the epidemic threat.

Academic discourses on plague in seventeenth-century Helmstedt have not been studied comprehensively so far. For the most part, modern research has focused on records of the social and political history of plague in the duchy of Braunschweig-Lüneburg, while leaving out a considerable part of the available records for the history of science and ideas for this particular academic milieu.[16] This disparity might be caused by the problematic assumption that records for the history of science and ideas would not reflect what was going on in reality, or might render an inaccurate representation of the historical situation. With this chapter I would like to take the opposite stand. As both recent and past epidemics suggest, the discussion of measures to be taken in times of epidemic threat can be patchy and inconsistent. Inversely, the fact that measures were taken does not imply their approval and acceptance by all authorities and experts. In early modern academic discourse, therefore, the question of what is right in times of plague was always a matter of dispute.

Plague, Libraries, and Scholarship between Wolfenbüttel and Helmstedt

When plague outbreaks in Leipzig and Wolfenbüttel threatened other areas in 1681, such as Helmstedt, the duchy of Braunschweig-Lüneburg was not completely unprepared.[17] Duke Rudolf August of Braunschweig-Lüneburg (1627–1704) and the municipality at Wolfenbüttel took measures, and the academic milieu in Wolfenbüttel and Helmstedt quickly addressed the problem. After the death of Duke August the Younger (1579–1666), the ducal library at Wolfenbüttel, the Bibliotheca Augusta, had become a public library. The duke's successor, Duke Rudolf August, installed the well-versed bibliophile and theologian David Hanisius (1630–81) as librarian, who held the position until his death in June 1681.[18] Hanisius realized the urgency of the epidemic threat and compiled two comprehensive catalogues of treatises on plague and other epidemic diseases, printed in Wolfenbüttel and Braunschweig in 1680.[19] Both catalogues are organized alphabetically by name—without title, but with date and format of the treatise—and thematically by diverse categories, such as "Ratschlagk" (advice), "Ordnung" (plague ordinances), "Medendi Methodi" (methods of cure), and "febris" (fever). Hanisius's second catalogue, the *Continuatio*, uses categories such as "Medici superioris seculi" (physicians of the previous century), "Medici praesentis seculi" (physicians of the present century), "Primi Medicinae parentes" (first, i.e. ancient, fathers of medicine), "Hebraeorum coryphaei" (Hebrew luminaries), "Arabum maximi" (most important Arabic writers), and many others. Together they form a diffuse array of authorities and texts concerned with plague or other epidemic diseases from the perspective of natural philosophy, medicine, law, and theology.

Indeed, the Latin congratulatory poem preceding Hanisius's *Catalogus* states that this list of treatises concerning plague and epidemic diseases is meant to serve the jurist, the theologian, and the physician (*medicus*) alike.[20] In one of the several other gratulatory poems concluding the *Continuatio*, its use in particular for the "ordo Medicorum," academically trained physicians and doctors, is made explicit:

> Now with Death fiercely threatening us, undaunted skill and science try to come together to you, my duke, and defy his [i.e. death's] armed weapons. … Many fall through plague, slaughtered by cruel death, as everyone knows living in Saxony these days. In order to not be harmed by the adjacent contagion, God's grace commands and medicine takes precautions. Your duty, physicians and doctors, is to prepare remedies against this pestilential mischief. But from where, you ask, should advice come? And help as well, you ask? Well, look: there is a most excellent authority at the library in Wolfenbüttel at hand. He [Hanisius] makes known and edits a treasure collected by meticulous study. Now is the time! So, be pleased to come here and use, I beg, the paths which this learned man opens up to follow. If due to his instructions things will once have turned out well, no one will fail to thank Hanisius. With how much praise this work is to be blessed everybody will learn who will undertake the same effort.[21]

This is an interesting plea for the relevance of book culture and academic reasoning in times of epidemic threat. In order to fight back plague, knowledge contained in books is supposed to be used. Libraries, universities, and their academic productions in natural philosophy, medicine, law, and theology would build core instruments in facing the deadly challenge; scholars and academics are even explicitly invited to come to the library at Wolfenbüttel in order to use its holdings. This rhetorical enthusiasm probably got dampened after the official announcement by the government at Wolfenbüttel in November 1680 that declared plague to be present in the duchy. In theory, it meant more severe border controls and a certain time of quarantine before entering the territory of Braunschweig-Lüneburg. This was not a popular choice, since restrictions like these often had a disastrous impact on local economies due to travel restrictions between towns. More typical in this case was to declare that plague was rampant only in the vicinity, giving the impression that one's own region was only threatened but not infected by the disease, so that the threat of plague appeared less problematic for residents of the ducal territory of Braunschweig-Wolfenbüttel. For instance, the number of recurring library visitors of the Bibliotheca Augusta at the ducal residence of Wolfenbüttel did not greatly fluctuate at this time: dukes, princes, academics, courtiers, privy councilors, even engineers and craftsmen, were using it just as they had before,[22] although the numbers were small enough to be quite manageable. However, slight changes in the borrowers' reading habits in favor of plague and related issues are notable, such as astronomical influences on earth, matters of anatomy, or more generally medical books on pestilential fevers.[23]

As the academic publications at the Academia Julia at Helmstedt between 1681 and 1683 show, the call initiated by Hanisius's two catalogues of plague treatises did not remain unechoed. Furthermore, the recurring threat of plague had been addressed already by Helmstedt scholars and their academic dissertations, such as by Hermann Conring (1606–81) or Heinrich Meibom (1638–1700), both respected professors of medicine. Already in 1659, Conring had written on plague under the stress of severe outbreaks in Braunschweig around 1658, and his dissertation was reissued without changes in 1678, probably provoked by the Great Plague of Vienna of 1678–79.[24] The events in Vienna around 1678 were reported in large parts of Europe in widely disseminated accounts. Paul de Sorbait, dean of the faculty of medicine at Vienna, in his *Consilium Medicum* (1679) reported on the severity of the plague outbreaks in Vienna, which served as a warning for many parts of the empire.[25] These outbreaks presumably motivated Heinrich Meibom's *De febribus malignis* (On malevolent fevers) of 1679, which was concerned in particular with severe forms of pestilence or plague.

Theories on the causes and spread of highly contagious diseases had been discussed intensely ever since the Black Death (1347–53). Especially following Girolamo Fracastoro's (ca. 1477–1533) works on syphilis and plague, theories of contagion experienced an upsurge, with a long-lasting echo into the seventeenth century.[26] Fracastoro set out three possible means of contagion: "by direct contact, by indirect contact through fomites, and at a distance."[27] It is this last form of contagion "at a distance" which had a particular career in the seventeenth century. For Aristotle, of course, effects *ad distans* (at a distance) were the least preferred ways how objects or subjects were thought to interact with each other. Hippocratic and Galenic medicine provided an ancient model to improve Aristotelian natural philosophy at this point with the much-debated concept of miasma, which had first been developed in the Hippocratic treatise *De flatibus* (On Breaths). In the seventeenth century, this miasma concept experienced a revival, not least initiated by plague treatises such as Isbrand van Diemerbroeck's (1609–74) often reissued *Tractatus de peste* (Treatise on Plague), first published in 1646.[28] According to the miasma theory, as displayed in *De flatibus*, so-called νοσηρά μιάσματα (unhealthy miasmas), i.e. "bad exhalations" of "bad miasmas," deriving from putrefying cadavers or marshes, can float through the air and cause many illnesses for mankind.[29] In Diemerbroeck's influential treatise, these Hippocratic miasmas were also translated into the Latin equivalent of *effluvia* (emanations, exhalations, respirations), which in the sense of particles flowing through air as a medium undoubtedly picked up what Fracastoro had already referred to as *effluxiones* (outpourings) by reassessing atomistic concepts from Empedocles and Lucretius.[30]

The term *effluvia* reoccurs most prominently in a slightly different context in the mechanical, physical, and chemical works of the English experimentalist Robert Boyle (1627–92). In his treatise *De mira subtilitate effluviorum* (On the Extraordinary Penetration of Effluvia) Boyle defined *effluvia* as extremely small and subtle particles, which could be approbated by Cartesians, Epicureans, and Aristotelians alike, regardless of contemporary philosophical quarrels.[31] This was a clever move, as it allowed Boyle to promote a corpuscular theory without operating with the rather vexed and problematic term of atoms (*atomi*), which were highly criticized by the mostly Aristotelian *Schulphilosophie* at the universities. Boyle even explicitly stated that *effluvia* were not the same as atoms, even though they might behave in the very same manner as neoatomists would describe.[32] In the end, *effluvia* were not indivisible, and that was all that mattered for traditionally trained Aristotelians. At the same time, the *effluvia* concept appeared highly acceptable through the Hippocratic miasma theory, deeply established in contemporary medical thought of the seventeenth century.

Natural Philosophy, Effluvia, and Corpuscular Theories in Helmstedt

In this setting of ideas, the phenomenon of *effluvia* was addressed by the philosophical faculty at Helmstedt. Only four months after the duchy officially declared the existence of plague in the territory in November 1680, the young professor for physics (*naturalis philosophia*) at the Academia Julia, Justus Cellarius (1649–89), published an academic disputation that revealed Boyle's influence already in the title: *Disputatio physica de penetrabili efficacia effluviorum in afficiendis corporibus animalium* (Physical Disputation on the Penetrating Virtue of Effluvia in Affecting Animal Bodies).[33] Cellarius came from a well-established scholarly family of Helmstedt. His father, Balthasar Cellarius (1614–71), taught theology in Helmstedt and enabled his son, who had also studied in Jena, to secure the physics chair at Helmstedt, which the young Cellarius took up shortly after his father's death in 1673.[34] However, the defending student (respondent) of Cellarius's disputation from 1681 was Konrad Barthold Behrens (1660–1736), who later became a respected doctor (even *Seuchenarzt*) and personal physician to Duke Anton Ulrich of Braunschweig-Wolfenbüttel.[35] He was also related to the councilor and court physician at Wolfenbüttel, Julius Georg Behrens, who from 1680 to 1683 had borrowed many medical, and in particular plague-related, books from the Bibliotheca Augusta and also exchanged letters with the Wolfenbüttel librarian David Hanisius. The disputation of Justus Cellarius and Konrad Barthold Behrens is also dedicated to Julius Georg Behrens, the personal physician of Duke Rudolph August. Even though the threat of contagion with plague is only implicitly present in the title of Cellarius's and the younger Behrens's disputation, the circulating reports of outbreaks at several spots of the empire most certainly formed the background for this academic text, particularly since Helmstedt was located on the very eastern periphery of the duchy, much closer to Magdeburg and Leipzig, where the plague had already been rampant.

Written in March 1681, their disputation was somewhat ahead of its time, given the location, since plague did not become an urgent threat for Helmstedt until July 1681, when it was brought there by troops and twenty houses had to be boarded up.[36] As the content of the disputation reveals, Cellarius and Behrens had good arguments for their early warning. As it seems, the two academics were anticipating a danger which was about to come and felt the need to work out this academic disputation before the disease had actually reached town.[37]

The content of the disputation is even more interesting. The title of the disputation, referring to the severe "penetrating virtue of effluvia," indicates the main thrust of the text: serious precautions against a threat that should not be underestimated. This concern about plague *effluvia* is addressed by Cellarius and Behrens, according to their fields of knowledge, in a natural philosophical manner, which encompassed physical as well as medical considerations. Even though the title claims to focus on animals, it becomes clear right away that mankind had to be cautioned against plague and its deadly *effluvia*.

The argument of the disputation represents a specific part of what around 1680 was discussed as *philosophia reformata* (reshaped or restituted philosophy), i.e. a kind of philosophy that was intended to negotiate between positions of ancient and more recent philosophy (*philosophia vetus et nova*).[38] As Cellarius and Behrens state right at the beginning, ancient testimonies already considered it to be common knowledge that the earth emits, both in microcosmic and in macrocosmic domains, most subtle corpuscles (*subtilia corpuscula*) into the surrounding air that we live in, giving cause to a variety of natural phenomena ranging from cosmology, to meteorology, down to meticulous physiological processes. These *effluvia* around us, as their name already reveals (lat. *effluere*, to flow out), flow through a medium, which is air, just as in a perpetually moving circle ("in perpetuo motu et veluti pericyclosi").[39] The basic idea, inspired especially by the works of Robert Boyle, is a mechanical one. Even though it challenges key positions of Aristotelian philosophy, such as on vacuum and on corpuscular (if not atomistic) theory, Cellarius and Behrens, just as Boyle, argue here for the consent of ancient and recent philosophy. Cartesians, Epicureans, or Aristotelians all can approbate these smallest corpuscles or particles as active in nature, since *effluvia* are not atoms. The authorities invoked by Cellarius and Behrens are of great interest here: Otto von Guericke, famous for his vacuum experiment of the Magdeburg hemispheres; Sebastian Wirdig and his *Nova Medicina spirituum curiosa* (1673), which garnered the professor from Tartu the suspicion of being a Rosicrucian and forced him to undergo an inquiry by the university of Wittenberg in 1683;[40] Kenelm Digby and his work on the famous "powder of sympathy" or "weapon salve" (*unguentum armarium*); and John Mayow's medico-physical works. All of them were scholars who in their own ways intended to extend or reform the established Aristotelian thinking on matters of natural philosophy.[41] In contrast to these currents of newer philosophy, references to Aristotle or Galen were placed much more sparsely.

One possible explanation why Cellarius and Behrens refer to so many contenders of the new and reformed philosophy seems to be that this appealed to a somewhat general academic trend within the second half of the seventeenth century. Another is that the imminent threat of plague and the incredible contagiousness of the disease required more detailed and precise explanations. The theory of *effluvia* and their subtle, often adverse, character seemed more than suited to explain the mystery of an almost supernatural disease with the help of new philosophy. The imminent threat of plague, one could argue, had a direct impact on discussions of what was considered right or probable within natural philosophical theory.

A key point here for Cellarius and Behrens appears to be a certain concept of experience, experiment, and evidence (*experientia, experimentum, evidentia*). In their disputation they never directly problematize the terms, but *ex negativo* we get a more or less clear impression from their chosen use of authorities, examples, and arguments. Crucial for this are the definitions which Cellarius and Behrens give for *effluvia*: nearly every animated or unanimated entity on this globe, as common experience would show, emits numerous *effluvia* in sizes that may be visible or invisible to the human eye. These are often very subtle and can penetrate the skin of animals and humans through pores.[42] This penetrability, they argue, can often range over very large distances, as Digby and Boyle report. The scent of rosemary, for instance, was still recognizable 30,000 paces ("tringinta milliarium") off the coast of Spain.[43] The same was reported of the smell of cinnamon and rubber transported through the wind for several miles off the Indian coast. These cases, Cellarius and Behrens argue, prove the *effluvia*'s incredible virtue at a distance. Recognizable odors and the ability to smell, Cellarius and Behrens continue, assure us that *effluvia* exist and that their "enduring tenacity" (*durabilis tenacitas*) has tremendous impact on their surroundings. In another argument borrowed from Boyle, Cellarius and Behrens argued that animals can smell each other during the rutting season over extremely long distances, which is impossible for human beings to do. To Cellarius and Behrens, these were proofs that some *effluvia* are so subtle that they are not even recognizable for us, even though they are undoubtedly present.[44]

Following these and other arguments, it appeared evident for Cellarius and Behrens to assume that contagion with plague and other infectious diseases works in a very similar manner to the behavior of these subtle *effluvia*. It seems more than likely, so Cellarius and Behrens believed, that direct or indirect contagion with plague takes place through certain plague seeds which flow out from infected bodies and carry the venom itself from one body to another. This point was not shared by all academically trained doctors at the time, a dissenter being Günther Christoph Schelhammer, Cellarius's colleague in the faculty of medicine at Helmstedt. As iatromechanics postulated, supported for instance by Giovanni Alfonso Borelli (1608–79), most creatures seemed to have the ability to smell plague—an odor that apparently did not derive from the malign breath and sweat of the infected body, but from "some other transpiration" as experiments would suggest ("quavis transpiratione alia experimentis probatum").[45] The main point and advice of Cellarius and Behrens was to beware of these severe plague *effluvia*. As it turns out, this was not an easy thing to do, as the following grim list of opportunities given by them illustrates. On animate as well as inanimate bodies, Cellarius and Behrens warn us, plague *effluvia* can be hidden for a fairly long time. As experience (*experientia*) shows, cats, dogs, pigeons, chicken, and even flies can function as carriers. The same goes for inanimate things, such as linen, feathers, clothes, leather and skins, tapestries, wools, beds, pottery, knives, swords, shoes, dust, spiderwebs, and even money—in short, basically everything around us, objects that physicians had many times identified as plague mediators.[46] Cellarius and Behrens retold the story related by the famous plague doctor Diemerbroeck that even after eight months of being exposed to severe weather, rain, and snow, a gurney on which an infected and deceased person was carried was itself still highly infectious. They claimed that a vendor of medicines (*pharmacopola*) who removed a bit of the litter with his foot shortly afterwards developed a carbuncle that took at least forty days to heal, as Cellarius and Behrens report, based on Diemerbroeck's account (c. XLI).[47]

The tone of Cellarius and Behrens's disputation is surprisingly gloomy, given the fact that plague was not even rampant in Helmstedt in March 1681 and was only evident in reports from neighboring territories and in historical accounts. Their core advice is to be cautious wherever one goes, wherever one breathes, and whatever one touches, because it might be infected. From this stark academic and natural philosophical point of view we get the impression that the scholarly milieu at Helmstedt, and probably elsewhere, was highly aware of the dangers of contagion. This sensibility and awareness, as it seems, later was only partly reflected in the political measures taken in the duchy, as differences between theory and actual practice were significant. What becomes clear from Cellarius and Behrens's disputation is the clear academic character of the text. The implicit recommendations or warnings were certainly not meant as a direct instruction for how to act. Due to its place within the faculty of philosophy, the main purpose of the disputation was to learn academic argumentation and rhetoric, and while doing so to prepare to obtain an academic degree. As we know, Konrad Barthold Behrens, the respondent, graduated *pro licentia* in the faculty of medicine in 1684 under Heinrich Meibom the Younger (1638–1700). Nevertheless, the arguments put forth by Cellarius and Behrens give us valuable insight into their thought concerning the prevention of contagion with plague, even though we cannot be certain to what extent their arguments were meant as concrete directives or just as a rhetorical word of warning. Unlike medicine, law, and theology, philosophical dissertations were much guided by the *libertas philosophandi*, the freedom of philosophizing, and were therefore not beholden to the same knowledge claims. In the end, we cannot determine for sure how literally Cellarius and Behrens's argument and their implicit advice is to be taken, although many aspects of their dissertation echo their later works on plague or other epidemic diseases.[48]

Medicine, Miasmas, and Fermentation in Helmstedt

The topic of plague in early modern times belonged in considerable part to the academic expertise of medicine. Official measures to prevent the spread of contagious diseases or to promote remedies to cure illnesses were usually disseminated and published by academically trained doctors and physicians rather than by practitioners, such as barbers, surgeons, or midwives.[49] After Cellarius and Behrens had published their disputation in spring 1681, the faculty of medicine at Helmstedt of course had to follow suit.[50] Early in 1682, only a few months after the death of the famous Helmstedt physician Hermann Conring, his son-in-law, Günther Christoph Schelhammer (1649–1716), Professor of Physiology, Pathology, and Botany at the Academia Julia, provided a dissertation with the simple and straightforward title *De Peste* (On Plague).[51] This academic text was clearly inspired by Conring's *Disputatio inauguralis medica de peste* (1659), which was reissued in Helmstedt in 1678, shortly before Conring's death in 1681.

With its one hundred pages, however, not only is Schelhammer's dissertation longer than Conring's, but also its knowledge base on plague and contagion is more current. It covers most important ancient sources, such as Hippocrates and Galen, but also medieval Arabic, Renaissance, and many early modern European authorities. The dissertation is accompanied by a dedicatory letter addressed to Anna Sophia of Hessen-Darmstadt (1638–83) and Anna Dorothea of Sachsen-Weimar (1657–1704) and signed by the responding student, Daniel Christoph Meineke. Meineke studied first at the *Gymnasium* at Magdeburg and went on to study at the University of Leipzig. In the dedicatory letter he portrays himself as Hercules, who had to choose between the path of virtue and the path of desire. Meineke's choice of path was between theology and medicine. While first choosing theology, he later settled for medicine because of his "natural love for this field of study."[52]

For the evaluation of this academic text it is worth noting that Meineke came to the university of Helmstedt from Leipzig, where in 1680 plague had been rampant. Schelhammer chose an ideal respondent for his dissertation who had studied under these circumstances of plague. This certainly gave the dissertation a sense of lived expertise, or at least a rhetorical advantage. As in the case of Cellarius and Behrens before, we can assume that Schelhammer and Meineke both have to be considered as authors of the dissertation. Apart from the dedicatory letter, the style and implied references in the text point more in the direction of Schelhammer as the primary author. Furthermore, it appears that this dissertation was first and foremost an opportunity for Schelhammer's self-fashioning as a young university professor and son-in-law of Hermann Conring, rather than for the student Daniel Christoph Meineke. For Schelhammer, not only was plague current and pressing, but he was also able to position himself as an emerging scholar who could step in for the recently deceased Conring and make a mark in the field.

During his academic journey through England in the 1670s, Schelhammer personally met Robert Boyle in London, where he became directly familiar with Boyle's work on the *effluvia*. It appears very likely that scholars and later colleagues in Helmstedt, such as Justus Cellarius, were informed about Boyle's theories not only through the printed and disseminated transactions of the Royal Society but also directly through Schelhammer, who was about to start a splendid career as physician, anatomist, and botanist in Helmstedt, and shortly after in Jena and Kiel.[53] Nevertheless, Schelhammer did not primarily promote the concept of *effluvia* but, rather, stuck with the medically more established Hippocratic and Galenic term of *miasmata*, even though the difference between both terms appears almost negligible, at least in the medical context of Helmstedt.[54] Here, the influence of Hermann Conring is felt, whose work on plague Schelhammer highlights at the beginning of his dissertation (Cap. I, § II). Furthermore, Schelhammer shows how well versed he is not only in authorities such as Diemerbroeck or Athanasius Kircher, but also in other current literature on plague, especially by English scholars like Nathaniel Hodges' *Loimologia* (1672), which was based on first-hand knowledge from Hodges' practice as a doctor during the Great Plague of London in 1665.

In many respects Schelhammer repeated and affirmed what Cellarius and Behrens had already stated a couple of months earlier. The most striking difference from Cellarius and Behrens appears to be that Schelhammer emphasizes that effluvia or miasmas alone do not necessarily lead to a contagion and that not everything which smells bad is automatically to be taken as a sign of plague.[55] Cellarius and Behrens gave the impression that effluvia or miasmas almost inevitably led to a contagion with plague when inhaled, and that only plague effluvia had the power to cause plague. As famously described by Lucretius, Cellarius and Behrens believed that bad plague particles were able to travel great distances through the air and across the oceans and rather indistinctively could affect every area and person.[56] Schelhammer, on the contrary, was clearly more wary and argued that the process of contagion with plague involved many more, yet poorly understood, factors. He illustrates this with an interesting example from Wouter Schouten's travelogue.[57] Schouten reported that an outbreak of plague occurred on a ship after a severe storm on the way to the East Indies, more than fifteen days after having left port. This outbreak, Schelhammer warned, occurred outside the commonly assumed period of incubation. It was not likely, therefore, that crew members had brought the disease on board. This raised the question of how this epidemic outbreak could be explained. He concluded that it was unlikely that plague effluvia or miasmas, as Cellarius and Behrens might have argued, had come that far by wind and storm and caused a uniform contagion among crew members. The "one and simple cause" of plague (its "unica et simplex causa"), Schelhammer was convinced, had to come from inside the body itself, from a certain disposition.[58] Vicissitudes seemed more likely to be responsible, he continued, as wind and storm as well as hard labor on board had weakened the crew's general health and made their bodies much more susceptible to contagion, serious illness, and epidemic. In Schelhammer's words:

> What is more obvious here? That plague itself emerged so quickly after the storm and was generated within the bodies of the crew themselves, because of their hard work, the vicissitudes, and the following wanderings of the sea, and that therefore plague step by step took its origin from the corrupted humors of the crew, or that maybe plague seeds came into their bodies through whirlwind coming from the heaven just like from some sort of cloud? However, the contagion

> was not brought there by the wind, otherwise all crew members would have been infected instantly. In fact, a burning fever preceded this outburst, as can easily be seen by the fact that the more volatile and pure humors of some started to boil instantly just like a flame in sudden inflammation, while the thicker and more impure blood of the others only slowly, but more fatally, began with fermentation, from which plague emerged afterwards.[59]

Schelhammer departed from the arguments by Cellarius and Behrens in significant ways. His argument that plague was not brought by wind or by some sort of cloud ("ex nube quadam") implicitly criticizes the corpuscular approach in the famous passage in Lucretius's *De rerum natura* (The Nature of Things).[60] The key process, Schelhammer said, is not the "actio in distans" of the effluvia or miasmas, which penetrate every body without distinction, but the process of fermentation (*fermentatio*) of humors in already predisposed bodies. It is obvious how diligently Schelhammer tries here to bring Galenic humoral pathology into agreement with the corpuscular concept of Hippocratic miasmas and Boylean effluvia, while avoiding a close affinity with Lucretian's corpuscular theory on the other hand. Just as Cellarius and Behrens, Schelhammer sought a consensus between ancient and more recent contenders of natural philosophy and medicine. Schelhammer's argumentation also provides a view that became increasingly accepted among contemporary doctors, namely that many simple fevers first had to become epidemic and only afterwards were able to turn into real plagues.

An important second part of the question of what is right when facing epidemic threats is that one should care not only about plague effluvia and miasmas, but first and foremost about one's own general state of health. A stronger and healthier body, Schelhammer argued, was much more capable of preventing and fighting epidemic threats. An apple a day, one is inclined to say, keeps the plague away. Schelhammer, basing his arguments on Arabic authorities, such as the Andalusian doctor Ibn Zuhr (1092–1161), Galen, or the Venetian doctor and anatomist Niccolò Massa (1489–1569), even suggested that pestilential fevers were able to derive from an intrinsic alteration of the body itself, without external contagion from the air ("ab alteratione intrinseca posse fieri, sine externi aeris contagione").[61] Schelhammer concluded that the origin and cause of epidemic threats of plague were not effluvia and miasmas per se, but mostly corrupted blood and the specific state of health of individuals or certain endangered groups, such as children or older people or people who generally live or have to live unhealthily.[62] There was, however, no doubt that the spread of epidemic diseases worked primarily through the air, even over fairly long distances between two places that had no commercial relationship or other forms of contact with each other. Still, what constituted plague was the "corruption of blood" (*corruptio sanguinis*) as the primary cause of the disease.[63]

This point is important for the academic discussions on plague around 1680. As Schelhammer put it, there were two conflicting opinions: the old ones (*veteres*) and the more recent ones (*recentiores*).[64] Some recent philosophers and physicians, he says, suggested that a toxin causing plague is transported through the air. Since antiquity, however, contagion was not viewed as a process of poisoning but as one of fermentation or putrefaction of the blood. The detection of many worms in plague-infected bodies, as recently found by Jesuits like Athanasius Kircher, supported this point.[65] Schelhammer tried to combine older and newer currents of natural philosophy and medicine, combining differing views into a unified perspective on plague. He approved the effluvia mechanism proposed by Boyle and others, and also the well-received works of Jesuits like Kircher and others.[66] At the same time, he directly referred to the famous Aristotelian Hermann Conring, who had written on fermentation and had also stressed the importance of this process during contagion with plague.[67] Furthermore, Schelhammer referred to Andrea Cesalpino (1519–1603), the famous Italian physician, philosopher, botanist, and promoter of Aristotelian philosophy, whom he attests to be "the most discerning among the Aristotelians" ("iudiciosissimus Aristotelicorum").[68] The very current event of epidemic threat at Helmstedt prompted Schelhammer to reconsider the probability of older and more recent concepts of natural philosophy and medicine and weigh their accounts on pestilential fevers against each other. This way, Schelhammer intended to settle for a middle ground between *philosophia vetus* and *philosophia nova*. It is not surprising that Schelhammer argued for the effectiveness of smoking tobacco to prevent infection with serious diseases. Galen too, Schelhammer wrote, used to preserve his body by dehydrating it when experiencing a pestilence in Rome. Schelhammer was convinced that Galen would have accepted the cleansing properties of smoking tobacco, had he known of it.[69] However, Schelhammer conceded, tobacco also weakens the body on other levels and heightens the chance that the body becomes more vulnerable to contagion. In sum, the question of what is right in times of plague for Schelhammer was a crucial issue of dietetic lifestyle and had to be closely linked to certain bodily predispositions, such as pre-existing illnesses or age, but also to certain established assumptions made by Galenic medicine, humoral pathology, and Aristotelian natural philosophy.[70]

Law, Plague Ordinances, and Aristotelianism in Helmstedt

In early modern legal texts, plague or pestilence frequently is framed as *bellum Dei* (war of God) against which human force is powerless, as the later Helmstedt professor Johannes Andreas Schmidt stated in his dissertation on *The Duty of the Magistrate in Times of Plague* (*De Officio Magistratus circa tempora pestis Dissertatio politica*) from 1680.[71] Public order needed to be stabilized, even if plague was seen as God's tribunal. Rulers were in need of plague ordinances and reached out for legal help from their universities and law professors. In legal terms, plague was considered a *casus fortuitus*, a case of fortuity and unpredictable calamity. Needless to say, the faculty of law at Helmstedt addressed the issue of plague according to their field of expertise.[72]

This was the approach of the Helmstedt law professor Georg Engelbrecht the Elder (1638–1705), who held the chair for law at the Academia Julia beginning in 1671/72. In 1683 he published his *Discursus iuridicus de peste et iuribus circa tempus pestis. Von dem was recht ist zu Pest-Zeiten* (Juridical Discourse on plague and on matters of law during times of plague. About what is right in times of plague).[73] The responding student, Christian Ulrich Blume, had an aristocratic background, as was not uncommon among students of law in seventeenth-century Germany. His relative and protégé, Julius Heinrich von Blume, an alumnus of the Academia Julia at Helmstedt who studied under the aegis of Hermann Conring, appears, beside Duke Rudolph August, as a dedicatee of the dissertation. Blume had converted to Catholicism at the Reichstag of Regensburg in 1653. Later, he served as an official in Prague in the service of Emperor Leopold I, who had commissioned the so-called *Kayserliche Infections-Ordnung*, the imperial plague ordinance for Vienna and its surrounding area. It seems likely that Professor Engelbrecht was primarily responsible for the content of the dissertation. The aristocratic student Blume is referred to as "autor" (author), but, as recent studies on early modern dissertations and disputations have revealed, this should not be taken as an indication of the student's sole authorship.[74]

Engelbrecht's outlook on law, politics, and moral philosophy was clearly Aristotelian. Debates on natural law, in the wake of Grotius, Pufendorf, and others, were critically important during his career as a law professor. Already in the first lines of his dissertation, Engelbrecht favored Aristotle over the political philosophers Thomas Hobbes and Jean Bodin:

> Man, this most noble creature, even though rich in everything, cannot live outside society, but naturally tends to it, as all of those who are sound in mind and learned do attest (which, of course, is completely denied by Hobbes, the English philosopher, in his *Elementa philosophica de cive*, ch. I, § 2 etc., and by Bodin in book I, ch. 6 of his books *De republica*, whose arguments have been refuted by the famous Eichel in his disputation *De iure civitatis*.[75] As far as it concerns the voice of the learned ones, Aristotle, the leader of all erudition, asserts with pressure in his *Nicomachean Ethics*, book 9, 9, 8, when saying that "no one wants to be rich in all goods under the condition to live alone, because man is a social being and made by nature to live within a society.[76]

In Engelbrecht's view, new currents of political philosophy, like Hobbes propagating that "Man is a wolf to man" (*homo homini lupus*), could not be more wrong, especially in times of plague. Societies under the stress of plague, according to Engelbrecht, clearly needed another kind of political and social ideology. Aristotle, he says, was right to rely on the social character of man and the dynamics into which his social behavior was able to develop. Stabilizing this social character, the state, and the society living in it, was, ideally speaking, the major task of authorities in times of plague. For this reason, Engelbrecht wanted to consider plague in terms of law (*pestem iuridice considerare*) and in terms of the rights which apply in these times.[77] His modus operandi is that of a legally trained expert: first, he will explain what plague is (*definitio*); second, he will identify the individuals related to or affected by it (*de personis*); third, he will focus on the things which plague concerns (*de rebus*); fourth, he will set out the mode (*de modo*) in which plague requires man to act; and fifth and finally, he will consider the effect (*de effectu*) of the measures taken against plague.

Like the other dissertations I have presented so far, Engelbrecht's text provides ample context. The dissertation covers a wide variety of aspects concerning plague in early modern Europe, such as: questions about the role of the magistrate and authorities; plague preachers and their controversial right to flee;[78] assemblies and services at church; doctors and nursing staff, such as plague physicians (*Stadtphysici*) and midwives; gravediggers, infected and locked-up houses and their marking with crosses on the doors;[79] cleansing infected houses with fur or even burning them after the death of their inhabitants; the rights of barber-surgeons without academic training; problems of testaments; the question of potential insurances against plague (*restitutio damni*);[80] regulations concerning quarantines (usually forty days); the appointment of *Oberleichenschreiber* (head coroners) who supervised the lockdown of houses and the recording of deaths; the restriction of commerce and trade; border controls and the appointment of so called *Passchreiber* (passport scribe) who were supposed to check the officially signed documents of travelers and passersby; long-term storage of grain supplies; cleansing coins with vinegar; keeping the streets free from personal garbage and filth; using only particular and designated streets; the expulsion of beggars and strangers; charities to calm potential riots among the poor;[81] and so on. For most of these and similar measures, Engelbrecht referred to particular plague ordinances, frequently quoting from them, such as the plague ordinances for Leipzig (1680) and Silesia (1680), the *Infections-Ordnung* authorized by Emperor Leopold I for Vienna (1679), or well-known treatises such as Ludwig von Hörnigk's *Würg-Engel* (1644).[82]

Engelbrecht's definition (*definitio*) of plague or pestilence did not reference the prolix discussions among physicians. His agreement with his late colleague Hermann Conring is noteworthy: "[plague] should be understood as an epidemic disease, most destructive, and for the most part lethal." This, of course, encompasses other epidemic and contagious diseases, such as severe fevers or dysentery. Yet, Engelbrecht argued, this definition was sufficient to deliver medical parameters for establishing legal and political measures. He clarified that his dissertation was not so much about medical terminology but, rather, about rights and legal issues (*de iuribus*) in times of ongoing plague outbreaks.[83] Yet, in the Helmstedt discussion we recognize an interesting overlap of discourses between medicine and law as was not uncommon in early modern treatises of plague.

The ruler or magistrate, Engelbrecht continues, is responsible for setting plague ordinances and official measures against plague, which are of critical importance. He even asks: "Shall the majesty or magistrate designate an economic monopoly to a certain person in times of plague?"[84] While monopolies, given to particular merchants, were not good for the economy, they were proven measures to restrict contacts and lower the risk of contagion, especially when trading with merchants from other jurisdictions. Regardless of the economic devastation, it appeared preferable to Engelbrecht in times of epidemic threats to hand over responsibility for supplies to one party or individual merchant who was capable of distributing supplies. The primary aim of this rather severe measure was to limit the number of contact persons travelling between different areas, to gain control over possible ways of transmission, and, most importantly, to avoid lock-downs of entire towns. Once plague was rampant, a whole city would depend on merchants from other areas, and an even more severe situation for the local economy would develop. While temporary monopolies had economic advantages for merchants holding them, they also represented a serious responsibility for providing the town with critical supplies.[85]

Burial practices were another area in need of regulation, especially once plague had reached the city. A common practice, long established since the beginnings of Europe's experience with the Black Death, was to bury plague victims outside the city walls in a separate cemetery so that, as Engelbrecht put it, "no pestilential illnesses could break forth from the filth of the dead and no vapors from the graves of putrefying bodies."[86] Protecting these cemeteries from wild animals or dogs in order to prevent the further dissemination of the disease was important as well. To lower the risk of contagious burial places, the bodies were covered with burnt lime. The burial of bodies was supposed to take place as quickly as possible. Only so called *bajulatores* and *vespillones*, corpse-bearers, who were distinguished by certain marks and clothes, were supposed to carry the dead bodies to the cemeteries, sometimes with the help of long white bars or poles. They were not allowed to speak to anybody or to be spoken to while on duty.[87]

The financial compensation of citizens who were not allowed to pursue their profession as usual was an important problem as well. Professors at the university, as for instance at the Academia Julia in Helmstedt, were not allowed to gather and teach audiences during times of severe plague, which heavily affected their income during a semester. In addition, students apparently began to flee Helmstedt as plague advanced in the summer of 1681 and therefore no longer paid for lectures by university professors.[88] However, the annual salary of Helmstedt professors was safe, at least on paper, and in case of death was paid for the whole year to his household, mostly to his widow.[89] Luckily enough for the dukes and the magistrates at Wolfenbüttel, there was no significant number of deaths in 1681 and 1682 that were directly linked to plague among Helmstedt professors. Christoph Schrader (1680) or Hermann Conring (1681) had simply died of old age.

Lastly, the right to flee epidemics was a major enduring issue. Especially for physicians and clergymen, the situation was often tricky, since they were supposed to help and stand by those in need. Plague not only corrupting to the health but was also threatening to the very essence of man's social character. Law, politics, and ethics, Engelbrecht believed, were supposed to restore and preserve the Aristotelian idea of man as a social being. Everything tends to the good, as Aristotle himself stated at the beginning of his *Nicomachean Ethics*. This led Engelbrecht, in accordance with Duke Rudolf August, to delineate a paternalistic ideology of public peace and order in 1683, at the tail end of recent threats of plague in Helmstedt. What subjects needed more than ever in times of pestilential threat was faith and trust in the goodness of human character. Mutual distrust and personal advantage, as Hobbes and others maintained, were not considered to be a good foundation for a functional society, a society that even worked under the severe stress of plague. Even though social realities could change dramatically in times of plague, the academic milieu of Helmstedt still needed a concept of what was good, an ideal that was worth emulating, namely a paternalistic Lutheran and Aristotelian trust in the goodness of the human character. The law and plague ordinances, at least on paper, were supposed to give form to this ideal.

Theology, *libertas philosophandi*, and the History of Burial and Mourning Practices in Helmstedt

In the previous section we have seen that, in particular, burial practices became a special issue in times of plague. Scripture teaches that human beings have been persecuted by plagues since biblical times.[90] Epidemic diseases were an important issue addressed by early modern European theology and had a considerable effect on religious burial as well as mourning practices. Especially from a theological point of view, burial in times of plague became a delicate matter.

A somewhat typical academic example might be Johann Wilhelm Baier's *Dissertatio theologica ad Psal. XCI. versum 5. & 6. quo Pestis diurna ac nocturna describi creditur* (Theological Dissertation on Psalms 91: 5 and 6, where it is believed that plague during day and night is described), published in Jena in 1683.[91] In prominent passages such as Psalm 91: 5–6, early modern theology found many hints regarding the nature and apt caution against comparable lethal threats under the recurring Hebrew term of דֶּבֶר (*deber*, plague, pestilence). In Luther's translation the passage goes: "(5) You will not fear the terror of the night, nor the arrow that flies by day / (6) nor the pestilence that stalks in the darkness, nor the destruction that wastes at noonday."[92] Based on the interpretation of this and many other biblical passages, early modern theology was convinced that plague or pestilence had to be considered as an arrow sent from above, a divine punishment and examination (*sagitta Dei*).[93] Such passages often gave occasion for physico-theological considerations, an intellectual tendency to interpret biblical accounts with respect to their physical, natural philosophical background. The "pestilence that stalks in the darkness" and "the destruction that wastes at noonday" of Psalm 91: 5–6 was therefore often seen as a display of the fundamental characteristics of plague: burial at night and, as experience showed, most severe fevers in the middle of the day.

It is striking that in the years 1681 to 1683, when the threat of plague was high, we have no dissertation titles with explicit reference to plague published by the faculty of theology. The topic was, of course, very present in sermons, services, academic speeches, or theological devotional writings.[94] Yet, there was a dissertation that tackled plague from a mostly theological perspective that was issued by the faculty of philosophy and thus supported by the *libertas philosophandi*, the freedom of philosophizing.

Only one year after his Boyle-inspired dissertation on the effluvia, Justus Cellarius, Professor of Physics, presided over a dissertation centered on another problem of what to do during times of plague or other pestilential diseases. However, this work did not take the perspective of natural philosophy, but more broadly assumed the viewpoint of *historia litteraria*, as the title reveals: *Exercitatio academica de antiquo funerum ritu* (Academic Exercise on the Ancient Rite of Burial).[95] While this text did not relate to Cellarius's core discipline, it served his ambitions to gain promotion to the faculty of theology at Helmstedt, a goal he achieved by holding private lectures on theology in 1683 and 1684. There is no doubt that Cellarius in his dissertation on ancient burial rites from 1682, specifically dedicated to Duke Rudolf August of Braunschweig-Lüneburg in the middle of a pestilential threat, wanted to promote his career ambitions as a young professor.

Was he the main author of the text? There are two reasons why Caspar Heinrich Sellen (1660–1709), who is referred to as *responsurus auctor* on the title page, should be considered as the second author. The first is the dedicatory letter by Sellen, who as a student belonged to the dinner party (*Tischgesellschaft*) at Cellarius's house in Helmstedt. Second, there are hints in the funeral oration held for Sellen in 1709, given by the famous polymath, theologian, and house-master of Georg Philipp Telemann, Caspar Calvör (1650–1725), who knew Sellen from his time in Helmstedt.[96] This would also match with the fact that Sellen, after graduating from the university of Helmstedt and later spending some time with the Pietist Philipp Jacob Spener in Dresden, took up a theological profession and became a minister at the mining town of Wildemann in the Upper Harz region in 1691. It would also explain why a physics professor with a strong physico-theological profile, such as Cellarius, presided over a philosophical dissertation on ancient burial practices.

The link between the current threat of plague at Helmstedt and the dissertation on ancient burial rites is made explicit by the student Sellen in the dedicatory letter directly addressed to Duke Rudolf August:

> The occasion to elaborate in particular on the present subject of burial is given by the miserable situation of our time, now that the pestilential contagion, while creeping through Germany coming from the East, has already affected our neighbors. It is rampant there with such a force that mixed burials are packed abundantly with old and young alike, so that the people there suffer from a most miserable and fatal tragedy. Therefore, on the occasion of such a fear of mischief in the vicinity and since all of us, while recalling the final necessity, justly consider death more profoundly at the moment, it seemed not in vain to me to set forth more deeply an argument on the ancient burial practices of the old ones, since out of them it is possible to establish among learned men an historical account of the noncommon death. … God, the omnipotent and greatest, makes it that the bad smelling poison [*virus*] of the pestilence, raging in the vicinity, drifts by no means forward to these regions here, but keeps it at a distance from here as long as possible, where during the most severe miseries of our neighbors the lands of our most serene dukes rejoice in the blossom of their favored situation and in the public tranquility luckily far off due to God's grace.[97]

This is a remarkable passage, since it gives extra evidence to a major focus of this chapter: the deep conviction of early modern scholars and academics at Helmstedt that they should and indeed could contribute useful insights for their learned peers towards society's battle against plague. Sellen specifically wanted to address the learned ones (*eruditi*) with his historical account on uncommon burial practices (*non vulgaris mortis memoria*). His reference to pestilence coming from the East (*ex Oriente*) is in line with early modern views that plague and other epidemic diseases were mainly imported through trading and war contacts with the Orient, particularly the Ottoman Empire. Yet the plague threatening Helmstedt in 1682 actually came from German territories lying east of the duchy of Braunschweig-Lüneburg, namely Leipzig and Magdeburg. As we know from Cellarius's dissertation on the effluvia one year before, the threat of plague was taken seriously. Furthermore, external evidence proves that the disease had reached Wolfenbüttel in 1681 and that Helmstedt had some reported cases as well. Sellen, and indirectly also Cellarius, seem to deny that plague had reached the duchy already. Such denials were common practice, as discussed above. It was important to maintain one's own uninfected status for as long as possible in order to avoid the total lock-down of towns and to keep alive trading contacts with neighboring areas.

Despite this cautious denial of an actual pestilential threat to Helmstedt, the dissertation by Cellarius and Sellen gives a completely different impression than the dedicatory letter. It is apparent, Cellarius and Sellen say, that the question of the soul (*anima*) and what happens to it after death belongs to the expertise of the *scientia theologica*, the "theological science." The body, on the other hand, gets buried and dissolved into its several elements ("in sua principia dissolve").[98] At the same time, Cellarius and Sellen claim that we find a tremendous variety of practices for burial of corpses in history. They list some disturbing and astonishing ones that they have collected from several descriptions from Lilio Gregorio Giraldi, Hermann Conring, Jan Swammerdamm, or Theodor Kerckring.[99]

In the first chapter of their dissertation, Cellarius and Sellen stated that all human concepts of natural law required that the bodies of the dead should not be exposed to wild animals or left to rot under the open sky. Just as Aristotle had commented on Sophocles' tragedy at the beginning of his *Rhetoric*, it was just of Antigone to bury Polynices, even though it was forbidden. It simply followed natural law.[100] Besides personal affection for the deceased, Cellarius and Sellen continue, the *ultima ratio* of this practice was the necessity to avoid the spread of unhealthy putrefaction from dead bodies.[101] Already in scripture, as in Kings, Ezechiel, or Jeremiah, the impious are severely punished for not following the burial rites.[102] It is here where we get a glimpse of the physico-theological dimension of Cellarius's and Sellen's dissertation, in the conviction that *realia* to be found in scripture have often concrete physical or natural philosophical backgrounds and reasons.[103]

As Cellarius and Sellen explain in the second long chapter of their dissertation, one of the most striking curiosities that sets apart the classical ancient pagan from the Christian way of burial is the practice of burning a body (*crematio, ustrinum*). While this was not a viable option for Christians, it is surprising how extensively they discussed cremation. They even censured the superstition (*superstitio*) of burning witches still practiced by fellow Christians of their own time.[104] Cellarius and Sellen did not go as far as opposing fumigation in order to clean houses from pestilential diseases or prevent their contamination, a practice that was commonly recommended at the time. Yet the mere juxtaposition of conflicting practices left many things open. While only providing a survey of practices as reflected in the *historia litteraria*, they were covered by the *libertas philosophandi* granted by the faculty of philosophy.

After their extensive consideration of several ancient practices of burning (*crematio*) and burying (*humatio*), Cellarius and Sellen concluded that under certain conditions the natural law of burying the dead was tested. This was especially the case when severe lethal threats, such as plagues, made the burial of dead corpses a dangerous and precarious challenge. Remarkable in respect to plague is that Cellarius and Sellen elaborated on the entire ceremony of burying, which encompasses what happens before, during, and after the burial. It is on several of these occasions that Cellarius and Sellen seemed to opt for a simpler and less opulent service. This matches common advice given by plague orders, that plague victims should be buried quickly after death, at night, and without a funeral procession to attract minimal attention. This helped prevent contagion among preachers, mourners, and pallbearers. They also rejected the idea of Christian burials within churchyards as an ancient relic of Christian belief. While this was still common practice, the authors were not prepared to judge if it was right, or even safe (*rectene, an secus*).[105] In particular the practice of elaborate and luxurious funeral feasts, the two Helmstedt scholars asserted, had spread over the years, leading to immoral acts, such as drunkenness and disputes, and detracting from the original rite.[106] It was also important to distinguish mere superstitious devotion towards the deceased from the true traditional and ancient rites. When plague was rampant, time at the cemetery should be cut short, and mourners instead should cherish the memory of the deceased in God. Living during plague made it clear to mourners that death was literally omnipresent.[107]

Epidemics: Catalyzing Tradition and Changing Knowledge

These case studies show that late seventeenth-century knowledge of plague was far more complex than the measures taken by the authorities might suggest. The academic discourse went beyond these bare political measures. Academics at early modern universities were confronted and concerned with plenty of possibilities to answer the question of what appears to be "right" in times of epidemic threats. Especially within academic milieus, threats of plague, such as in Helmstedt around 1681, were crucial events that catalyzed discussions on knowledge and on what was considered "right" or "wrong." The academics at Helmstedt, as we have seen, arrived at comparable, but also different, conclusions according to their respective discipline and expertise.

Starting with physics and medicine at Helmstedt, we have seen that certain corpuscular theories played a role in explaining the spread of plague and the process of contagion. In physics the theory of effluvia, promoted by

Fracastoro, Kircher, Digby, and Boyle, was taken increasingly into consideration to explain the spread of contagious diseases. In medicine, however, the ancient Hippocratic and Galenic concept of miasma prevailed. Both concepts offered similar answers to the spread of contagion. Scholars in Helmstedt had also no problem with making these corpuscular approaches compatible with early modern Aristotelian and Peripatetic positions, which, by doctrine, were mostly skeptical about any slightly Epicurean or Lucretian and neo-atomistic positions. Terms like *effluvia* avoided the neo-atomistic appeal and made corpuscular theory useable also for university scholars mostly driven by Aristotelianism. While the concepts of effluvia and miasma had several overlaps and similar assumptions, it becomes clear that physics and natural philosophy were much more inclined to use these corpuscular concepts to describe plague with the aid of new currents of philosophy, such as Boyle, Digby, or Borelli. However, the faculty of medicine in Helmstedt, as we have seen, admonished that effluvia and miasmas were only one half of the explanation, since they would only explain the spread, but not the actual processes taking place during a contagion. Effluvia or miasmas, the ranks of doctors in Helmstedt were convinced, should not be considered as carriers of poison which would without distinction affect every living being in the same way. Here, the faculty of medicine in Helmstedt showed its huge indebtedness to traditional Galenic humoral pathology by highlighting fermentation processes in predisposed bodies as a major factor enabling plague to infect these living beings in the first place.

The chair of law at Helmstedt presented itself as a strong fortress of Aristotelianism and traditional ideas on civil rights. In strong contrast to political philosophers such as Hobbes or Bodin, law professors at Helmstedt promoted the optimistic Aristotelian view, as displayed in the *Nicomachean Ethics* and in *Politics*, that man is a social being and that everything tends to the good. Exceptionally severe times of plague required the mutual trust and empathy of the members of a society. Mutual distrust and seeking only one's personal advantage, as Hobbes maintained, were not a political ideology apt for the paternalistic approach pursued by the dukes of Braunschweig-Lüneburg. Especially during times of plague, members of society had to follow their social roles and professions. For the sake of preventing contagions those merchants who were best equipped were obliged to take care of trading supplies. Rulers had to ensure that enough provisions were available. One of the main tasks to get society under control in times of plague was to offer a reasonable and agreeable ideology of mutual trust and peace. Interesting as well appears to be the fact that plague gave Lutheran law professors in Helmstedt the opportunity to criticize newer currents of political philosophy, such as Thomas Hobbes and others.

Finally, in the faculty of philosophy we have seen the discussion of burial practices during times of plague that also extended to theological questions and considerations. Despite the fact that the core objective of theology was to save the Christian soul (*anima*), there were also practical considerations, such as how to best bury the dead in times of plague. As the case of Helmstedt has shown, Lutheran scholars at the Academia Julia, in the wake of physico-theology and Pietist tendencies, opted for a reduced and more internalized funeral service rooted in traditional Christian beliefs. The Helmstedt scholars under discussion argued that scripture contained evidence that early burial practices protected the living from putrefying bodies that were often responsible for plagues and pestilences. Plague was, of course, considered to be a divine punishment, but also, being part of the divine creation, a natural disease.[108]

The case of Helmstedt and its academic milieu shows that book culture and the use of libraries, public or private, had an important influence on the scholars who took up their pens to fight pestilential illnesses. By using their libraries, sorting, browsing, and citing the books, they guarded the tradition of knowledge, but were at the same time catalyzing this tradition through several strands of transmission into new and reformed concepts of knowledge. This, inevitably, also transformed traditional academic knowledge about plague at universities such as Helmstedt that were mostly driven by Aristotelian and Galenic concepts. This development changed how academics in Helmstedt looked at plague and other pestilences, not least because these epidemic outbreaks undeniably burst into everybody's life and family. For professors in Helmstedt, as elsewhere, the fight against plague around 1680 began with academic reasoning and the consulting of knowledge contained in books.

Benjamin Wallura (né Hübbe) studied Classics and History at Freie Universität Berlin from 2008 to 2014. He continued his PhD in Berlin and Jyväskylä, Finland and is currently finalizing his thesis on the plants and animals of scripture as discussed by Bible philology and sciences in seventeenth- and eighteenth-century Europe. He has worked on several projects, such as "Encounters with the Orient in Early Modern Scholarship" (EOS) funded by Humanities in the European Research Area from 2013 to 2016, and "Der Aristotelismus in Helmstedt. Die Karriere eines europäischen Paradigmas" based at the Herzog August Library and Freie Universität funded by the Deutsche Forschungsgemeinschaft from 2017 to 2020. He is a researcher and honorary lecturer at Freie Universität Berlin. His research interests cover early modern science and medicine, history of philology, history of universities, early modern Latin disputations and dissertations, as well as the history of books and libraries. On all of these subject matters he has co-edited volumes and published several articles.

Notes

1. This interchangeable use of "plague," "pestilence," and "epidemic" occurs already in the sources relevant for this chapter, see Conring, *De peste*, c. V, who refers to Massaria's *De peste libri duo* (Venice, 1579). See also Christensen, *Politics and the Plague*, 61–66, esp. 63.
2. Varlık, "Rethinking the History of Plague," 285–93; Blum, "Epidemic and the Individual," 53–68.
3. Eisenberg, "Uses of History during the First Nine Months of Covid," 421.
4. See Green, *Pandemic Disease in the Medieval World*; Bergdolt, "Die Pest im 16. und 17. Jahrhundert," 25–35.
5. The literature on this most confusing relation of "knowledge" and "validity/authority" is extremely dense and complex, not least because of the several semantic fields and their connotations in different languages. I refer here just to one of many recent publications: Kaiser et al., "Einleitung—Wissen und Geltung," 11–25. For a relevant older discussion see Fleck, *Entstehung und Entwicklung*, 31–70; for a critical review of Fleck's ideas, see Zittel, "Ludwik Fleck."
6. For differing concepts of health and illness in the early modern period, see Salatowsky, "Wer heilt mich?" 13–23.
7. For a useful approach to the terms "contagion" and "infection" in late medieval and early modern southern German towns, see Kinzelbach, "Infection, Contagion, and Public Health," 369–89.
8. For the reception of Hippocratic miasma theory through Galen, see Jouanna, "Air, Miasma, and Contagion," 121–36.
9. For a discussion of the variety of medical practitioners in seventeenth-century Central Europe, such as physicians, surgeons, barber surgeons, laymen doctors, midwifes, etc., see Christensen, *Politics and the Plague*, 52–61; Salatowsky and Stolberg, "Einleitung," 8–9. The group most relevant for my study are university professors with a chair for medicine, anatomy, or botany or fully academically trained physicians.
10. See e.g.: Mayow, *Opera omnia medico-physica*; Zacchia, *Quaestiones medico-legales*; Castro, *Medicus Politicus*.
11. See recent research on this topic: Omodeo and Volkhard, *Natural Knowledge and Aristotelianism*; Beyer et al., *Alte und neue Philosophie*.
12. The faculty of law even did so in very explicit terms, see Engelbrecht and Blume, *Von dem was recht ist zu Pest-Zeiten*.
13. Herz, "Die Pest," 49–57.
14. According to Christensen, *Politics and the Plague*, 222, the plague in 1681 was rampant in Braunschweig, Quedlingburg, and Blankenburg, where the disease caused about four hundred deaths. It was also brought to Helmstedt by troops, where twenty houses were closed as a precaution. Nevertheless, no deaths seem to be recorded in this case. Officially, Helmstedt was not out of imminent danger of plague until 30 May 1684.
15. This approach methodologically owes a lot to: Mulsow and Stamm, *Konstellationsforschung*, 7–12.
16. For a discussion of archival records and printed sources Christensen, *Politics and the Plague*. Most scholarship, however, has neglected to discuss the academic sources.
17. Christensen, *Politics and Plague*.
18. Otto, "Zu David Hanisius"; Raabe, *Die Fürstliche Bibliothek zu Wolfenbüttel*, 36–38.
19. Hanisius, *Catalogus*.

20. Hanisius, *Catalogus*, fol. 4v.
21. All English translations are mine, unless noted otherwise. For the original Latin text of the poem, see Hanisius, *Catalogus*, 15.
22. According to Raabe, *Leser und Lektüre*, the average number of users per year from 1678 to 1682 is more or less stable with no significant drops in visitors during the years 1680–82.
23. Raabe, *Leser und Lektüre*, provides a comprehensive overview of all the borrowings between 1680 and 1683.
24. Conring, *De Peste*.
25. Sorbait, *Consilium Medicum*. On the plague in Vienna around 1678/79, see Schmölzer, *Die Pest in Wien*.
26. Fracastoro, *Syphilis*. On Fracastoro and his works on contagion, see Nutton, "The Reception of Fracastoro's Theory of Contagion," 196–234; Strasser, "Ansteckungstheorien der Pest in der Frühen Neuzeit," 69–76.
27. Nutton, "The Reception of Fracastoro's Theory of Contagion," 200.
28. Diemerbroeck, *De peste libri quattuor*.
29. Hippocrates, *Des vents*, 108–9. For a comprehensive account on the reception of this miasma theory since antiquity, see Jouanna, "Air, Miasma, and Contagion," 121–36.
30. Diemerbroeck, *Tractatus de peste*, c. X, § VI, 64; Fracastoro, *De sympathia et antipathia rerum*, c. 5.
31. Boyle, "De mira subtilitate effluviorum," c. I, 3–4. The polymath and Jesuit Athansius Kircher spoke of "Effluenz" in his treatise on plague as well; see Strasser, "Ansteckungstheorien der Pest," 74. The English scholar Kenelm Digby picked up the term as well.
32. Boyle, "De mira subtilitate effluviorum," c. I, 3–4.
33. Cellarius and Behrens, *De penetrabili efficacia effluviroum*.
34. On Justus Cellarius, see Ahrens, *Lehrkräfte*, 49; Bruning, *Innovation*, 198–99; Klein, *Les Chaires*, esp. 49–51, 59–60, and 243–45. On Cellarius' significiance for the natural philosophy at Helmstedt, see with further literature: Wallura, "Oszillierende Schulphilosophie," 247–72.
35. The academically trained physician Konrad Barthold Behrens remained under the influence of miasma theory, for instance Behrens, *Medicus Legalis*.
36. See Christensen, *Politics and the Plague*, 143 and 222.
37. On the question whether the presiding professor or the responding student or both have to be considered authors see Friedenthal et al., "Introduction," in *Early Modern Disputations*, 1–33. There are indications that Cellarius and Behrens shared authorship of their dissertation.
38. See Mercer, "Leibniz and His Master," 10–46, for a discussion of *philosophia reformata* in the letters of the Helmstedt professor Hermann Conring, the philosopher Gottfried Wilhelm Leibniz, and the Leipzig professor Jacob Thomasius.
39. Cellarius and Behrens, *De penetrabili efficacia effluviroum*, c. I, fol. A2r–v.
40. See Wirdig, *Victrix veritas*, 86–96.
41. Guericke, *Experimenta nova Magdeburgica*; Wirdig, *Nova Medicina Spirituum*; Digby, *Demonstratio immortalitatis animae rationalis*; Mayow, *Opera omnia medico-physica*.
42. Cellarius—Behrens, *De penetrabili efficacia effluviroum*, th. V–VIII and th. XIV–XVI, fol. A3v–B1r.
43. Cellarius—Behrens, *De penetrabili efficacia effluviroum*, th. X, fol. B2r.
44. Cellarius—Behrens, *De penetrabili efficacia effluviroum*, th. XII, fol. B2v–B3r.

45. Cellarius—Behrens, *De penetrabili efficacia effluviroum*, th. XXVI, fol. D1r.
46. Cellarius—Behrens, *De penetrabili efficacia effluviroum*, th. XL, fol. E2r–E2v.
47. Cellarius—Behrens, *De penetrabili efficacia effluviroum*, th. XLI, fol. E2v–E3r.
48. Behrens, *Consilium*.
49. See, for instance, the 1680 plague tract by the Braunschweig *Stadtphysikus* Lorenz Gieseler, *Kurtze, aber nöthige Anweisung*, 31–32, which contains a list of valuable ingredients to prepare remedies against plague.
50. On the faculty of medicine at Helmstedt, see Triebs, *Die medizinische Fakultät*; Kloth and Aumüller, *Geschichte der Anatomie*.
51. Schelhammer and Meineke, *De Peste*.
52. Schelhammer and Meineke, *De Peste*.
53. On Schelhammer, see Scheffel, *Epistolae selectiores*; Ahrens, *Lehrkräfte*, 202–3.
54. See, Conring, *De peste*, c. XXIX, fol. D2v. See also Bötticher, *Disputatio medica de peste*, § V, 6–7 (1712). Note that for Bötticher it seemed much easier to refer to effluvia and miasmas under the rather vexed term of 'atoms.'
55. Schelhammer, *De Peste*, Cap. III, § X, 19–20.
56. See the famous passage in Lucretius (6, 1141–44) inspired by Thucydides' account on the plague of Athens.
57. Schelhammer referred to Schouten, *Oost-Indische voyagie*.
58. Schelhammer, *De Peste*, Cap. III, § IX, 18–19. Kinzelbach, "Infection, Contagion, and Public Health," 383, argues that similar ideas occurred in the German territories already since the late sixteenth century.
59. Schelhammer, *De Peste*, Cap. III, § XII, 22–23.
60. Cf. Lucr. 6, 1098–1102.
61. Schelhammer, *De Peste*, Cap. III, § XIV, 25.
62. Ibid., Cap. III, § XVII, 27.
63. Ibid., Cap. IV, § I, 32.
64. Ibid.
65. Ibid., Cap. IV, § III, 35.
66. See Kircher, *Scrutinium pestis*; for the German translation published in 1680, see Kircher, *Natürliche und Medicinalische Durchgründung*.
67. Conring and Behrens (resp.), *Disputatio de fermentation*. Note that the respondent is a relative of Konrad Barthold Behrens, who later become a student and respondent of Justus Cellarius in Helmstedt. See also Conring, *De peste*.
68. Schelhammer and Meineke, *De Peste*, Cap. IV, § III, 35.
69. For this argument, also promoted by Diemerbroeck, see Schelhammer and Meineke, *De Peste*, Cap. VIII, § VIII, 81.
70. This particular issue remained important for Schelhammer's entire medical career, see Schelhammer, *De genuina febres curandi methodo dissertatio*; Schelhammer—Waltsgott (resp.), *Disputatio inauguralis de morbis aetatum*.
71. See, for instance, Schmidt, *De Officio Magistratus circa tempora pestis*, § 10, fol. A2r–A2v. Schmidt in 1695 became a professor of theology in Helmstedt; he had strong interests in natural philosophy. See Roling, "Mechanik und Mirakel," 211–45.
72. Behse, *Die juristische Fakultät der Universität Helmstedt*.
73. Engelbrecht—Blume, *Discursus iuridicus*, § XXIX, fol. F2. "About what is right" in the title of the dissertation points to a general tone of "right," but at the same time refers more directly to the strict sense of "legally right." Both moral and legal connotation appear to be implied.

74. Friedenthal et al., "Introduction," in *Early Modern Disputations*, 1–33.
75. The reference is to Johann Eichel von Rautenkron (1621–88) whose disputation *De iure civitatis/Vom Bürgerrecht* was published in 1662.
76. Engelbrecht, *Von dem was recht ist zu Pest-Zeiten*, § I, fol. Ar, where references to Aristotle's *Politics* and to Samuel Pufendorf's well-known *De iure belli et pacis* are made.
77. Engelbrecht, *Von dem was recht ist zu Pest-Zeiten*, § II, fol. A2v.
78. See, for example: Hohmuth and Hellwich (resp.), *An fuga tempore pestis sit licita?*
79. See, for instance, Saltzmann and Fasterling (resp.), *De claudendis aedibus peste infectorum*.
80. See, for instance, Mylius and Einert (resp.), *De testamento tempore pestis condito*.
81. Carmichael, *Plague and the Poor*.
82. Anon., *Der Stadt Leipzig Verneuerte und verbesserte Pest-Ordnung*; Anon., *Neue schlesische Infections-Ordnung*; Anon., *Neüe Infections-Ordnung*; Hörnigk, *Würg-Engel*.
83. Engelbrecht, *Von dem was recht ist zu Pest-Zeiten*, § IV, fol. A3v. See also Conring, *De peste*, c. XII.
84. Engelbrecht, *Von dem was recht ist zu Pest-Zeiten*, § XVI, fol. C3v.
85. For further aspects see Engelbrecht, *Von dem was recht ist zu Pest-Zeiten*, § XVI, fol. C3v.
86. Engelbrecht, *Von dem was recht ist zu Pest-Zeiten*, § XXI, fol. D2r.
87. Engelbrecht, *Von dem was recht ist zu Pest-Zeiten*, § XXII, fol. D3r–v.
88. Breithaupt and Leporin, *Memoria Caplatoniana*, 49–50.
89. Engelbrecht, *Von dem was recht ist zu Pest-Zeiten*, § XXIX, fol. Fv.
90. See for instance Lev. 26:16, 26:25; Num. 14:12; Deut. 28:59; Jer. 14:29, 14:34; Ezech. 14 and 23; Ex. 9; 2 Sam. 24; Ps 34:1–2; Col. 1:24; Phil. II:30; 2 Joh. III:16.
91. Baier—Beyer (resp.), *Dissertatio theologica*.
92. Luther, *Die Bibel*, Ps 91:5–6. See Baier, *Pestis diurna ac nocturna*, fol. Ar–v.
93. See, for instance: Gecser, "Doctors and Preachers against the Plague," 78–102.
94. See, for instance, Buroner, *Pest-Büchlein*.
95. Cellarius—Sellen (resp.), *De antiquo funerum ritu*.
96. Calvör, "Personalia," in Calvör, *Unaußlöschliche Ehe- und Liebes-Flamme*, fol. 1v.
97. Cellarius and Sellen (resp.), *De antiquo funerum ritu*, fol. 2r–3r.
98. Cellarius and Sellen (resp.), *De antiquo funerum ritu*, fol. A2r.
99. Giraldi, *De sepulchris et vario sepeliendi ritu*; Conring, *Dissertationes medicae de nonullis*, esp. c. V, 367–76: *Sepultura Christi et condicndorum cadaverum ritus*. Reference to it is made in Cellarius—Sellen (resp.), *De antiquo funerum ritu*, c. III, § 6, fol. D3v.
100. Cellarius—Sellen (resp.), *De antiquo funerum ritu*, fol. c. I, § IV, fol. A3v.
101. Cellarius—Sellen (resp.), *De antiquo funerum ritu*, c. I, § I, fol. A2v.
102. Cellarius—Sellen (resp.), *De antiquo funerum ritu*, c. I, § XV, fol. B4r–v.
103. Cellarius early on in his career gave private lectures in Helmstedt that were entitled with the very same term of *lectiones physico-sacras*. See Wallura, "Oszillierende Schulphilosophie."
104. Cellarius—Sellen (resp.), *De antiquo funerum ritu*, c. I, § XVII–XIIX, Cv–r.
105. Cellarius—Sellen (resp.), *De antiquo funerum ritu*, c. VI, § VII, fol. Hr.
106. Cellarius—Sellen (resp.), *De antiquo funerum ritu*, c. VII, § IX, fol. Kv.
107. See also Wallura, "Oszillierende Schulphilosophie," 269–70.
108. Behrens, *Gründlicher Bericht*, c. XX, 13–14, provides very interesting and comprehensive aspects of plague discussed around 1700.

Bibliography

Primary Sources

Anon. *E. E. Hochweisen Raths der Stadt Leipzig Verneuerte und verbesserte Pest-Ordnung ….* Leipzig: Johann Grossen und Consorten, 1680.

Anon. *Neue schlesische Infections-Ordnung und Medicinisches Consilium abgefasset und entworffen Anno 1680.* Dresden: Johann Christoph Miethen, 1680.

Anon. *Der Römischen Kayserlich / auch zu Ungarn und Böhaimb / [et]c. Königlichen Majestätt / Leopold Deß Ersten / [et]c. Ertz-Herzogens zu Oesterreich / [et]c. Unsers Allermächtigsten Herrn / Neüe Infections-Ordnung.* Wien: Leopold Voigt, 1679.

Baier, Johann Wilhelm—Beyer, Johannes Carl (resp.). *Dissertatio theologica ad Psal. XCI. versum 5. & 6. quo pestis diurna ac nocturna describi creditur.* Jena: Samuel Krebs, 1683.

Behrens, Konrad Barthold. *Consilium, Oder Rähtliches Gutachten, wie ein Soldat im Felde für Kranckheiten sich hüten und denselben zur Noht begegenen könne.* Hildesheim: Johann Leonhard Schlegel, 1689.

Behrens, Konrad Barthold. *Medicus Legalis, oder: Gesetzmäßige Bestell- und Ausübung Der Artzney-Kunst.* Frankfurt, Leipzig, Helmstedt: Paul Zeising, 1696.

Behrens, Konrad Barthold. *Gründlicher Bericht von der Natur, Eigenschafft und wahren Uhrsprung* [sic] *der Pest, auch wie dieselbe auf alle Weise praecaviret und am sichersten curiret werde.* Braunschweig: Johann Georg Zilliger and Ludolph Schröder, 1714.

Bohnstedt, Andreas. *Eigentliche und wahre Beschreibung der jetziger Zeit graßierenden Pest, welche in gründlicher Unterricht- und Anweisung fürstellet.* Helmstedt: Johann Lüderwalt, 1681.

Bötticher, Andreas Julius, and Justus Andreas Richers (resp.). *Disputatio medica de peste, quam auspicio sacro sanctae triados ex veterum et recentiorum observationibus collectam.* Helmstedt: Georg Wolfgang Hamm, 1712.

Boyle, Robert. "De mira subtilitate effluviorum." In *Exercitationes de athmosphaeris corporum consistentium.* London: William Godbid and Moses Pitt, 1673.

Breithaupt, Joachim Justus, and Christian Polycarp Leporin. *Memoria Caplatoniana, oder Lebensbeschreibung Zweener Breithaupten.* Quedlinburg: self-publishing, 1725.

Buroner, Leonhard Ulrich. *Pest-Büchlein. Mein Christ, hie findestu wider die Gifftige Pest-plag den allerbesten Rath: Num. XXI Durch Gottes Gnade angewiesen.* Helmstedt: Friedrich Lüderwald, 1683.

Calvör, Caspar. *Unaußlöschliche Ehe- und Liebes-Flamme. / Als Des frommen und getreuen Ehe-Paars / Des Weyland Herrn Casparis Henrici Sellen …* , Clausthal: Wilckische Schrifften 1709.

Castro, Rodrigo de. *Medicus Politicus, sive de Officiis Medico-Politicis Tractatus, quattuor distinctus libris ….* Hamburg: Georg Ludwig Froben, 1614.

Cellarius, Justus—Behrens, Konrad Barthold (resp.). *Disputatio physica de penetrabili efficacia effluviorum in afficiendis corporibus animalium.* Helmstedt: Heinrich David Müller, 1681.

Cellarius, Justus—Sellen, Caspar Heinrich (resp.). *Exercitatio academica de antiquo funerum ritu.* Helmstedt: Georg Wolfgang Hamm, 1682.

Conring, Hermann. *Dissertationes medicae de nonullis quae circa passionem et mortem Domini contigerunt.* In *Christliche Passions-Andachten …* , edited by Johannes Albrecht, 265–376. Hildesheim: Albrecht Weißkopf and Johann Ludolf Ebel, 1674.

Conring, Hermann—Matthaeus, Theophilus (resp.). *Disputatio inauguralis medica de peste.* Helmstedt: Johann Georg Täger and Martin Vogel, 1659.

Conring, Hermann—Matthaeus, Theophilus (resp.). *Disputatio inauguralis medica de peste.* Helmstedt: Heinrich David Müller, 1678.

Diemerbroeck, Isbrand van. *De peste libri quatuor, truculentissimi morbi historiam ratione et experientia confirmatam exhibentes.* Arnheim: Johannes Jacob, 1646.

Diemerbroeck, Isbrand van. *Tractatus de peste in quattuor libros distinctus, ruculentissimi morbi historiam ratione et experientia confirmatam exhibens.* Amsterdam: Johannes Blaeu, 1665.

Digby, Kenelm. *Demonstratio immortalitatis animae rationalis … .* Paris: Jacob Villery and Georg Iosse, 1651.

Engelbrecht, Georg—Blume, Christian Ulrich (resp.). *Discursus iuridicus de peste et iuribus circa tempus pestis. Von dem was recht ist zu Pest-Zeiten.* Helmstedt: Georg Wolfgang Hamm, 1683.

Fracastoro, Girolamo. *Syphilis sive morbus Gallicus.* Verona: Stefano dei Nicolini da Sabbio, 1530.

Fracastoro, Girolamo. *De sympathia et antipathia rerum.* Venice: Luca Antonio Giunta, 1546.

Fracastoro, Girolamo. *De contagione et contagiosis morbis et eorum curatione libri tres,* Venice: Luca Antonio Giunta, 1546.

Gieseler, Lorenz. *Kurtze, aber nöthige Anweisung, wie sich ein jeder bey dieser sehr sorgsamen und gefährlichen und weit umb sich greifenden Pest-Seuche fürsehen, praeserviren und curiren sol.* Braunschweig: Johann Heinrich Duncker, 1680.

Giraldi Lilio, Gregorio. *De sepulchris et vario sepeliendi ritu.* Basel: Michael Isengrin, 1539.

Gosky, Martin. *Ptripsema seu Fuga Luis Pestiferae. Das ist: Die Erste und kurtze ordentliche Verhütung und Chur der Pestilentz.* Helmstedt: Jacob Lucius, 1625.

Guericke, Otto von. *Experimenta nova (ut vocantur) Magdeburgica de vacuo spatio.* Amsterdam: Johann Janssonius van Waesberge, 1672.

Hanisius, David. *Catalogus scriptorum et tractatuum de peste.* Wolfenbüttel: Kaspar Johann Bißmarck, 1680.

Hanisius, David. *Continuatio Catalogi scriptorum et tractatuum des peste.* Braunschweig: Christoph Friedrich Zilliger, 1680.

Hippocrates. *Des vents,* edited and translated by Jacques Jouanna. Paris: Belles Lettres, 1988.

Hohmuth, Andreas—Hellwich, Joachim (resp.). *Problema morale, an fuga tempore pestis sit licita?* Wittenberg: Christian Schrödter, 1681.

Hörnigk, Ludwig von. *Würg-Engel: Von der Pestilentz Namen, Eigenschafft, Ursachen, Zeichen, Praeservation, Zufällen, Curation, etc. … .* Frankfurt am Main: Christoph Le Blon, 1644.

Kircher, Athanasius. *Scrutinium physicum-medicum contagiosae luis, quae pestis dicitur.* Rome: Typis Mascardi, 1658.

Kircher, Athanasius. *Natürliche und Medicinalische Durchgründung der leidigen ansteckenden Sucht und so genanten Pestilentz.* Augsburg: Jacob Koppmayer, 1680.

Luther, Martin. *Die Bibel—The Bible. Lutherübersetzung 2017—English Standard Version.* Stuttgart: Deutsche Bibelgesellschaft, 2018.

Mayow, John. *Opera omnia medico-physica, tractatibus quinque comprehensa.* Den Haag: Arnout Leers, 1681.

Mylius, Andreas—Einert, Nicolaus (resp.). *De testamento tempore pestis condito. Von dem testament, so zur zeit der Pest auffgerichtet wird.* Leipzig: Johann Georg, 1680.

Saltzmann, Johann Philipp—Fasterling, Martin Luther (resp.). *De claudendis aedibus peste infectorum*. Altorf: Heinrich Meyer, 1681.
Scheffel, Christian Stephan. *Virorum Clarissimorum ad Guntherum Christophorum Schelhammerum Epistolae selectiores, rem litterariam, philosophiam naturalem ac medicinam potissimum ...* . Wismar, Stralsund: Samuel Gottlieb Lochmann, 1727.
Schelhammer, Günther Christoph. *De genuina febres curandi methodo dissertatio inter tres partes divisa ...* . Jena: Johann Bielcke, 1693.
Schelhammer, Günther Christoph, and Daniel Christoph Meinecke (resp.). *De Peste*. Helmstedt: Georg Wolfgang Hamm, 1682.
Schelhammer, Günther Christoph—Waltsgott, Johann Ernst (resp.). *Disputatio inauguralis de morbis aetatum*. Jena: Johann Zacharias Nisius, 1694.
Schmidt, Johannes Andreas—Posner, Heinrich Friedrich (resp.). *De Officio Magistratus circa tempora pestis dissertatio politica*. Jena: Johann David Werther, 1680.
Schouten, Wouter. *Oost-Indische voyagie; vervattende veel voorname voorvallen en ongemeene oreemde geschiedenissen, bloedige zee- en landtgevechten tegen de Portugeesen en Makassaren ...* . Amsterdam: Jacob van Meurs, 1676.
Sorbait, Paul de. *Consilium Medicum, Dialogus, oder freundliches Gespräch über den betrübten und armseligen Zustand der Kayserl. Residentz- und Haupt-Statt Wienn in Oesterreich, bey diser gefärhlichen und vorhero nie erhörten contagion ...* . Vienna: Johann von Gehlen, 1679.
Wirdig, Sebastian. *Nova Medicina Spirituum: curiosa scientia et doctrina, unanimiter hucusque neglecta et a nemine merito exculta, Medicis tamen et Physicis utilissima ...* . Hamburg: Gottfried Schultze, 1673.
Wirdig, Sebatian. *Victrix veritas in censuris theologico-medicis de Nova Spirituum Medicina ...* . Güstrow: Johannes Spierling, 1684.
Zacchia, Paolo. *Quaestiones medico-legales*. 3 vols. Leipzig: Elias Rehefeld, 1630.

Secondary Sources

Ahrens, Sabine. *Die Lehrkräfte der Universität Helmstedt*. Helmstedt: Landkreis Helmstedt, Kreismuseen, 2004.
Behse, Arthur. *Die juristische Fakultät der Universität Helmstedt im Zeitalter des Naturrechts*. Wolfenbüttel: Julius Zwißler Verlag, 1920.
Bergdolt, Klaus. "Die Pest im 16. und 17. Jahrhundert." In *Eine göttliche Kunst. Medizin und Krankheit in der Frühen Neuzeit*, edited by Sascha Salatowsky and Michael Stolberg, 25–35. Erfurt: Universität Erfurt, Veröffentlichungen der Forschungsbibliothek Gotha, 2019.
Beyer, Hartmut, Sinem Kılıç, et al., eds. *Alte und neue Philosophie. Aristotelismus und protestantische Gelehrsamkeit in Helmstedt und Europa (1600–1700)*. Wiesbaden: Harrassowitz, 2023.
Blum, Paul Richard. "Epidemic and the Individual: Renaissance Understandings of the Plague in View of Modern Experiences." *Roczniki Kulturoznawcze* 3 (2020): 53–68.
Bruning, Jens. *Innovation in Forschung und Lehre. Die Philosophische Fakultät der Universität Helmstedt in der Frühaufklärung 1680–1740*. Wiesbaden: Harrasowitz, 2012.
Carmichael, Ann G. *Plague and the Poor in Renaissance Florence*. Cambridge: Cambridge University Press, 2014.
Christensen, Daniel. *Politics and the Plague in Early Modern Germany. Political Efforts to Combat Epidemics in the Duchy of Braunschweig-Wolfenbüttel during the Seventeenth Century*. Saarbrücken: VDM Verlag Dr. Müller, 2008.

Eisenberg, Merle. "Uses of History during the First Nine Months of Covid." *Perspectives in Biology and Medicine* 64, no. 3 (2021): 421–35.

Feuerstein-Herz, Petra, ed. *Gotts verhengnis und seine straffe—Zur Geschichte der Seuchen in der Frühen Neuzeit*. Wolfenbüttel: Herzog August Bibliothek, 2005.

Fleck, Ludwik. *Entstehung und Entwicklung einer wissenschaftlichen Tatsache. Einführung in die Lehre vom Denkstil und Denkkollektiv*. Frankfurt am Main: Suhrkamp, 1980 [first: 1935].

Friedenthal, Meelis, Hanspeter Marti, and Robert Seidel, eds. *Early Modern Disputations and Dissertations in an Interdisciplinary European Context*. London, Boston: Brill, 2021.

Gecser, Ottó. "Doctors and Preachers against the Plague: Attitudes towards Disease in Late Medieval Plague Tracts and Plague Sermons." In *The Sacred and the Secular in Medieval Healing. Sites, Objects, and Texts*, edited by Barbara Bowers and Linda Migl Keyser, 78–102. London, New York: Routledge, 2016.

Green, Monica H., ed. *Pandemic Disease in the Medieval World. Rethinking the Black Death*. Leeds: Arc Humanities Press, 2015.

Herz, Andreas. "Die Pest in Selbstzeugnissen aus der Zeit des Dreißigjährigen Krieges." In *Gotts verhengnis und seine straffe—Zur Geschichte der Seuchen in der Frühen Neuzeit*, edited by Petra Feuerstein-Herz, 49–57. Wiesbaden: Harrasowitz, 2005.

Jouanna, Jacques. "Air, Miasma, and Contagion in the Time of Hippocrates and the Survival of Miamsas in Post-Hippocratic Medicine (Rufus of Ephesus, Galen, and Palladius)." In *Greek Medicine from Hippocrates to Galen: Selected Papers*, edited by Philip van der Eijk, 121–36. Leiden, Boston: Brill, 2012.

Kaiser, Ronny, and Frank Noll, et al., eds. *Wissen und Geltung. Interdisziplinäre Beiträge zur Dynamik kulturellen Wissens in Mittelalter und Neuzeit*, Göttingen: V&R unipress, 2020.

Kinzelbach, Annemarie. "Infection, Contagion, and Public Health in Late Medieval and Early Modern German Imperial Towns." *Journal of the History of Medicine and Allied Sciences* 61, no. 3 (2006): 369–89.

Klein, Boris. *Les Chaires et L'Esprit. Organisation et transmission des savoirs au sein d'une université germanique au xviie siècle*. Lyon: Presses universitaires de Lyon, 2017.

Kloth, Wiebke, and Gerhard Aumüller. *Geschichte der Anatomie und der Botanik an der Medizinischen Fakultät der Academia Julia zu Helmstedt*. Helmstedt: Landkreis Helmstedt, Kreismuseen, 2018.

Mercer, Christia. "Leibniz and His Master. The Correspondence with Thomasius." In *Leibniz and His Correspondents*, edited by Paul Lodge, 10–46. Cambridge: Cambridge University Press, 2004.

Mulsow, Martin, and Marcelo Stamm, eds. *Konstellationsforschung*. Frankfurt: Suhrkamp, 2005.

Namouchi, Amine, Guellil, Meriam, et al. "Integrative Approach Using Yersinia pestis Genomes to Revisit the Historical Landscape of Plague during the Medieval Period." *Proceedings of the National Academy of Science of the United States of America* 115, no. 50 (2018): E11790–97.

Nutton, Vivian. "The Reception of Fracastoro's Theory of Contagion. The Seed that Fell among Thorns?" *Osiris* 6 (1990): 196–234.

Omodeo, Pietro Daniel, and Volkhard Wels, eds. *Natural Knowledge and Aristotelianism at Early Modern Protestant Universities*. Wiesbaden: Harrasowitz, 2019.

Otto Jr., Karl F. "Zu David Hanisius, dem unbekannten Bibliothekar." In *Wolfenbütteler Beiträge. Aus den Schätzen der Herzog August Bibliothek*, vol. 3, edited by Paul Raabe, 283–99. Frankfurt am Main: Klostermann, 1978.

Raabe, Mechthild. *Leser und Lektüre vom 17. zum 19. Jahrhundert: Die Ausleihbücher der Herzog August Bibliothek Wolfenbüttel 1664–1806*. 4 vols. Munich: Saur, 1989–1998.

Raabe, Mechthild. *Die Fürstliche Bibliothek zu Wolfenbüttel und ihre Leser. Zur Geschichte des institutionellen Lesens in einer norddeutschen Residenz 1664–1806*. Wolfenbüttel: self-published, 1997.

Roling, Bernd. "Mechanik und Mirakel: Johannes Andreas Schmidt (1652–1726) und die technischen Grenzen des Wunders in Helmstedt." In *Was als wissenschaftlich gelten darf—Praktiken der Grenzziehung in Gelehrtenmilieus der Vormoderne*, edited by Rexroth, Frank and Martin Mulsow, 211–45. Frankfurt am Main, New York: Campus Verlag, 2014.

Salatowsky, Sascha, and Michael Stolberg, eds. *Eine göttliche Kunst. Medizin und Krankheit in der Frühen Neuzeit*. Katalog zur Ausstellung der Forschungsbibliothek Gotha und des Instituts für die Geschichte der Medizin der Julius-Maximilians-Universität Würzburg vom 14. April bis 23. Juni 2019. Gotha: Forschungsbibliothek Gotha, 2019.

Salatowsky, Sascha. "Wer heilt mich? Konzepte von Gesundheit und Krankheit in der Frühen Neuzeit." In *Eine göttliche Kunst. Medizin und Krankheit in der Frühen Neuzeit*, edited by Sascha Salatowsky and Michael Stolberg, 13–23. Gotha: Forschungsbibliothek Gotha, 2019.

Schmölzer, Hilde. *Die Pest in Wien. 'Deß wütenden Todts eine umbständig Beschreibung.'* Berlin: Verlag der Nation, 1988.

Strasser, Gerhard F. "Ansteckungstheorien der Pest in der Frühen Neuzeit am Beispiel von Girolamo Fracastoro und Athanasius Kircher." In *Gotts verhengnis und seine straffe*, edited by Petra Feuerstein-Herz, 69–76. Wolfenbüttel: Herzog August Bibliothek, 2005.

Triebs, Michaela. *Die medizinische Fakultät der Universität Helmstedt (1576–1810). Eine Studie zu ihrer Geschichte unter besonderer Berücksichtigung der Promotions- und Übungsdisputationen*. Wiesbaden: Harrasowitz, 1995.

Varlık, Nükhet. "'Oriental Plague' or Epidemiological Orientalism? Revisiting the Plague Episteme of the Early Modern Mediterranean." In *Plague and Contagion in the Islamic Mediterranean*, edited by Nükhet Varlık, 57–88. Newark: Arc Humanities Press, 2017.

Varlık, Nükhet. "Rethinking the History of Plague in the Time of COVID-19." *Centarus* 62, no. 2 (2020): 285–93.

Vries, Malte de. "Pestepidemien im Braunschweig des 16. und 17. Jahrhunderts. Alltag in Zeiten einer 'Gottesstrafe.'" *Braunschweigisches Jahrbuch für Landesgeschichte* 101 (2020): 27–50.

Wallura, Benjamin. "Oszillierende Schulphilosophie. Heinrich Rixner, Justus Cellarius und der Helmstedter Physikunterrichte zwischen Aristoteles-Exegese und neuerer Philosophie (1663–83)." In *Alte und neue Philosophie. Aristotelismus und protestantische Gelehrsamkeit in Helmstedt und Europa (1600–1700)*, edited by Hartmut Beyer, Sinem Kilic, et al., 227–72. Wiesbaden: Harrasowitz, 2023.

Zittel, Claus. "Ludwik Fleck and the Concept of Style in the Natural Sciences." *Studies in East European Thought* 64, no. 1–2: *Origins of Social Theories of Knowledge* (2012): 53–79.

CHAPTER 9

Diseases as a Threat to the Human and Animal World

Interdependencies of Early Modern Contagion Discourses in Central Europe

ANSGAR SCHANBACHER, PHILIP KNÄBLE, AND MALTE DE VRIES

Introduction: Interwoven Destinies

Born in the imperial city of Speyer, Johann Joachim Becher (1635–82) lived a restless but academically productive life. His career brought him to Munich as personal physician of the elector and an author of books in the fields of natural philosophy, pedagogics, and politics, to Vienna as a councilor of Emperor Leopold I, and eventually to England and the Netherlands, providing a migratory life between these countries. Especially renowned for his cameralistic concepts and his experiments in alchemy, Becher also published a partly rhymed work on the medical effects of animals and plants and a reference book for the early modern household economy.[1] The works of this polymath show the broad interests of early modern scholars and provide examples where historical evidence on the triangular relationship between humans, animals, and pathogens can be found.

Printed sources such as Becher's tracts, as well as ordinances and archival sources, serve to explore this triangle and to follow three research questions.[2] First, we will explore what role animals played during the occurrence of epidemics such as the plague. Here, the differentiation between useful and useless animals as well as their liminality comes into play.[3] Second, we will take an overview of still poorly researched transmissible animal diseases and major outbreaks during the sixteenth and seventeenth centuries, which in the words of the economic historian Friedrich-Wilhelm Henning "were widespread and destroyed time and again the livestock of whole villages."[4] Third, we will observe how people interpreted, dealt with, and tried to control such animal diseases in cities and territories of the Holy Roman Empire, both on the level of scientific discourses and in practical reality. The time frame includes the sixteenth and seventeenth centuries, still neglected by historical research on animal diseases, and reaches into the eighteenth century, when cattle diseases as rinderpest, also known as cattle plague, began to trigger and dominate a fast-growing discourse on animal health. We argue that the early modern period saw a high convergence between human and animal diseases, both with regard to their interpretation, preventive measures, and medical treatment. It therefore seems important to research the history of transmissible diseases in an integrated, interspecies way.

To begin with, we have to clarify the different terminology used for transmissible diseases in the human and animal realms. Parallel to epidemics and pandemics, which are defined respectively as human diseases with temporarily high prevalence and a wide geographical spread, epizootics and panzootics regard transmissible animal diseases.[5] Parallels between human and animal epidemics are far from unknown in history. After lying dormant for generations, a deadly cattle panzootic, originating in Bohemia, erupted in Europe in the fourteenth century. Similar to the plague that reached Germany around 1350, the disease was not new, but, due to ecological factors, expanded suddenly at the beginning of the fourteenth century.[6] Despite this apparent connection, there is scarce literature on epizootics before 1700. Rare exceptions are studies by Bruce Campbell and Philip Slavin, both focusing on the fourteenth century.[7] Still, the main emphasis of historical research lies on the development of veterinary science and on knowledge concerning animal diseases that occurred in the nineteenth century, with precursors in the eighteenth century, in the context of global movement of animals and their pathogens as well as the establishment of state veterinary services.[8] For eighteenth-century Germany, the work of Carsten Stühring with its focus on the Electorate of Bavaria, and of Dominik Hünniger, who investigates crisis management in the face of the rinderpest in Schleswig and Holstein mainly in the 1740s and 1750s, is important for the understanding of how contemporaries interpreted these panzootic waves and how they reacted to these challenges.[9] Further, in several articles Jutta Nowosadtko analyzes how early modern societies dealt with animal diseases and their control.[10] Moreover, several veterinary studies and dissertations observe animal diseases in a historical context, mainly with an emphasis on the spread of the diseases, their identification, and control measures.[11] As a rule, these works omit the sixteenth and seventeenth centuries as a period with seemingly minor scientific progress, and focus on earlier periods and on the eighteenth century, although the centuries in between saw further discussions and developments on the level of scientific and practical discourses. Before focusing on maladies, a short overview in the next section contextualizes farm animals in early modern German society.

The Role of Livestock in Early Modern Germany

Animals were an integral part of early modern agriculture.[12] Aside from horses, which were used in particular as draft animals and often suffered as a result, cattle, pigs, sheep, and goats were important domestic animals that contributed to the social and economic existence of premodern humans, even becoming part of tradition and culture, for example in ecclesiastical architecture, on coats of arms, or in trials.[13]

The animals that were companions and often housemates of the premodern inhabitants of Central Europe (Figure 9.1) reflected the contemporary food preferences, varying craftsmanship, the muscle power needed, but also wealth and the social order. Moreover, the climate influenced animal husbandry. While the sixteenth century has been termed a "pleasant century," the following century saw hard winters, wet and cool summers leading to fodder shortages, the greater importance of farming, and a lower number of animals. Livestock numbers usually correlated positively with the area of particular estates, but few data exist with regard to larger political entities.[14] This lack of data leads to mainly qualitative assumptions about animal husbandry.

Poultry were present on any farm and provided peasants with eggs, meat, and feathers for duvets or quills.[15] Goats were usually tax exempt and popular in hilly regions and in the Alps, where they fed on marginal food like twigs and leaves.[16] The keeping of undemanding goats that delivered milk and meat was an indicator of the owner's relative poverty, while the meat-producing hogs were kept in well-to-do households.[17] Similar to goats, sheep were reckoned to be animals both easy to keep and profitable. They delivered wool, about 0.8 to 1 kilogram annually per animal, but also milk and meat. Sheep interacted well with farming by reducing weeds and producing manure, which resulted in larger flocks but also in environmental changes, especially in Northern Germany.[18] The profits which could be gained from sheep husbandry made this field of livestock farming of particular interest for territorial lords. In the sixteenth century, the landgrave of Hesse possessed the exclusive right to use the commons, which resulted in manorial sheep farms containing up to seven hundred animals.[19]

Owning two hogs was enough to see a family through the winter, and in many regions there was easy access for fodder, whether in the form of garbage or simply found in the forests where the animals were supervised jointly by the village inhabitants. While this feeding method extended the fattening period, it allowed the owners of the animals to minimize the use of valuable grain.[20]

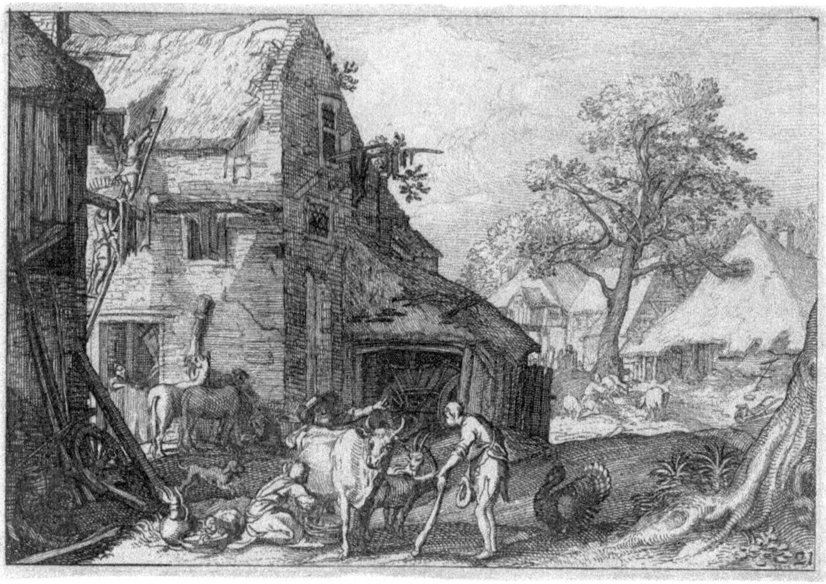

Figure 9.1. Claes Jansz. Visscher, 1620: *Boerenerf met mensen en vee*. Rijksmuseum Amsterdam RP-P-1889-A-14967 (public domain). Source: https://commons.m.wikimedia.org/wiki/File:Boerenerf_met_mensen_en_vee_Landschappen_met_boerderijen_(serietitel),_RP-P-1889-A-14967.jpg.

Consequently, pigs that on average weighed sixty kilograms did not compete with cattle for food but could help maintain a fertile soil. This and the fertility of the sows, which could give birth to about eight piglets annually, made them a valuable factor in efforts to mitigate the regularly occurring early modern shortages of food.[21] In the sixteenth century, the keeping of hogs partly depended on the proximity of oak and beech forests, which led to irregular patterns in the distribution of these animals in Germany—approximately fifteen thousand hogs were pastured in the Solling mountains near Hanover in 1598—and subsequently to an interregional hog trade with all its sanitary risks.[22]

Cattle bred in Germany or imported from Denmark, Poland, or Hungary had many uses, including for meat, bones, milk, but also leather, and consequently were highly esteemed by early modern authors.[23] Especially in the sixteenth century, population growth led to an increasing demand for meat, which resulted in tens of thousands of animals on the move annually in Central Europe, potentially spreading diseases at the same time.[24] Until the eighteenth century, efforts to standardize the features of cattle such as color, weight, size, and milk yield were somewhat unsuccessful, but for the sixteenth and seventeenth centuries there at least exist average weights of cows (200 kilograms), calves (20–35 kilograms), and oxen (375 kilograms).[25] The milk yield of cows depended on fodder quality and quantity. A single cow could eat four kilograms of hay daily, and especially in winter supplementary feeding was necessary. In the first half of the seventeenth century, the milk yield ranged from 440 liters on the domains of the Principality of Brunswick to 1,600 liters on the fertile marshlands of the count of Oldenburg. Usually, cows were primiparous at the age of three years and had a life expectancy of nine to ten years. On domains in Northwest Germany, 80 percent of the cows gave birth to a healthy calf annually, so that numbers following cattle diseases took some time to be restored.[26] Consequently, epizootics resulted in financial losses for the owners of animals, but also threatened the livelihood and health of ordinary people, destabilized the agricultural system, and harmed the individual animals themselves. But animals also directly interacted with humans during epidemics.

Epidemics and Animals

During the early modern period the plague and other epidemics had significant influence on economic, social, and religious practices, which is a main subject of historical research.[27] But infectious diseases also changed and influenced the relationship between humans and animals. This refers to livestock, but also to domestic and feral animals with connections to human settlements.

The abundance of several animal species, such as mice, rats, snakes, flies, caterpillars, and worms, were considered signs of the beginning of an epidemic because they leave rotten soil that is prone to emit miasmas.[28] Such signs also could be epizootics themselves. In 1599, an applicant for the position of municipal doctor in the imperial city of Esslingen warned against a plague and explained this was due to a widespread livestock disease ("starckhe pestilentzische viehkrankheit") caused by bad air that was intensified by the presence of carcasses.[29] Epidemics such as the plague spared horses, cattle, and sheep, but could infect cats, dogs, and other animals.[30]

Similar to the development of other branches of knowledge, antiquity provided a blueprint for early modern discourses. Lucretius (ca. 94–55 BCE), for instance, whose work was reprinted and translated throughout Europe in the sixteenth and seventeenth centuries, had already connected the plague with animal disease: "Few Birds appear'd, no wing could serve for flight; The Beasts scarce dar'd to trust themselves to Night: The Plague walkt thro the Woods, in every Den They lay and figh'd, and groan'd, and dy'd like Men."[31] Infected animals, however, were also feared as vectors of disease, consequently limiting their numbers or killing them was an important hygienic measure, in addition to repentance and other religious practices.[32] In 1498, the city council of Schwäbisch Hall prohibited hog imports from several places and obliged their owners to swear to the health of their animals; and in 1652 and 1654 the city council of Regensburg permitted only a limited number of hog trades.[33] When the plague occurred, brutal interactions between humans and animals could arise, both to fight the epidemic and as a symbolic warning to the population, described by Mark Jenner as the "large-scale slaughter of dogs and cats."[34] Such events also occurred in Britain and Italy in the sixteenth and seventeenth centuries.[35]

In central Europe, humans similarly feared contagion from infected furs of cats and dogs, and experts recommended the killing of these animals.[36] In 1657, for instance, Brunswick authorities linked the transmission of a disease that affected humans and livestock to infected cats and dogs and recommended their killing.[37] Other examples show the difficulties in enforcing such regulations. In the small principality of Sayn-Hachenburg near Koblenz, the authorities ordered the killing of all cats, dogs, and doves and the expulsion of hogs in one parish in 1666, but the edict was probably ignored by the villagers.[38]

Not only living animals or their body parts were regarded as vectors of disease. As in many other cities, in sixteenth- and seventeenth-century Brunswick manure heaps and other organic waste were banned from the streets to avoid the allegedly poisonous stench, although with questionable effect. Around 1500, the council of the small imperial city of Nördlingen attempted to at least reduce the number of hogs and to speed up the removal of manure heaps from the streets.[39] One hundred years later, in Schwäbisch Hall, the trade in hogs was limited again, due to the same reason.[40] On the other hand, animals also were expected to help against epidemic diseases. Slaughtered but still warm animals, such as lambs, grown sheep, or goatlings were said to suck the poison out of plague spots, as did plucked butts of living chicken or doves held against the swelling.[41] Johann Joachim Becher even recommended using stones from the entrails of horses against the dreaded poison that accompanied epidemic diseases.[42] While playing their part in human diseases and possibly even mitigating the effects of some epidemics, animals themselves regularly suffered from contagious diseases.

Animal Contagious Diseases

In the fifth biblical plague of Egypt, livestock diseases afflicted the animals of the Egyptians: "Behold, the hand of the LORD is upon thy cattle which is in the field, upon the horses, upon the asses, upon the camels, upon the oxen, and upon the sheep: there shall be a very grievous murrain." (Exodus 9: 3). The immense damage animal diseases caused to their owners and the prevailing interpretation of such plagues as divine punishment are referenced in prayers to Catholic saints such as St. Blasius, St. Leonhard, and St. Wendelin.[43] With regard to animal diseases, modern veterinary medicine differentiates between obligate infectious diseases, triggered by highly infectious pathogens that are adapted to the respective species, and facultative infectious diseases that benefit from environmental factors unfavorable for the animals.[44] Many pathogens are not confined to animals or humans, and there are more than two hundred known diseases that are triggered by viruses, bacteria, fungi, arthropods, and more, which can be transmitted reciprocally (*zoonosis*).[45]

Before the eighteenth century, there was no focus on veterinary medicine of livestock. Early modern veterinary thought was mostly confined to horses, as these were highly important both for the military and for the social position of their owners. Particular theories were influenced by knowledge from Italy, for example by Pasquale Caracciolo's *La Gloria del Cavallo* (1566), although animal diseases such as rinderpest (*Rinderpest*), anthrax (*Milzbrand*), sheep pox (*Schafpocken*), and foot and mouth disease (*Maul- und Klauenseuche*) regularly threatened livestock.[46] To treat sick animals, their owners consulted illiterate farriers, shepherds, knackers, or wise women, rather than veterinarians.[47] The knowledge and experience of such laypersons should not be underestimated. In the case of shepherds, a broad range of cures can be found in the sources, including effective ones such as inoculation against sheep pox.[48] Throughout the sixteenth and seventeenth centuries, different animal diseases occurred in all parts of Europe (Table 9.1), often as byproduct of military campaigns.[49] Only in the eighteenth century did rinderpest become the most dangerous and prominent threat to cattle.

As in the case of the plague and other epidemics, early modern authors and practitioners followed models from antiquity and blamed astral influences, especially bad air (miasmas) and, increasingly, contagions, for the emergence of cattle diseases.[50] Since medical treatment often was limited to bloodletting or traditional drugs, the separation of diseased animals—with the help of certificates and rigorous controls as in Switzerland in the seventeenth century—was the most efficient way to slow down the spread of disease. Additionally, the fumigation of stables and barns and the burning and burying of carcasses was thought to help against it.[51] An anonymous pamphlet from 1682, issued in Hildesheim, is regarded as one of the first instructions for prevention of the transmission of infectious diseases in animals. After they had dealt with infected animals, people should wash their hands and burn all used materials and use citron, juniper juice, or vinegar to prevent further infection.[52] Next to such tangible measures, religious and magical practices abounded, as will be discussed below.

The different animal diseases had varying impacts on the early modern societies of Central Europe and were interpreted differently. While anthrax regularly harmed livestock, it also was a hazard for people who worked and lived near sick animals because of its potential to infect humans.[53] Rinderpest

Table 9.1. Major epizootics of the sixteenth and seventeenth centuries; Schwarz, "Schweinepest," 45; Spinage, *Cattle Plague*, 96, 98, 100; Blancou, *History*, 46, 73, 99, 155, 172, 214.

Year	Region	Disease
1499–1505	Saxony	Cattle plague
1504	Germany	Anthrax
1514	Italy	Cattle plague; foot and mouth disease
1515	France	Sheep pox
1552	France, Italy	Anthrax
1559	Prussia (Magdeburg)	Cattle plague
1567/68	France	Sheep pox
1578	Western Europe	Rabies
1586	Western Europe	Rabies
1590	France, Italy	Anthrax
1598/99	Germany, France, Italy	Cattle plague
1604	Lyons	Rinderpest
1609/10	Palatinate, Alsace, Saxony, Bavaria	Anthrax; cattle plague
1617	France, Spain	Anthrax
1643	-	Rinderpest
1662–1680s	Western Europe	Foot and mouth disease
1671	France, Italy	Anthrax
1679	Austria	Cattle disease
1679	Hungary	Anthrax
1682–1691	Italy, Switzerland, France, Germany	Anthrax
1690	Italy	Different animal diseases
1693	Hesse	Contagious bovine pleuropneumonia
1695	Western Europe	Foot and mouth disease
1698	Germany	Sheep pox (first occurrence)

(*pestis bovina*), which had been described already in antiquity, is a highly contagious and deadly cattle disease. Especially between 1700 and 1720, millions of animals fell victim to it. Local studies show the positive correlation between the indoor housing of animals in winter and the spread of the disease. The only effective preventive measure turned out to be the separation of infected cattle.[54] As early as 1682, Christian Albrecht, duke of Schleswig and Holstein, prohibited the entry of cattle into pastures or other barns without a valid health certificate and ordered quarantine for sick animals, which provided a model for the following century.[55]

Cattle plague is the most thoroughly researched premodern epizootic and its different varieties are regularly documented in archival sources. This provides us an opportunity to observe modes of disease interpretation by ordinary people, which can then be transferred to other species and to earlier centuries. In eighteenth-century Rothenburg ob der Tauber, a small imperial city near Nuremberg, townspeople from different social strata held frozen grass, wet and cold weather, heat and dust, mildew, insect stings, as well as the malevolence of particular inhabitants responsible for the death of their cattle.[56] In the sixteenth and seventeenth centuries, bovine tuberculosis (*Perlsucht*) was incorrectly considered a variant of syphilis, an epidemic known as *Morbus gallicus*, and experts believed in its transmission via sodomy from humans to cattle.[57] Moreover, rabies (*Lyssa/toller Hundebiß*) not only struck dogs but also could harm cattle, hogs, sheep and horses.[58] This overview shows how manifold epizootics threatened livestock and gives first hints as to their interpretation and possible reactions.

The Discourses of the Learned in the Sixteenth and Seventeenth Centuries

Early modern authors regularly referred to authorities of Greek and Roman antiquity, as was common in other fields of knowledge as well. One of these was Vegetius (383–450 CE), who wrote a detailed work on animal diseases that was published in a German translation in 1532. For Vegetius it was commonplace to fear the infection of the whole herd when one individual had caught a disease, which is why he recommended the isolation of sick animals.[59] This argument was also followed by early modern authors. In his book on animals (*Thierbuch*), the Swiss polymath Conrad Gessner (1516–65), who died of the plague, among other things discussed transmissible cattle diseases and deduced that "when one animal in the herd is infected, the whole herd dies."[60] Contemporary authors for whom diseases were direct consequences of the sinful behavior of men made no differentiation between humans and their animals. David Herlitz (1557–1636), astrologer and municipal doctor (*Stadtphysicus*) in Lübeck, deduced that divine wrath resulted in comets that in turn ignited the air, and "after that men and livestock receive poison and infection ... which provokes the plague."[61]

In the course of the early modern period different groups of actors and different types of publications cover the interpretation of animal diseases.

As stated above, animal diseases in the sixteenth century were mainly dealt with in manuals on horse keeping and horse diseases, *Rossarzneibücher* (horse medicine books) written by equerries.[62] The importance of horses is evident in the title page of the printed translation of Vegetius' work, which portrays the medical treatment of a sick horse following the instructions of a medical book (Figure 9.2). In the seventeenth century a new category of handbooks, the *Viehbüchlein* (cattle book) or *Vieharznei* (cattle medicine) expanded the subject to all kinds of livestock such as cattle, pigs, sheep, and poultry, and to some extent to dogs and cats. With the great cattle plagues at the beginning of the eighteenth century, physicians and veterinarians entered the discourse on animal diseases.

"Hence men and horses are very similar," the equerry Caspar Reuschlein von Hagenau points out in his *Hippiatria* from 1593, as they suffer from similar diseases. However, the treatment of horses required special knowledge that all stable masters should have. The horse medicine books contain detailed collections of prescriptions against equine diseases. They follow the medieval tradition that concentrates on horses, dogs, and falcons as companions for hunting and status symbols of aristocrats, while neglecting other animals.[63] The focus of these books is on illnesses and diseases, while epizootics are rarely mentioned, and only a few prescriptions deal with contagious diseases.

The growing economic importance of cattle as working animals and providers of meat, dairy produce, and manure in early modern Europe led to a closer look at the health of these animals. The cattle medicine books from the seventeenth century are compilations of ancient natural history writings, the *Rossarzneibücher* of the sixteenth century, and older cattle books. The manuals represent the hierarchy of animals, starting with horses, then dealing with oxen and cows, and closing with remarks on sheep and pigs. They also contain collections of prescriptions and practical information on the treatment of diseases and epizootics.[64] A cattle book from 1697 mentions *Stertz* disease and smallpox among the diseases of cattle. To cure smallpox, the author describes the following procedure: "Cut or bite their tongue a little, take them by their feet, roll them from one side to the other that they might roll over on their back. Afterwards take a strap of leather and hit them four times on the body; they will soon get better."[65]

Aside from these handbooks that address animal diseases, most books of the *Hausväterliteratur* (paterfamilias literature) include chapters dealing with the subject.[66] They addressed nobles, landowners, and wealthy farmers. Following the ancient tradition of the ideal of rural life, these books place special emphasis on efficient farming and agriculture. In their view, the head of the house is responsible for all economic and moral aspects of his manor, including the education of his wife and children, handling beggars, or curing sick animals.[67]

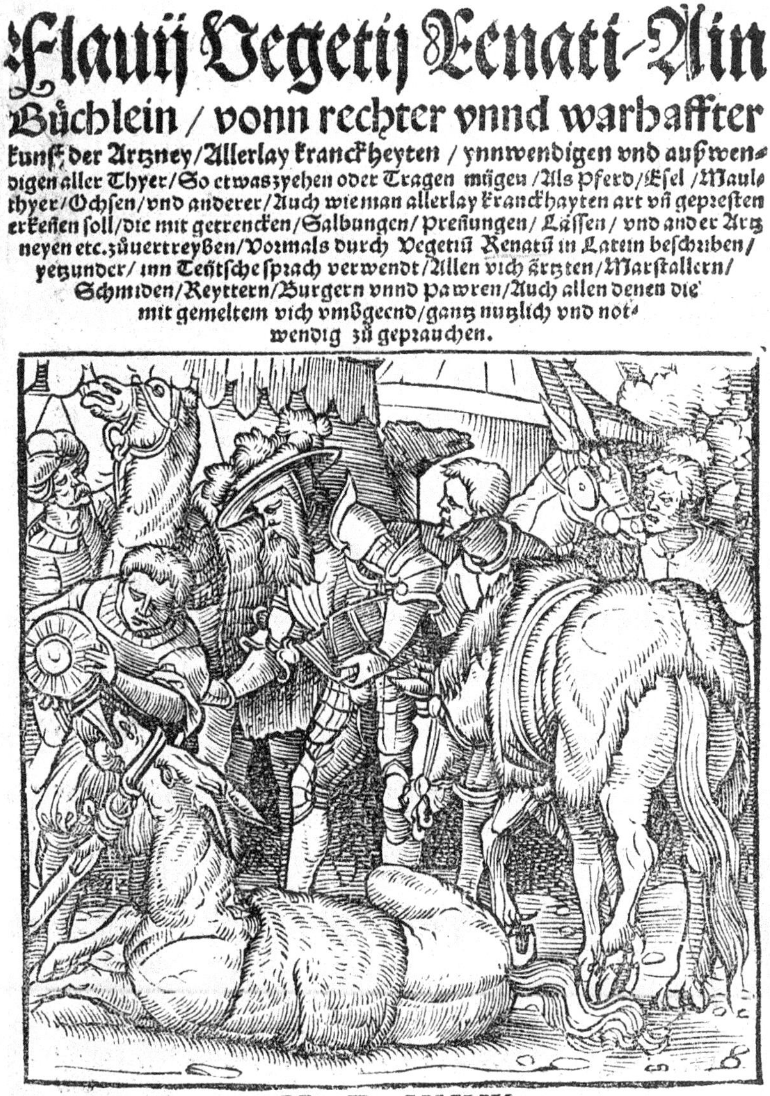

Flauij Vegetij Renati-Ain
Bůchlein / vonn rechter vnnd warhaffter
kunst der Artzney/Allerlay kranckheyten / ynnwendigen vnd außwen-
digen aller Thyer/So etwas zyehen oder Tragen mügen /Als Pferd/Esel /Maul-
thyer/Ochsen/vnd anderer/Auch wieman allerlay kranckhayten art vñ geprestẽ
erkeñen soll/die mit getrencken/Salbungen/ Preñungen/ Lässen / vnd ander Artz
neyen etc. zůuertreyben/Vormals durch Vegetiũ Renatũ in Latein beschriben/
yetzunder/ inn Teütsche sprach verwendt/Allen vich ärtzten/Marstallern/
Schmiden/Reyttern/Burgern vnnd pawren/Auch allen denen die
mit gemeltem vich vmbgeend/gantz nutzlich vnd not-
wendig zů geprauchen.

M. D. XXXII.

Figure 9.2. Vegetius, *Ain Büchlein*, title page (detail). Vegetius, Flavius. *Ain Büchlein / vonn rechter vnnd warhaffter kunst der Artzney / Allerlay kranckheyten / ynnwendigen vnd außwendigen aller Thyer* . . . . Augspurg: Steiner, 1532.

Johann Joachim Becher (1635–82), known today as Germany's most famous mercantilist, in the third chapter of his manual recommends numerous recipes to the house father and—which is rare in the seventeenth century—to the house mother as well. He emphasizes that all recipes are from his own experience and, in true mercantilist fashion, that they save labor and money. Becher dedicates more than hundred of eight hundred pages of his book to the cure of animal diseases, illustrating how to add certain plants to the fodder to protect the animals from epidemics, magic, and the devil.[68] His collection contains both detailed prescriptions and very simple recipes, such as "Feed feverfew to the cattle / it drives away the nasty plague, panting, swelling, and is very cleansing."[69]

As another general preventive against diseases, many books recommended that cows should be kept in barns in winter so that they are protected from the cold. Standing close in the barn is seen as beneficial, as too much movement of the animals would increase the risk of fever.[70] The indices of recipes show various ingredients and dosage forms. In the case of an unspecified pig disease (*Schweinenseuche*), the animals should be given a medicine made from hellebore, laurel, cress seeds, and Venetian soap, mixed with sweet milk.[71] Another *Viehbüchlein* mentions theriac, saltpeter, and other ingredients mixed in beer to cure sick cattle, especially against the plague.[72] The cavalry colonel Alexander von Neuneck zu Madenburg gives a long list of recipes in 1631, useful for both humans and animals: "this is followed by a number of fine and proven prescriptions useful for man and cattle. Powder for dying cattle, for illnesses of lung and liver, even pestilence."[73] The fact that it was not necessary to differentiate between recipes for humans and animals could well be due to the military context of the Thirty Years' War.

A focus on practical instructions and recipes can also be found in some treatises against the plague in the sixteenth and seventeenth centuries. Shorter treatises, in particular, forego a detailed historical and theological classification and are limited to collections of prescriptions and healing methods.[74]

Since animal diseases similar to the plague were widely interpreted as God's punishment for the sinful behavior of people, religious practices are important for ending the epizootics, as discussed below: prayer and penance in Lutheran territories and supplicatory processions and blessings of animals in Catholic ones. This also is reflected in theological tracts. In 1575, the Protestant superintendent Christoph Vischer from Schmalkalden criticized these pious practices as the superstition of the "papists." He especially spoke against blessings for the well-being of humans and animals and the appeal for help to the devil.[75] For his part, Vischer is not interested in practical aspects of curing maladies but, rather, in a detailed theological legitimization of his rejection. As a Lutheran pastor he enlists God's help to eliminate infections, as the title of his other plague treatise also indicates.[76] The reason for writing such tracts was rarely purely medical. Stable masters tried to hold onto or expand their courtly positions and preachers used animal diseases as an opportunity to present their own dogmatic ideas.

Generally, during the sixteenth and seventeenth centuries, animal diseases are treated much less frequently than human epidemics, a circumstance that changed in the eighteenth century with the occurrence of the great waves of cattle plague and the appearance of new, widespread animal diseases.

Practical Measures against Epizootics before 1700

The fight against contagious animal diseases was by no means waged only on paper and in theory. There were many different ways in which premodern authorities could react against livestock plagues, but only a few of these were frequently used. The practical measures mostly resembled strategies used to protect areas from pestilence or other human epidemics, as we will see below.

As soon as governments became aware of a nearby outbreak of an epizootic, they warned all officials within their territory. In 1682, for instance, the landgrave of Hesse-Kassel announced that the territories of Lorraine, Strasbourg, Upper and Lower Swabia, as well as Bavaria, had recently been struck by substantial livestock deaths ("graßirenden Vieh-Seuchen"). Once infected, the cattle would die within a few hours if no remedy was given. The landgrave therefore ordered his officials and magistrates to keep an eye on farmers and traders and not allow them to let "any horse, ox or cattle [from the infected areas] on their pasture or in their stable" and strictly forbid them "to lead them into our territory for slaughter."[77] Such written notifications nearly always came together with prohibitions on trading cattle from affected areas. As in the case of human plagues, the authorities tried to quarantine those districts that had been recently infected. To achieve that, they had to stop larger cattle movements within principalities. The Lower Saxon city of Peine near Hanover cancelled its annual livestock market in 1638 because "an evil, poisonous cattle plague has broken out in many places," in order "to prevent the calamity, mentioned above, as good as possible." For this reason, the magistrate decided not to allow any foreign cattle into the city.[78] During the same plague, the city council of Brunswick noted in 1637 that many "foul, reeking, and useless" skins of infected cattle had been brought and sold within the city.[79] The gatekeepers were therefore told not to let carts with smelling or rotten skins pass through the gates, to avoid infections. The citizens of Hildesheim even had to dispose of the milk of infected cows after they had been struck by a heavy plague in 1582.[80]

Of course, those measures and warnings alone were scarcely sufficient, and the governments knew that. The most common way to support the people was to help them in dealing with the plague on site.[81] In order to do that, the edicts mostly contained a recipe instructing the local offices and house fathers how to cure the infected animals. In the seventeenth century, these recipes were very similar to each other, sometimes even literally, and so it can be assumed that governments were in contact with each other and exchanged prescriptions. In August 1682, for instance, Duke Rudolf August of Brunswick-Wolfenbüttel called his published recipe a "proven remedy" ("bewehrtes Mittel"), which had been "recommended by other neighbors" ("von andern Benachbahrn recommendiertes Recept").[82] In fact, the recipe was a word-for-word copy of a recommendation that had also been used by the elector of Mainz one month earlier.[83] As the same text circulated in other territories as well,[84] it seems to have been a common recipe against the plague around 1682.

But what advice did this public recipe include? First, it was recommended to keep all livestock locked inside the barns for eight days as soon as any infection was noticed nearby. In the mornings and evenings, the farmers were supposed to scratch the tongues of the animals with a special silver instrument, since the infection was known to show itself by little bubbles on the surface of the tongue.[85] In order to remove the bubbles, all municipal administrations were asked to craft at least one of these silver instruments. An illustration of the "scraper" at the end of the edict usually showed the reader what it looked like (Figure 9.3).

If there was not enough money or material to make this tool, the governments sometimes also suggested to use a "Braunschweiger Mariengroschen" (a rough, not really valuable coin from Brunswick) as a tongue-scraper.[86] Of course, many more actions were recommended besides the few mentioned here. The duke of Saxe-Weimar, for instance, ordered his subjects in 1682 to fumigate the infected barns with juniper[87]—a measure similar to those taken in times of bubonic plague. Moreover, many authorities also suggested the cure-all "theriac" as remedy.[88] In Lucerne, the city council had understood the danger of contagion and in 1682 ordered persons with contact with sick animals to wash their hands with fresh water, forbid the use of milk from sick cows, and bury carcasses deep in the ground.[89] Frederick William, the Great Elector of Brandenburg, told his knackers in 1684 to fetch the skins of dead cattle within twenty-four hours and bury them deep in the ground to avoid further spread of the infection.[90] In addition, people were supposed to provide all dead animals to the knackers within one day's time. However, governments always had to keep in mind that local authorities and the inhabitants had to accept and understand these instructions. Otherwise, the people might just have ignored the orders, as can be seen in some records.[91]

Aside from governmental measures, traditional religious and magical practices to mitigate epizootics endured. For instance, wood from gallows and execution wheels was ignited and the animals were chased through the fire and fed

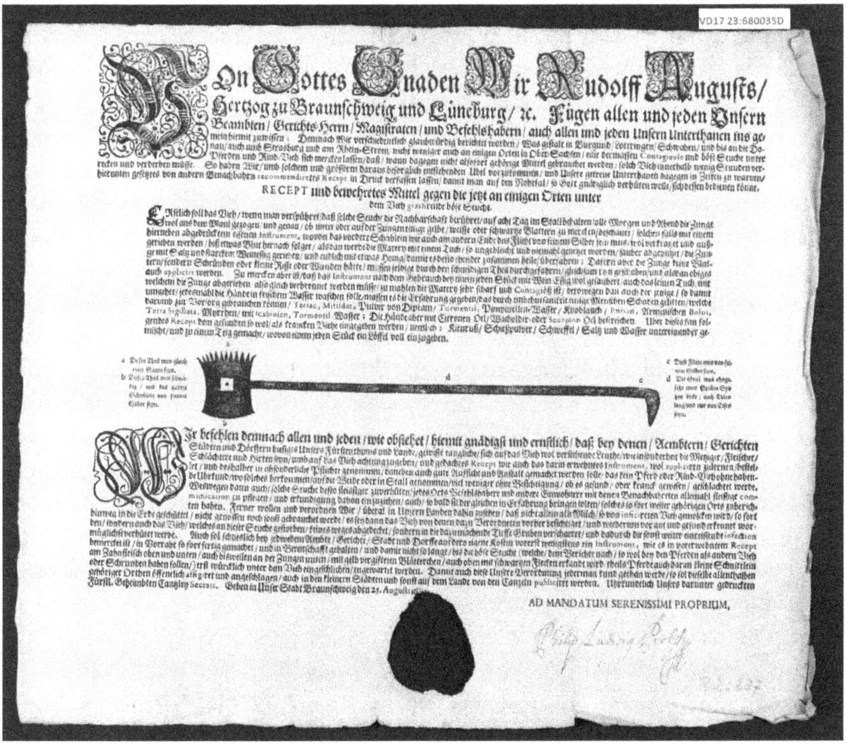
VD17 23:680035D
Von Gottes Gnaden Wir Rudolff Augusts/
Hertzog zu Braunschweig und Lüneburg/ etc. Fügen allen und jeden Unsern
RECEPT und bewehretes Mittel gegen die jetzt an einigen Orten unter
AD MANDATUM SERENISSIMI PROPRIUM.

Figure 9.3. Illustration of a so-called fleam ("Fliete")—a scraper against cattle plague bubbles. Edict of August 25, 1682 [VD17 23:680035D], Herzog August Bibliothek Wolfenbüttel: R2:287. See Spinage, *Cattle Plague*, 101 for a similar instrument.

with the ash to fight diseases.[92] In Catholic regions, governments and common people held processions to fend off cattle plagues[93] and provided votive offerings. When people got sick, a common reaction was to go on a typically local pilgrimage and give votive offerings to the saints, since medical care in rural areas was lacking until the nineteenth century.[94] Those offerings were usually made after a supplication for recovery appeared to be successful, but also could be given earlier to help initiate the healing process.[95] The same procedure was used when livestock became sick, especially in the case of epizootics. Contrary to the common assumption, even of many historians, votive offerings were not limited to the "plain," rural people. In fact, even princes used them.

In 1631, Bavaria was haunted by an intense livestock plague. The Elector Maximilian I decided to sacrifice a horse with his own hands to end the crisis.[96] He took the best horse from his stables in Schleißheim near Munich, as well as his own riding horse, and led them to the pilgrimage church of St. Leonhard in

Inchenhofen near Augsburg. There, he sacrificed both animals to St. Leonard, one of the common saints against livestock plagues and mental illnesses. After that, a horse from the elector's stables (*Marstall*) was presented to St. Leonard every year, a tradition maintained until 1779.[97]

With such a noble role model it is not surprising that the Bavarians adopted these measures as well, although unlike their elector they did not usually sacrifice living animals. Most of the votive offerings were figurines in the shape of the specific animal that the petitioner wished to be healed.[98] In 1672, the inhabitants of Vierkirchen north of Munich promised a votive offering and a large wax candle to stop the further spread of the livestock plague.[99] Similar sacrifices were made by the citizens of Altomünster in 1682, when they donated six florins and held a holy mass to prevent the epizootic from spreading.[100] The miracle book (*Mirakelbuch*) from the monastery Maria Stern in Taxa, which contains entries from 1654 until 1753, contains 85 supplication texts in case of cattle plague and 103 in case of horse diseases. In 1666, for example, the inhabitants of nearby Dachau came to the monastery to pray for the end of an epizootic which possibly was foot and mouth disease.[101] Thus it seems that these religious measures against livestock plagues and diseases were quite common, at least in Catholic regions.

Lutherans of course did not approve of processions or votive offerings, but until the eighteenth century they responded with their own public prayers.[102] Although the Lutheran governments usually did not tolerate popular devotion, they were not totally free from superstition either. As with human diseases, people often searched for the supernatural causes of a plague and sometimes found them in the persons of Jews or witches and sorcerers. Between 1562 and 1563, for example, several alleged witches in Wiesensteig near Augsburg were burned because they were said to have killed many people and sixty-six horses.[103] A few years later, in 1599, two Jews in Württemberg were blamed for the deaths of "many thousands of animals."[104] After they had been arrested, they confessed under torture to be sorcerers who had bewitched all the livestock with the devil's help.[105] Both Jews were executed, and the plague vanished, so it seemed. A similar process was held during the great livestock plague of 1682. Several alleged sorcerers were blamed for bewitching the animals and were soon captured and tortured. As a pamphlet from Coburg approved by the authorities argues, the judges and the government had tried to get more information from the defendants how to stop the disease.[106] The accused testified under torture that there was only one way to cure the ill animals, namely scraping off the bubbles on the tongue with a silver instrument, in almost the same procedure described above.

It has become evident that there were many similarities between the practical measures against human and livestock plagues. In both cases, the authorities reacted with quarantines as well as with medical treatment, fumigation of infected houses and barns, and prayers or sacrifices to God. These results correspond to the findings of Jutta Nowosadtko, who has pointed out that human and animal plagues provoked very similar reactions: "To fight against contagious animal diseases, the governments resorted to measures and experiences they had gained and improved earlier by dealing with human epidemics. Thus, there was a close relation between the ordinances against livestock plague of the late seventeenth century and those of prior human plagues."[107]

New Horizons—the Cattle Plagues of the Eighteenth Century

In the 1680s the first signs of a new cattle epizootic were reported in Germany. An anonymous tract from Brunswick gave a detailed account of a contagious disease that allegedly was caused by sorcerers in Milan and spread rapidly to other regions.[108] A few years later, at the beginning of the eighteenth century, the academic discourse about animal diseases was changing significantly. This was mainly due to the fact that the first major wave of cattle diseases occurred from 1711 to 1717, which contemporaries perceived as a new crisis.[109] At the same time, one of the last great waves of plague took place in the Holy Roman Empire, from 1709 to 1713, and so farmers, theologians, state administrators, and doctors were able observe the disease and death of humans and animals in Central Europe simultaneously. The massive number of animal deaths and the associated economic consequences ensured that doctors became increasingly concerned with animal diseases.

An edict published by the Prussian government in 1711 deplored the fact that the causes of the epizootics and their healing methods were largely unclear, "because Medici or Physici, as those who should have a thorough knowledge in natural things, worry little about such damage."[110]

The first German-language publications by physicians about the *Hornviehseuche* (horned cattle disease) still show learned doctors' unease with the subject. The Halle (Saale) medical professor Friedrich Hoffmann and Johann Kanold, who got his doctorate in medicine in Halle and later practiced in his native city of Breslau (Wrocław), emphasized that renowned contemporary doctors from Italy had already dealt with the subject and had referred to ancient authorities to justify their research. Following a cameralist line of argumentation, both authors also underlined that the disease was an economic problem. Hoffmann saw the epizootics as a threat to the "community,"[111] which required the intervention of medical professionals. Kanold explained that "these animals (*Bruta*) account for a large part of the blessing and the necessities of a country."[112] The two trained doctors had prior experience with epidemics and had already published about them. Hoffmann pointed out that some

Italian physicians considered the new animal disease comparable to the human smallpox.[113] Seven years later Johann Wilhelm Roeseler and Anton Philipp Bornemann, doctors in Halberstadt in the Harz region, stressed the similarity of human and animal diseases: "The fates of men and animals are similar, when the latter dies, so does the first. … Consequently, one can make arguments and deductions from human diseases to epizootics and vice versa."[114] Thus they proposed using methods already approved for treating epidemics. The theories of contagion and miasma, which had been developed in the late Middle Ages after the great waves of plague and remained influential throughout the early modern period, were also used to explain the death of animals.[115] Doctors who believed in miasmas considered poisonous fumes that threatened the animals in the meadows to be responsible for the pandemic. The solution was to put the cattle in clean, healthy barns—which in fact could facilitate infections.

Anatomical practices to examine the corpses of humans, used already since the Renaissance, were transferred to dead animals. The authors recommended that individual organs of animals that had died from the disease be examined for changes, using autopsies. With the new findings from the anatomical examinations, the doctors provided extensive descriptions of symptoms. Influenced by the new academic culture of the early Enlightenment, Hoffmann emphasized that *vernunft* (reason) and *experienz* (experience) were the guidelines for his methods of treatment.[116] Like many of his colleagues, he added a list of recipes, repeating some of the recipes from the older cattle medicine books.[117] Plague treatises usually offered two types of recipes for successfully combating the disease: general recipes and recipes for the poor, who were urged to use cheaper alternatives, such as juniper berries soaked in vinegar.[118] The treatises on animal diseases share this dualism. Roeseler and Bornemann give a recipe for theriac, which required costly ingredients. Hoffmann, on the other hand, argued that it made little sense to use particularly exotic or expensive ingredients that were not available to farmers. To the contrary, he argued "that we are not restricted to precious ingredients and things that are hard to get, rather that the most simple and plain items and herbs that can be found easily and everywhere, have the best powers and effects to cure diseases."[119] Even at the beginning of the eighteenth century, extensive prescription collections remained an important part of medical publications. By the middle of the eighteenth century, recipes to fend off both human plague and animal diseases made up almost half of the corresponding entry in Zedler's *Universallexikon*.[120]

The common idea in the medical works, namely that sick animals should immediately be brought into barns and stables, was consistently developed in the Agricultural Enlightenment (*Agraraufklärung*) of the eighteenth century. Moreover, cattle should be kept indoors all year round, instead of only in winter or when sick. Farmers should grow clover as fodder in fallow fields in order to achieve intensive animal husbandry with high gains. The model estates (*Mustergüter*) of enlightened aristocrats put the new ideas into practice and should present the new forms of agriculture to the farmers in the area as models worth emulating.[121] The reformers characterized the pastures used until now as unhealthy places, responsible for numerous animal diseases and epidemics, as Johann Friedrich Mayer, pastor and member of the Swiss Economic Society, explained: "Wind, frost, fog, rain, heat, swamp water, lack of water, wide shoots, dense shrubbery, hilly ground, unhealthy grass ... disgusting places besmirched with feces and urine, trampled and polluted grass, ... are all things that are disadvantageous, dangerous, and harmful to the health of the cattle, that are against the constitution of their body, insofar cold, frost, rain, and heat cause epidemics and diseases."[122] Mayer notes that in the places where stable husbandry was introduced in preference to pasture husbandry, there has not been an epizootic in the last seventy years. The primary task of animal husbandry is to maintain the state of health of the animals and to protect them from diseases and epizootics, "because all profit depends on this."[123]

Both the treatises on the plague and the treatises on animal diseases always emphasized that the epidemics were a "foreign enemy" coming into the territory from outside. The report of Brunswick from 1682 underlined that the cattle plague "sneaked out in a short time from distant lands, namely from the territory of Milan,"[124] to the region of Brunswick. In the eighteenth century the agrarian innovator Friedrich Mayer observed that there would be no cattle plague "if not due to the long war the Hungarian cattle came to us and infected our cattle."[125] By blaming an external threat the authorities were able to draw a line between "them" and "us" in order to conceal their own failures and to channel fear and anger in the population onto already stigmatized marginal groups such as Jewish traders and "gypsies."[126]

Conclusion

Different pathogens and their impact on living beings were omnipresent in early modern Central Europe. During epidemics, animals had different functions. Partly, they frightened experts and ordinary people as alleged vectors of disease. On the other hand, domestic animals, which were highly important for trade and livelihood, sometimes were thought to cure epidemics such as the plague. In premodern societies the fate of humans and animals in the face of contagious diseases was surprisingly similar. In many cases, epizootics and epidemics spread parallel to each other, due to trading and military activities. Before and during the epidemiological transition of the eighteenth century, which was linked to a decreasing influence of epidemics on population growth,[127] most individuals, both animal and human, had a high vulnerability to transmissible diseases. Bearing in mind the new concepts of human–animal history that recognized the value and agency of animals themselves,[128] it is necessary to stress the human responsibility for animal suffering and death, both in premodern societies and today. With regard to the interpretation of epizootics and reactions to them, both recommended and realized, the similarities to epidemics are conspicuous. Usually, they both were interpreted as divine punishments or threats from outside, often brought in by dubious individuals. With some exceptions, for instance the famous tongue-scraper, recipes and preventive measures against such diseases were similar and included fumigation, separation of individual animals, which supported the idea of indoor housing during the eighteenth century, quarantine for sick animals, as well as the prohibition on trading allegedly contagious animal products, especially skins. Similarly, religious and magical practices existed and persisted as measures against epidemics and epizootics.

Ansgar Schanbacher is a visiting scholar at the Institute for Historical Regional Research at the University of Göttingen. He is especially interested in environmental and urban history of the early modern period. After studies in Leipzig and Lublin (Poland), he became a member of the Research Training Group "Interdisciplinary Environmental History" at the University of Göttingen, where he completed his dissertation on the famine of the 1840s in northwest Germany in 2015. Between 2016 and 2020 he was scientific coordinator in the research program "Sustainability as an Argument" at the University of Göttingen. After research stays in Brno (Czech Republic) and Poznań (Poland), he has recently published a book on natural hazards and resource management in early modern cities, especially in Braunschweig, Würzburg, and Utrecht.

Philip Knäble is Research Associate at the University of Göttingen. He studied history and social sciences at the universities of Bielefeld and Paris VII. Philip Knäble received his PhD from the University of Bielefeld in 2014. His research interests include medieval dance history and early modern religious and economic history. His ongoing research explores the economic practices of Jesuit missionaries in Paraguay (1600–1750) under the perspective of a Catholic ethic and the spirit of capitalism.

Malte de Vries is an archivist at the Niedersachsen Federal State Archives in Stade. His work is mainly focused on the history of "Gute Policey" in early modern times. His 2020 dissertation in history examines the implementation of the Reformation in Brunswick. During his doctoral studies he also worked as a research assistant at the Herzog August Bibliothek Wolfenbüttel (2018–19). Furthermore, he researched the development of historic road networks in different parts of northern Germany for the project "Map of the Chausees in Lower Saxony, 1764–1843" at the Institute for Historical Regional Research Göttingen. His recent publications include "Zwischen Autonomie und landesherrlichem Kirchenregiment" as well as "Hebammenausbildung in den Herzogtümern Bremen und Verden."

Notes

1. Hassinger, "Becher"; Smith, *Business*, 69–70; Becher, *Kluger Hauß-Vater*; Becher, *Parnassus Illustratus*.
2. The primary sources cited mostly are accessible online via www.vd16.de, www.vd17.de, and www.vd18.de.
3. Steinbrecher, "Hunde," 210; Wischermann and Howell, "Liminality"; Schanbacher, "Tiere," 7–8.
4. Henning, *Landwirtschaft*, 202. All English translations are ours unless noted otherwise.
5. Encyclopedia Britannica, "Epidemic." Retrieved 14 April 2021 from https://www.britannica.com/science/epidemic.
6. Campbell, "Panzootics," 182–84, 194. For the connection between epidemics and environment see Bergdolt, "Seuchentheorie."
7. Campbell, "Panzootics"; Slavin, "Fifth Rider."
8. Brown and Gilfoyle, "Introduction," 2–3, 8.
9. Stühring, *Seuche*; Hünniger, *Viehseuche*; Hünniger, "Policing Epizootics."
10. Nowosadtko, "Milzbrand"; Nowosadtko, "Die policirte Fauna."
11. Blancou, *History*; Wilkinson, *Animals*; Stähle, "Verlauf"; Schnurrer, "Tierseuchenbekämpfung"; Schwarz, "Schweinepest."
12. van Dülmen, *Dorf und Stadt*, 31.
13. Reinhard, *Lebensformen*, 406–8; Schumann, "Tiere"; Lux, "Agrargeschichte," 394; Oeser, *Pferd*, 141–42. Especially horses exceeded merely economic uses by confirming the social, political, and military power of their owners; Roche, *Culture*, 23.
14. Niemann, *Wirtschaftsgeschichte*, 83; Nowosadtko, "Ausbeutung," 253, 267, 270–71.
15. van Dülmen, *Dorf und Stadt*, 36.
16. Troßbach, "Tierhaltung," 102.
17. Regnath, *Schwein*, 270.
18. Achilles, "Landwirtschaft," 191; Troßbach, "Tierhaltung," 106–7; Jacobeit, *Schafhaltung*, 21–31; Radkau, *Natur*, 37–38.
19. Lerch, *Agrargeschichte*, 117.
20. Regnath, *Schwein*, 270; Achilles, "Landwirtschaft," 192–93.
21. Regnath, *Schwein*, 269–70; Troßbach, "Tierhaltung," 102; Lux, "Agrargeschichte," 392.
22. Troßbach, "Tierhaltung," 105.
23. Gessner, *Thierbuch*, 116.
24. Orłowska, "Spuren"; Mathis, *Deutsche Wirtschaft*, 25–26, 117; Stadelmann, "Schlachtvieh"; Abel, *Landwirtschaft*, 179–81.
25. Troßbach, "Tierhaltung," 98–99; Henning, *Landwirtschaft*, 199.
26. Troßbach, "Tierhaltung." 100–1.
27. Jütte, *Krankheit*, 30–31, 34.

28. Feuerstein-Herz, *Gotts verhengnis*, 228. For the connection between diseases and insects see Kircher, *Durchgründung*, 50–51.
29. Sturm, *Leben*, 88.
30. Reinhard, *Lebensformen*, 159; Vasold, *Grippe*, 61.
31. Lucretius, *De Rervm Natvra*; English translation: Lucretius, *Six Books*, 221; Latin original: "nec tamen omnino temere illis solibus ulla comparebatavis, nectristia saeclaferarum exibant silvis; languebant pleraque morbo et moriebantur." Lukrez, *De rerum natura*, VI, 1219–22.
32. Seelbach, *Maßnahmen*, 201.
33. Sturm, *Leben*, 403; Kellner, *Pesthauch*, 166.
34. Jenner, "Massacre," 45.
35. Jenner, "Massacre," 45–49, 56.
36. Wendler, "Tiere." 44–45.
37. City Archives Braunschweig, B I 3 Nr. 21, 2, fol. 768–69.
38. Seelbach, *Maßnahmen*, 217.
39. Vries, "Pestepidemien," 33–34; Sturm, *Leben*, 125–26.
40. Sturm, *Leben*, 388.
41. Wendler, "Tiere," 48–50.
42. Becher, *Parnassus Medicinalis Illustratus*, I, 25: "Der Stein den man bißweil in Därm und Magen findt / Er gleicht dem Bezoar / das Gifft er überwindt."
43. Jürgens, *Tierseuchen*, 2–3. Naturally, not only animals but also crop plants such as grains and potatoes were damaged by diseases. Also see Schanbacher, *Kartoffelkrankheit*, 48–50.
44. Hoy, "Tierhygiene," 246.
45. Driesch and Peters, *Geschichte*, 157.
46. Schwarz, "Schweinepest," 41–42; Driesch and Peters, *Geschichte*, 91.
47. Schwarz, "Schweinepest," 47.
48. Jacobeit, *Schafhaltung*, 258, 262.
49. Driesch and Peters, *Geschichte*, 159.
50. Stühring, *Seuche*, 42, 52; Hünniger, *Viehseuche*, 81; Spinage, *Cattle Plague*, 98.
51. Schwarz, "Schweinepest," 54, Driesch and Peters, *Geschichte*, 158; Spinage, *Cattle Plague*, 98.
52. Spinage, *Cattle Plague*, 100.
53. Driesch and Peters, *Geschichte*, 160.
54. Driesch and Peters, *Geschichte*, 164–65; Stähle, *Verlauf*, 23.
55. Hünniger "Epizootics," 79, 81.
56. Schnurrer, *Tierseuchenbekämpfung*, 15–16.
57. Driesch and Peters, *Geschichte*, 176.
58. Nowak, "Beitrag," 50, 53, 59.
59. Vegetius, *Ain Büchlein*, LVII: "vnd wenn sy [die Kranckheit] ein thier begreiffen / gangen sie gar bald zu allen / vnd also machen sie sterblichheit einer ganntzen gesunden herd oder schar / oder allen gezämptten / Derhalbenn sollen die thier welche ein mal berürt seind worden / mit allem fleiß abgesündert werden."
60. Gessner, *Thierbuch*, 119: "so eins vnder der herd angestossen so verderben sie ein gantze herd."
61. Quoted after Feuerstein-Herz, *Gotts verhengnis*, 216.
62. Reuschlein von Hagenau, *Hippiatria*, 57.
63. Driesch and Peters, *Geschichte*, 85–109.

64. Saris, "*Von Schafen*," 59.
65. "Schneid oder beiß ihnen ein wenig von der Zunge/ nimm sie bey den Füssen/ wältze sie von einer Seiten zur andern/ daß sie sich wohl auf den Rücken wältze/ hernach nimm einen Riemen von Leder/ und schlage sie viermal auf den Leib/ so wird ihnen bald besser." *Neu-vermehrt-nutzlich Vieh-büchlein* 1697, 59; Böhme, *Vieh-Arztney*, 2.
66. Driesch and Peters, *Geschichte*, 158f.
67. Rössner, *Wirtschaftsgeschichte*, 244f.
68. Nowosadtko, "Milzbrand," 84.
69. Becher, *Kluger Haus-Vater*, 614: "Mutter-Kraut dem Viehe zu essen gegeben/ vertreibet diese böße Seuche/ das Keichen/ Auffblehen/ Geschwulst/ und reiniget sehr."
70. *Neu-vermehrt-nutzlich Vieh-büchlein* 1697, 57.
71. *Neu-vermehrt-nutzlich Vieh-büchlein* 1697, 126.
72. Saris, *Von Schafen*, 66.
73. Alexander von Neuneck, *Roßarzneibuch*, quoted by Saris, *Von Schafen*, 47: "hernach folgen etliche schöne vnd bewehrte recept vor menschen vndt viehe zugebrauchen. pulver im viehsterbendt, vor lung vndt lebersucht auch pestilentz."
74. For example *Kurze Pestordnung*, Hildesheim 1609, *Kurze Pestordnung*, Wolfenbüttel 1611.
75. Vischer, *Bericht* [50–51].
76. Vischer, *Kurtzer unterricht*.
77. Apell, *Sammlung*, 212–13: They should not allow "einiges Pferd= Ochsen= oder Rind= Vieh bey sich in die Weide oder uffn Stall zu nehmen, viel weniger zum Schlachten in Unser Lande zu bringen."
78. City Archives Braunschweig, B I 3 Nr. 19, 391: "[Es sei] eine böse gifftige seuche an vielen orten eingerißen [... weshalb das Vieh] obangedachtem vnheill so viel müglich vorzukommen, vor diesmahl daselbst in der stadt nicht verstattet" werden solle.
79. City Archives Braunschweig, B I 3 Nr. 19, 378.
80. Hänselmann, *Brandis Diarium*, 191.
81. Nowosadtko, "Milzbrand," 82.
82. *Edict of 25 August 1682* [VD17 23:680035D].
83. *Edict of 19 July 1682* [VD17 12:626805K].
84. "Recipe against current cattle plague" ("Recept. Für gegenwärtige Seuch deß Viehs") [VD17 12652197N]. "Wohlbewehrt- und approbirte Recept oder Mittel/ Welche für die ietzt graszierende Vieh-Kranckheit/ Ihro Churfl. D. in Bayern/ gnädigst publiciren lassen" [VD17 15:745996L].
85. In 1682, an anthrax epizootic affected cattle in France, Germany, and Switzerland. The tumors appearing on the tongue were also scraped with silver spoons. Since the spoons were contagious after the procedure, infections of humans who used them happened, too; Blancou, *History*, 95.
86. *Verordnung wie es wegen der in der Nachbarschafft*, 4.
87. *Verordnung wie es wegen der in der Nachbarschafft*, 3.
88. *Verordnung wie es wegen der in der Nachbarschafft*, 4.
89. Schwarz, "Schweinepest," 54.
90. *Edict of 24 July 1684*, in: Mylius, *Corpus Consistutionum*, 427–28.
91. Nowosadtko, "Milzbrand," 82.
92. Jürgens, *Tierseuchen*, 3.
93. See for further information: Nowosadtko, "Milzbrand," 83, and Nowosadtko, "Policirte Fauna," 322–23.

94. Selheim, "Votivgaben," 36.
95. Kasparek, "Votivgaben," 85–94.
96. Andree, *Votive und Weihgaben*, 148.
97. Böck, "Kult und Brauch," 30. See also Andree, *Votive und Votivgaben*, 148.
98. For pictures of those sacrificed figures see Kasparek, "Votivgaben," 91–94.
99. Böck, "Kult und Brauch," 30.
100. Böck, "Kult und Brauch," 30.
101. Böck, "Kult und Brauch," 31; Jordan, *Viehseuchen*, 7.
102. Hünemörder, "Rinderpestbekämpfung," 28.
103. Riezer, *Hexenprozesse in Bayern*, 143.
104. *Zwo Newe Zeitungen*, fol. Aiir.
105. *Zwo Newe Zeitungen*, fol. Aiiir.
106. *Nöthiger Unterricht.*
107. Nowosadtko, "Milzbrand," 95: "Die Regierungen griffen bei der Bekämpfung von ansteckenden Tierkrankheiten auf Instrumente und Erfahrungen zurück, die sie im Umgang mit menschlichen Epidemien entwickelt und erworben hatten. Bei den seit der zweiten Hälfte des 17. Jahrhunderts wegen der Viehseuchen erlassenen Verordnungen bestand insofern eine enge Beziehung zu den zeitlich vorhergegangenen Pestordnungen."
108. *Bericht der an etlichen Orten eingerissenen Vieh-Seuche betreffend* … . Braunschweig: Zilliger, 1682, [1–2].
109. Hünniger, *Rinderseuche*, 9.
110. Mylius, *Corpus*, 433: "weil Medici oder Physici, als diejenigen, welche eine gründliche Wissenschaft in denen natürlichen Dingen besitzen sollen, sich um dergleichen Schaden wenig bekümmern."
111. Hoffmann, *Vorschläge*, 4.
112. Kanold, *Relation*, Vorrede: "daß diese Bruta einen großen Theil des Seegens und der Nothwendigkeiten von einem Lande ausmachen." See also Hünniger, *Rinderseuche*, 65–67.
113. Hoffmann, *Vorschläge*, 9.
114. Roeseler and Bornemann, *Nachrichten*, 369r: "Es gehet dem Menschen wie dem Vieh, wie dies stirbt, so stirbt auch das. … als daß von menschlichen Krankheiten auf Vieh-Seuchen & vice-versa, gar wohl zu argumentiren und zu schliessen stehe."
115. Cf. Driesch and Peters, *Geschichte*, 158; Stühring, *Seuche*, 40f.
116. Cf. Hoffmann, *Vorschläge*, 11.
117. Cf. Saris, *Von Schafen*, 170–81.
118. Cf. Cravelius, *Pestordnung*, 74–76.
119. Hoffmann, *Vorschläge*, 11: "…daß wir nicht solche Mittel und Dinge, welche kostbar, und nicht wohl zu haben sind, gebunden, sondern, daß vielmehr die simplesten, schlechtesten Sachen und Kräuter, die gar leicht und überall zu bekommen sind, die besten Kräffte und Wirckungen in Heilungen der Sichten bey sich halten."
120. Zedler, "Pest."
121. Cf. Nisly, "Mustergüter," 47.
122. Mayer, *Fortsetzung*, 112: "Wind, Frost, Nebel, Regen, Hitze, Sumpfwasser, Mangel an Wasser, weite Triebe, dorichte, höckerichte Gegenden, ungesundes Gras, … eckelhafte mit Koth und Harn verschleppte Plätze, zertrettenes, besudeltes Gras, … sind lauter solche Dinge, welche der Gesundheit des Viehes nachtheilig, gefährlich und

schädlich sein müssen, welche, gegen die Constitution ihres Körpers gehalten, zumal Kälte, Frost, Regen und Hitze, drohen allemal Seuchen und Krankheiten."

123. Mayer, *Fortsetzung*, 111: "dann hievon hangt aller Gewinn ab."
124. *Bericht der an etlichen Orten eingerissenen Vieh-Seuche betreffend*, 2r: "… welche in kurzer Zeit von fernen Landen / und zwar aus dem Mayländischen Gebiet / sich heraus geschlichen … ."
125. Mayer, *Fortsetzung*, 113: "… wann nicht das Ungarische Vieh durch den anhaltenden Krieg zu uns gekommen wäre, und das unsrige angesteckt hätte." For the link to antiquity see Gessner, *Thierbuch*, 117.
126. Cf. Dinges, "Pest," 284; Höhl, *Pest*, 158.
127. Reinhard, *Lebensformen*, 161.
128. Cf. Howell and Kean, "Writing," 5–7; Breittruck, *Flügelschlag*, 10–21.

Bibliography

Primary Sources

Apell, Christian Gerhard. *Sammlung Fürstlich=Hessischer Landes=Ordnungen und Ausschreiben nebst dahin gehörigen Erläuterungs= und anderen Rescripten, Resolutionen, Abschieden, gemeinen Bescheiden und dergleichen*. Part 3. Kassel: Seiberts Erben, 1777.

Becher, Johann Joachim. *Kluger Hauß-Vater, verständige Hauß-Mutter, vollkommener Land-Medicus, wie auch wohlerfahrner Roß- und Viehe-Artzt*. Leipzig: Groschuff, 1698.

Becher, Johann Joachim. *Parnassus Medicinalis Illustratus. Oder: Ein neues/ und dergestalt/ vormahln noch nie gesehenes Thier- Kräuter- Und Berg-Buch Sampt der Salernischen Schul*. Ulm: Görlin, 1663.

Bericht der an etlichen Orten eingerissenen Vieh-Seuche betreffend … . Braunschweig: Zilliger, 1682.

Böhme, Michael: *Kurtze doch bewährte Vieh-Artzney …* . s.l., 1682.

City Archives Braunschweig, B I 3 Nr. 19.

Cravelius, Johann. *Pestordnung / Oder Gründlicher Bericht …* . Goslar: Johann Vogt, 1625.

Edict of 19 July 1682, Braunschweig-Wolfenbüttel [VD17 12:626805K].

Edict of 25 August 1682, Braunschweig-Wolfenbüttel [VD17 23:680035D].

Gessner, Conrad. *Thierbuch / Das ist / Ausführliche beschreibung / und lebendige ja auch eigentliche Contrafactur und Abmahlung aller Vierfüssigen thieren …* . Heidelberg: Cambier, 1606.

Hänselmann, Ludwig, ed. *Joachim Brandis' des Jüngeren Diarium. Ergänzt aus Tilo Brandis' Annalen 1528–1609*. Hildesheim: C. A. Schwetschke und Sohn, 1902.

Hoffmann, Friedrich. *Heilsame Vorschläge wie der Graßirenden Seuche unter dem Horn-Vieh vorzubauen, und was vor Mittel dazu dienlich*. Halle: Rengerische Buchhandlung, 1716.

Kanold, Johann. *Historische Relation der Pestilentz des Horn-Viehes, Welche Anno 1711. und 1712. in Schlesien … starck grassiret*. Breslau: Fellgiebel, 1713.

Kircher, Athanasius. *Natürliche und Medicinalische Durchgründung Der laidigen ansteckenden Sucht/ und so genanten Pestilentz …* . Augsburg: Brandan, 1680.

Kurze Pestordnung unnd Verzeichnuß der Artzneyen. Hildesheim: s.n., 1609.

Kurze Pestordnung unnd Verzeichnuß der Artzneyen. Wolfenbüttel: s.n., 1611.

Lucretius, Titus. *His Six Books De Natura Rerum. Done into English Verse With Notes*. Oxford: L. Lichfield, 1683.

Lucretius, Titus. *De Rervm Natvra Libri Sex*. Frankfurt am Main: Fitzer, 1631.

Lukrez. *De rerum natura. Welt aus Atomen*. Stuttgart: Reclam, 2020.

Mayer, Johann Friedrich. *Fortsetzung der Beyträge und Abhandlungen zur Aufnahme der Land- und Hauswirthschaft nach den Grundsätzen der Naturlehre und der Erfahrung entworfen*. Frankfurt am Main: Andreaische Buchhandlung, 1770.

Mylius, Christian Otto. *Corpus Consistutionum Marchicarum, oder Königl. Preußis. und Chrufürstl. Brandenburgische in der Chur= und Marck Brandenburg, auch incorporierten Landen publicirte und ergangene Ordnungen, Edicta, Mandata, Rescripta ...* . Berlin, Halle: Buchladen des Weisenhauses, 1736.

Neu-vermehrt-nutzlich- und vollkommenes Vieh-Büchlein: Darinnen Die eigentliche Beschreibung der fürnehmsten Kranckheiten/ und derer darwider dienenden Artzneyen/ der Pferde/ Maulthier/ Esel/ wie auch der Rinder/ Schafe/ Ziegen/ Schweine/ Hunde/ Hün.../ zu grossen Nutzen ... zusammen getragen. Nürnberg: Endter, 1697.

Nöthiger Unterricht/ Die An etlichen Orthen eingerissene Viehe=Seuche betreffend. Coburg, s.n., 1682 [VD17 3:304709N].

Recept. Für gegenwärtige Seuch deß Viehs, 1682 [VD17 12652197N].

Reuschlein von Hagenau, Caspar. *Hippiatria. Gründlicher und eigentlicher Bericht von Art und Eygenschafften der Pferde ...* . Straßburg: Bernhard Jobin, 1593.

Roeseler, Johann Wilhelm, and Anton Philpp Bornemann. *Nachdem bishero so wohl Nachrichten eingelauffen, als auch durch unterschiedene öffentliche Schrifften bekannt worden, daß ... unter denen Pferden, Horn- und andern Viehe eine solche ansteckende Seuche eingerissen ...* . s.l., 1723.

Vegetius, Flavius. *Ain Büchlein / vonn rechter vnnd warhaffter kunst der Artzney / Allerlay kranckheyten / ynnwendigen vnd außwendigen aller Thyer ...* . Augsburg: Steiner, 1532.

Verordnung wie es wegen der in der Nachbarschafft eingerißenen und befahrenden Vieh=Seuche in dem Fürstenthum Weimar zu halten. Weimar: Müller, 1682 (SUB Göttingen, 8 J STAT II, 5523).

Vischer, Christoph. *Einfeltiger vnd in der heiligen Götlichen schrifft wolgegründter Bericht ...* . Schmalkalden: Michael Schmuck, 1575.

Vischer, Christoph. *Kurtzer unterricht / Wie man sich mit Gottes huelffe vor der Pestilentzischen vergifftung bewaren*. Schmalkalden: Michael Schmuck, 1566.

Wohlbewehrt- und approbirte Recept oder Mittel/ Welche für die ietzt graszierende Vieh-Kranckheit/ Ihro Churfl. D. in Bayern/ gnädigst publiciren lassen, 1682 [VD17 15:745996L].

Zedler, Johann Heinrich. "Pest, Viehpest, Schelm, Viehseuche, Viehsterben, Umfall." In *Zedlers Universallexikon*, vol. 27, 773–80. Halle, Leipzig: Zedler, 1741.

Zwo Newe Zeitungen/ Die erste/ welcher gestalt zween falsche Juden/ durch Zauberey zuwegen gebracht/ daß vil tausent Stück Vihe hingefallen und gestorben ist. Vienna: Johann Formick, 1599 [VD16 N 1023].

Secondary Sources

Abel, Wilhelm. *Geschichte der deutschen Landwirtschaft vom frühen Mittelalter bis zum 19. Jahrhundert*. Stuttgart: Eugen Ulmer, 1978.

Achilles, Walter. "Die Landwirtschaft." In *Die Wirtschafts- und Sozialgeschichte des Braunschweigischen Landes vom Mittelalter bis zur Gegenwart. Vol. 2: Frühneuzeit*, edited by Karl Heinrich Kaufhold, Jörg Leuschner, and Claudia Märtl, 139–314. Hildesheim: Georg Olms Verlag, 2008.

Andree, Richard. *Votive und Weihgaben des katholischen Volks in Süddeutschland.* Braunschweig: F. Vieweg und Sohn, 1904.

Bergdolt, Klaus. "Seuchentheorie und Umwelt in der Frühen Neuzeit." In *Natur als Grenzerfahrung. Europäische Perspektiven der Mensch-Natur-Beziehung in Mittelalter und Neuzeit: Ressourcennutzung, Entdeckungen, Naturkatastrophen*, edited by Lars Kreye, Carsten Stühring, and Tanja Zwingelberg, 221–34. Göttingen: Universitätsverlag Göttingen, 2009.

Blancou, Jean. *History of the Surveillance and Control of Transmissible Animal Diseases.* Paris: Office International des epizooties, 2003.

Böck, Robert. "Kult und Brauch im Amperland. St. Leonhardsverehrung, Rosskulte, Umritte und Leonhardifahrten—Pferde- und Fußrennen." In *Bayerisches Jahrbuch für Volkskunde* 65 (2015): 19–60.

Breittruck, Julia. *Ein Flügelschlag in der Pariser Aufklärung. Zur Geschichte der Beziehungen zwischen Menschen und ihren Vögeln.* München: Universitätsbibliothek Ludwig-Maximilians-Universität München, 2021.

Brown, Karen, and Daniel Gilfoyle. "Introduction." In *Healing the Herds. Disease, Livestock Economies, and the Globalization of Veterinary Medicine*, edited by Karen Brown and Daniel Gilfoyle, 1–18. Athens: Ohio University Press, 2010.

Campbell, Bruce M. S. "Panzootics, Pandemics and the Climatic Anomalies in the Fourteenth Century." In *Beiträge zum Göttinger Umwelthistorischen Kolloquium 2010–2011*, edited by Bernd Herrmann, 177–215. Göttingen: Universitätsverlag Göttingen, 2011.

Dinges, Martin, "Pest und Politik in der europäischen Neuzeit." In *Pest. Die Geschichte eines Menschheitstraumas*, edited by Mischa Meier, 283–313. Stuttgart: Klett-Cotta, 2005.

Driesch, Angela von den, and Joris Peters. *Geschichte der Tiermedizin. 5000 Jahre Tierheilkunde.* Stuttgart, New York: Schattauer, 2003.

Feuerstein-Herz, Petra, ed. *Gotts verhengnis und seine straffe. Zur Geschichte der Seuchen in der Frühen Neuzeit.* Wiesbaden: Harrassowitz Verlag, 2005.

Hassinger, Herbert. "Becher, Johann Joachim." In *Neue Deutsche Biographie*, retrieved 10 May 2021 from https://www.deutsche-biographie.de/pnd118507923.html#ndbcontent.

Henning, Friedrich-Wilhelm. *Landwirtschaft und ländliche Gesellschaft in Deutschland. Vol. 1. 800 bis 1750.* Paderborn: Ferdinand Schöningh, 1979.

Höhl, Monika. *Die Pest in Hildesheim. Krankheit als Krisenfaktor im städtischen Leben des Mittelalters und der Frühen Neuzeit (1350–1750).* Bielefeld: Verlag für Regionalgeschichte, 2002.

Howell, Philip and Hilda Kean. "Writing in Animals in History." In *The Routledge Companion to Animal–Human History*, edited by Hilda Kean and Philip Howell, 3–27. London/New York: Routledge, 2019.

Hoy, Steffen. "Tierhygiene." In *Nutztierhaltung und -hygiene* by Steffen Hoy, Matthias Gauly, and Joachim Krieter, 187–297. Stuttgart: Eugen Ulmer, 2016.

Hünemörder, Kai F. "Zwischen 'abergläubischem Abwehrzauber' und der 'Inokulation der Hornviehseuche.' Entwicklungslinien der Rinderpestbekämpfung im 18. Jahrhundert." In *Beten, Impfen, Sammeln. Zur Viehseuchen- und Schädlingsbekämpfung in der Frühen Neuzeit*, edited by Katharina Engelken, Dominik Hünniger, and Steffi Windelen, 21–56. Göttingen: Universitätsverlag Göttingen, 2007.

Hünniger, Dominik. *Die Viehseuche von 1744–52. Deutungen und Herrschaftspraxis in Krisenzeiten.* Neumünster: Wachholtz Verlag, 2011.

Hünniger, Dominik. "Policing Epizootics. Legislation and Administration during Outbreaks of Cattle Plague in Eighteenth-Century Northern Germany as Continuous

Crisis Management." In *Healing the Herds. Disease, Livestock Economies, and the Globalization of Veterinary Medicine*, edited by Karen Brown and Daniel Gilfoyle, 76–91. Athens: Ohio University Press, 2010.

Jacobeit, Wolfgang. *Schafhaltung und Schäfer in Zentraleuropa bis zum Beginn des 20. Jahrhunderts*. Berlin: Akademie-Verlag, 1987.

Jenner, Mark S. R. "The Great Dog Massacre." In *Fear in Early Modern Society*, edited by William G. Naphy and Penny Roberts, 44–61. Manchester, New York: Manchester University Press, 1997.

Jordan, Winfried. "Viehseuchen im bayerisch-schwäbischen Voralpengebiet während des 17., 18. und 19. Jahrhunderts." Dissertation. LMU Munich, 1951.

Jürgens, Karin. *Tierseuchen in der Landwirtschaft. Die psychosozialen Folgen der Schweinepest für betroffene Familien—untersucht an Fallbeispielen in Nordwestdeutschland*. Würzburg: Ergon, 2002.

Jütte, Robert. *Krankheit und Gesundheit in der Frühen Neuzeit*. Stuttgart: W. Kohlhammer, 2013.

Kasparek, Max Udo. "Votivgaben und Mirakelbücher als Quellen der Haustierforschung mit besonderer Berücksichtigung Niederbayerns." In *Bericht des Naturwissenschaftlichen Vereins Landshut* 24 (1964): 85–94.

Kellner, Katharina. *Pesthauch über Regensburg. Seuchenbekämpfung und Hygiene im 18. Jahrhundert*. Regensburg: Friedrich Pustet, 2005.

Lerch, Hans. *Hessische Agrargeschichte des 17. und 18. Jahrhunderts*. Hersfeld: Hans Ott-Verlag, 1926.

Lux, Thomas. "Agrargeschichte bis zum Ende der bergischen Zeit." In *Geschichte des bergischen Landes. Bis zum Ende des alten Herzogtums 1806*, edited by Stefan Gorißen, Horst Sassin, and Kurt Wesoly, 359–404. Bielefeld: Verlag für Regionalgeschichte, 2014.

Mathis, Franz. *Die deutsche Wirtschaft im 16. Jahrhundert*. Munich: Oldenbourg, 1992.

Niemann, Hans-Werner. *Europäische Wirtschaftsgeschichte. Vom Mittelalter bis heute*. Darmstadt: WBG, 2009.

Nisly, Jadon, "Mustergüter als Utopie der agrarökonomischen Aufklärung." In *Utopie Landwirtschaft*, edited by Max Böhm et al., 47–62. Ingolstadt: Stadt Ingolstadt, 2018.

Nowak, Karl-Heinz. "Beitrag zur Geschichte der Haustiertollwut unter besonderer Berücksichtigung von Pferd und Klauentieren." Dissertation. FU Berlin, 2002.

Nowosadtko, Jutta. "Milzbrand, Tollwut, Wölfe, Spatzen und Maikäfer. Die gesellschaftliche Verteilung von Zuständigkeiten bei der Bekämpfung von Viehseuchen und schädlichen Tieren in der Frühen Neuzeit." In *Beten, Impfen, Sammeln. Zur Viehseuchen- und Schädlingsbekämpfung in der Frühen Neuzeit*, edited by Katharina Engelken, Dominik Hünniger, and Steffi Windelen, 79–98. Göttingen: Universitätsverlag Göttingen, 2007.

Nowosadtko, Jutta. "Die policirte Fauna in Theorie und Praxis. Frühneuzeitliche Tierhaltung, Seuchen- und Schädlingsbekämpfung im Spiegel der Policeyvorschriften." In *Policey und frühneuzeitliche Gesellschaft*, edited by Karl Härter, 297–340. Frankfurt am Main: Vittorio Klostermann, 2000.

Nowosadtko, Jutta. "Zwischen Ausbeutung und Tabu. Nutztiere in der Frühen Neuzeit." In *Tiere und Menschen. Geschichte und Aktualität eines prekären Verhältnisses*, edited by Paul Münch and Rainer Walz, 247–74. Paderborn: Ferdinand Schöningh, 1999.

Oeser, Erhard. *Pferd und Mensch. Die Geschichte einer Beziehung*. Darmstadt: WBG, 2007.

Orłowska, Anna Paulina. "Spuren des Ochsenhandels in den großpolnischen Städten des 16. Jahrhunderts." *Forum Stadt* 1 (2021): 29–38.

Radkau, Joachim. *Natur und Macht. Eine Weltgeschichte der Umwelt*. Munich: C. H. Beck, 2012.
Regnath, R. Johanna. *Das Schwein im Wald. Vormoderne Schweinehaltung zwischen Herrschaftsstrukturen, ständischer Ordnung und Subsistenzökonomie*. Ostfildern: Jan Thorbecke Verlag, 2008.
Reinhard, Wolfgang. *Lebensformen Europas. Eine historische Kulturanthropologie*. Munich: C. H. Beck, 2006.
Riezer, Sigmund von. *Geschichte der Hexenprozesse in Bayern*. Stuttgart: J. G. Cotta, 1896.
Roche, Daniel. *La culture équestre de l'Occident. XVIe–XIXe siècle. L'ombre du cheval*. Paris: Fayard, 2008.
Rössner, Philipp. *Wirtschaftsgeschichte neu denken. Mit einer Darstellung der Ursprünge moderner ökonomischer Theorien*. Stuttgart: Schäffer-Poeschel Verlag, 2017.
Saris, Tomke. "*Von Schafen, Bienen, Ochsen und anderm lieblichen Viehe." Die Rezepte für landwirtschaftliche Nutztiere in Rossarzneihandschriften des 15. bis 18. Jahrhunderts*. Gießen: Deutsche Veterinärmedizinische Gesellschaft Service GmbH, 2018.
Schanbacher, Ansgar. "Tiere und Pflanzen in der Stadt der Frühen Neuzeit." *Forum Stadt* 1 (2021): 3–10.
Schanbacher, Ansgar. *Kartoffelkrankheit und Nahrungskrise in Nordwestdeutschland 1845–1848*. Göttingen: Wallstein, 2016.
Schnurrer, Barbara. "Die Tierseuchenbekämpfung im Territorium der freien Reichsstadt Rothenburg ob der Tauber im 18. Jahrhundert." Dissertation. LMU Munich, 1991.
Schumann, Eva. "'Tiere sind keine Sachen.' Zur Personifizierung von Tieren im mittelalterlichen Recht." In *Natur als Grenzerfahrung. Europäische Perspektiven der Mensch-Natur-Beziehung in Mittelalter und Neuzeit: Ressourcennutzung, Entdeckungen, Naturkatastrophen*, edited by Lars Kreye, Carsten Stühring, and Tanja Zwingelberg, 23–49. Göttingen: Universitätsverlag Göttingen, 2009.
Schwarz, Diana-Kerstin. "Schweinepest. Ein Beitrag zur Geschichte der Tierkrankheiten." Dissertation. FU Berlin, 2005.
Seelbach, Kirsten Renate. *In dieser harten und sterbenden Zeit. Maßnahmen gegen die Pest 1620–1750*. Marburg: Tectum, 2007.
Selheim, Claudia. "Votivgaben mit medizinischen Motiven aus Neuzeit und Gegenwart." In *Asklepios. Heilgott und Heilkult*, edited by Claudia Selheim and Thomas Schnalke, 34–37. Erlangen: Primed, 1990.
Slavin, Philip. "The Fifth Rider of the Apocalypse. The Great Cattle Plague in England and Wales and its Economic Consequences, 1319–1350." In *Le interazioni fra economia e ambiente biologic nell'Europa preindustriale secc. XIII-XVIII* edited by Simonetta Cavaciocchi, 165–80. Florence: Firenze University Press, 2010.
Smith, Pamela H. *The Business of Alchemy. Science and Culture in the Holy Roman Empire*. Princeton: Princeton University Press, 1994.
Spinage, C. A. *Cattle Plague. A History*. New York: Kluwer Academic, 2003.
Stadelmann, Nicole. "Vom Schlachtvieh bis um Schuh. Die Produktionslinie von Leder in der frühneuzeitlichen Stadt St. Gallen und die Austauschbeziehungen zwischen städtischen Handwerkern und dem Umland." In *Reichsstadt und Landwirtschaft*, edited by Stefan Sonderegger, Helge Wittmann, and Dorothee Guggenheimer, 227–53. Petersberg: Michael Imhof Verlag, 2020.
Stähle, Reinhard. "Verlauf und Verbreitung der Rinderpest im Herzogtum Bremen und Verden von 1715 bis 1781." Dissertation. TH Hannover, 1981.

Steinbrecher, Aline. "Hunde und Menschen. Ein Grenzen auslotender Blick auf ihr Zusammenleben (1750–1850)." *Historische Anthropologie. Schwerpunktheft* 2 (2011): 192–210.

Stühring, Carsten. *Der Seuche begegnen. Deutung und Bewältigung von Rinderseuchen im Kurfürstentum Bayern des 18. Jahrhunderts.* Frankfurt am Main: Peter Lang, 2011.

Sturm, Patrick. *Leben mit dem Tod in den Reichsstädten Esslingen, Nördlingen und Schwäbisch Hall. Epidemien und deren Auswirkungen vom frühen 15. bis zum frühen 17. Jahrhundert.* Ostfildern: Jan Thorbecke Verlag, 2014.

Troßbach, Werner. "Tierhaltung." In *Grundzüge der Agrargeschichte. Vol. 1: Vom Spätmittelalter bis zum Dreißigjährigen Krieg,* edited by Rolf Kießling, Frank Konersmann, and Werner Troßbach, 98–108. Cologne: Böhlau Verlag, 2016.

van Dülmen, Richard. *Kultur und Alltag in der Frühen Neuzeit. Dorf und Stadt.* Munich: C. H. Beck, 2005.

Vasold, Manfred. *Grippe, Pest und Cholera. Eine Geschichte der Seuchen in Europa.* Stuttgart: Franz Steiner Verlag, 2008.

Vries, Malte de. "Pestepidemien im Braunschweig des 16. und 17. Jahrhunderts. Alltag in Zeiten einer 'Gottesstrafe.'" *Braunschweigisches Jahrbuch für Landesgeschichte* 101 (2020): 27–50.

Wendler, Ulf. "Tiere, Menschen und Iatromagie in deutschsprachigen Pestschriften 1565–1713." *Forum Stadt* 1 (2021): 39–53.

Wilkinson, Lise. *Animals and Disease. An Introduction to the History of Comparative Medicine.* Cambridge: Cambridge University Press, 1992.

Wischermann, Clemens and Philip Howell. "Liminality: A Governing Category in Animate History." In *Animal History in the Modern City. Exploring Liminality,* edited by Clemens Wischermann, Aline Steinbrecher, and Philip Howell, 1–24. London: Bloomsbury Academic, 2019.

CHAPTER 10

Plague Cemeteries in Early Modern German Towns

MARTIN CHRIST

Introduction

Whenever an epidemic broke out, magistrates, councilors, and rulers were faced with a range of difficult questions.[1] These included isolating infected people, ensuring the supply of goods, and administrative issues arising from the deaths of council members and officials.[2] Clerics also had to make difficult decisions, as visiting the sick was an important part of their work but increased the risk of spreading disease further.[3] Other members of the community also had to adapt their approaches to accommodate for the drastic changes that epidemics like the plague brought, for example guilds and fraternities, who had to pray for the sick and the souls of the dead, or women involved in washing the corpses of the dead.[4] During such times of disease, and especially during outbreaks of plague, in the words of Paul Slack, towns developed "sophisticated mechanisms intended to control the spread of epidemic disease and to mitigate its effects."[5]

The sudden and significant increase of death during plague epidemics meant that a town could be flooded with dead bodies, making this one of the most pressing issues during an epidemic. Considering the treatment of the plague dead enables scholars to investigate the pandemic-conditioned interactions between families, magistrates, clergy, and the populace at large during a pandemic emergency. When there was no outbreak of disease, the dead received specific treatment by clerics and family members, which could not be performed during pandemics. Family members and loved ones might wish for their dead to be buried in a proper way, but urban magistrates and clerics wanted to enforce quick burials, without elaborate ceremonies, to reduce the risk of further contagion. Magistrates and hygiene experts feared that if the dead were not buried quickly, the disease might spread further, especially as vapors could pollute the air.[6] One way to counteract the spread of diseases and ensure quick burial was the establishment of burial sites reserved for the plague dead.

This chapter considers the opening and multiple meanings of these plague cemeteries (*Pestfriedhöfe*) in early modern Germany. It provides examples of this kind of burial ground and traces the distinctive features of the cemeteries, such as mass graves and special burial procedures. It asks how these cemeteries shaped urban life and focuses on the ways in which urban and religious dignitaries interacted in their creation and administration. The chapter also shows that while many cities had to respond to outbreaks of plague, the burial locations could vary, depending on the time and precise circumstances. While extramural burial grounds were one possibility, it was just as common to try to bury people in the cities, especially in the sixteenth century. It was also possible for plague cemeteries to be turned into regular cemeteries, as was the case in Munich, but this could lead to resistance against the urban decrees and instructions that forced people to be buried there. This case study of plague cemeteries shows the complex ways in which urban populations, town magistrates, physicians and other medical experts, and clerics interacted during pandemics in early modern Germany.

The establishment of cemeteries specifically for victims of plague is hard to trace, in terms both of the archaeological evidence and of references in contemporaneous sources.[7] Churchyards in the medieval and early modern period had a wide range of functions, and only one of them was their use as a burial space.[8] Many serious outbreaks of plague led to quick responses by urban magistrates. Therefore burials can appear random, particularly as plague did not leave any definitive osteo-archaeological evidence. Burial grounds for other diseases, like leprosy, could also be established and further complicate an already complex situation, as they might leave similar traces in the written or archaeological evidence. Indeed, what constitutes a "plague cemetery" is unclear, as the concept of an ordered, clearly demarcated space for the dead is a modern one.[9] In the Middle Ages and early modern period, many dead were buried around the church, with the spots marked with simple wooden crosses or not at all.[10] Further burial spaces, for example for dishonorable individuals or members of so-called defiled trades, could be even less regulated, for instance if corpses were left under the gallows, outside the town center. For these reasons it can be hard to trace plague cemeteries, yet a focus on these spaces and their use can offer revealing insight into the impact of epidemics on early modern polities.

This chapter first provides an overview of the treatment of the plague dead in early modern Germany before focusing on three case studies that illustrate different responses to serious outbreaks of plague. In Nuremberg, urban magistrates established plague cemeteries, against the resistance of the local clergy.

The establishment of the two cemeteries in 1517/18 was comparatively early. Soon after the establishment of the spaces as plague cemeteries, they became the town's main cemeteries but remained on the outskirts of the town. In Munich, the second case study, a former plague cemetery was also turned into the main urban burial space, but the process took much longer than in Nuremberg. In the case of Munich, the change in necrogeography signified the changing meaning of the urban periphery from a dishonorable space to one that belonged to the town.[11] A final set of examples explores responses of small town and village magistrates to serious outbreaks of plague. They illustrate that the opening of plague cemeteries was not just an urban phenomenon. The diverse responses show that while establishing plague cemeteries was one option, magistrates also had a range of other possibilities. Whether a plague cemetery was opened and what happened with it after the plague was highly dependent on local circumstances and even individual preferences.

Plague and the Dead in Early Modern Germany

Dealing with the plague dead was not a specifically early modern problem. In the Middle Ages, the establishment of plague cemeteries was normally connected to concerns about the space for the dead and the lack of space in cemeteries, rather than concerns about hygiene. In fourteenth-century Zürich, there were reports about corpses of the plague dead piled on top of each other.[12] Already in the fifteenth and early sixteenth centuries, some towns established extramural burial grounds outside the city walls, for example Coburg in 1494, Freiburg in 1510, even against the will of the university and clerics, and Eichstätt in 1535–36, after initial negotiations in 1511.[13] The reasons given for the movement were not always linked to plague explicitly but could be connected to other concerns, including complaints about bad smell or the state of cemeteries more generally.

But while there were already concerns about the plague dead and their bodies in the Middle Ages, it was only in the early modern period that a discourse around the plague dead and the spread of diseases, usually connected to ideas about "foul air," gained currency, and the number of measures against the spread of diseases also increased in this period.[14] Many of the earlier plague cemeteries were still inside the city walls, fitting this lack of concern about hygiene and the bad air dead bodies supposedly spread. The number of plague cemeteries increased in the sixteenth and seventeenth centuries, possibly also linked to increasing population numbers and urban density.

Almost all settlements in early modern Germany experienced serious outbreaks of plague, leading to efforts to regulate the disease and its spread. In the early modern period, the miasma theory articulated that diseases spread through "foul air," meaning that victims of serious diseases had to be buried quickly.[15] Urban magistrates and medics recognized the challenges that the outbreaks of plague posed, as the increasing number of bodies could lead to administrative systems being overwhelmed and often adapted in order to avoid even more serious problems. From the middle of the sixteenth century, physicians and magistrates published plague ordinances (*Pestordnungen*) in towns across German-speaking Europe.[16] Danzig's town physician, Bartholomeus Wagner, recommended in 1565 that "the plague dead should not be kept in the houses for one night, but should be buried in the earth in deep graves, and as far as possible outside the city."[17] The fear that those who died in their own bedchambers might be left there clearly worried urban magistrates and they wanted to counteract the spread of any disease by taking measures to limit the time corpses spent in private houses.[18] This included washing clothes of the deceased outside of the city, marking and locking the houses of those who had died of plague, and avoiding anyone who had been in contact with the deceased.[19]

The most common response of urban magistrates to the increasing number of corpses was to continue regular burials for as long as possible.[20] In most cases, the plague dead continued to be buried in regular cemeteries for as long as there was space. The establishment of a separate cemetery outside the city walls was only a last resort, if the regular urban churchyards no longer had the capacity to take dead bodies. Only during such times of acute crisis did urban magistrates open plague pits or mass graves, where gravediggers or day laborers buried the dead quickly and without many of the clerical ceremonies usually associated with burials.[21] Using part of an already existing burial space for the plague dead was not as complex as opening a new cemetery. This practice was particularly common in important urban centers during the Middle Ages. In Lübeck, a mass grave was opened in the main cemetery in 1350, while in Cologne there were similar pits during the plague epidemic of 1451. The evidence suggests that these plague pits may have been even more common in other countries, for example in England.[22] In many cases, outbreaks of plague were included in narratives about a town's history. It appears that in German lands it was more common to open plague pits in regular cemeteries in medieval times than in the early modern period, suggesting that growing urban density and scarcity of space may have forced magistrates to open extramural plague cemeteries. Moreover, as the population of towns grew, so did the number of dead bodies. The burial spaces did not always keep up with the population growth, and so the number of corpses could increase beyond the capacity of urban churchyards.

In some cases, the initiative to move a cemetery came from rulers who were concerned about the health in their towns. In 1518, Emperor Maximilian I (1459–1519) encouraged the inhabitants of Nuremberg to move their cemeteries outside of the city walls, something he likely also advocated in towns like Freiburg, Vienna, Constance, and Graz.[23] In other instances, it was the urban magistrates who pushed for the quick removal of the plague dead into specific burial spaces. While rulers hoped to improve a town's general health and hygiene, urban magistrates by contrast normally ordered to move cemeteries in response to specific circumstances, such as a recent epidemic. In many cases, it was the urban magistrates who were in charge of the plague cemeteries, and not clerical actors. Therefore it was very rare that clergy are recorded as favoring opening plague cemeteries. Urban burial sites in hospitals (*Spitäler* or *Hospitäler*) that were run by clergy or religious orders could also be supplemented by the new extramural burial spaces, a move that was resisted by many of the clergy in charge of the hospitals.[24] Additionally, there was popular resistance against the payment of cemetery fees and the abandonment of family tombs.[25]

In many cases, the opening of new cemeteries was motivated by reasons of urban population growth and concerns about the spread of diseases. In 1525, Königsberg magistrates considered moving the cemetery due to the increasing population numbers and the resulting hygiene problems.[26] In Pfalz-Neuburg, the instructions from 1576 argued that the presence of the dead could no longer be tolerated as it "scared the young people and created bad air, even outside the towns and villages."[27]

The opening of regular cemeteries involved a range of rituals and sacramentals that could include consecration of the ground or the building and blessing of a chapel.[28] If the main cemeteries were churchyards, as was the case for much of the early modern period, many of these rituals were connected to the church itself, and the building of a new church included the establishment of the burial space around the church. Later, there were demands to wall in such areas, as we know from frequent complaints about animals or thieves disturbing the graves.[29] When it came to the opening of plague cemeteries, many of these processes were abandoned or performed later. In some cases, burials started before the ground was consecrated.

Other rituals and customs were adapted in a similar manner to prioritize speed over ritual uniformity. The cemetery of St. Prokulus in Tyrol (Austria) can serve as an example. It was established in 1636–37 and is one of the examples of a plague cemetery that enables us to draw some conclusions about the treatment of the plague dead. As we know from excavations, at first, grave goods were still contained in graves. However, when burials had to be performed at a faster pace, grave goods were no longer added. Other adaptations included a lack of funeral sermons, and the graves themselves could contain additional materials, such as slaked lime or herbal remedies against plague, which were less common during regular times.[30]

The establishment of plague cemeteries was not only important for the urban topography, but could also result in changes to liturgies. There are some indications that preachers delivered sermons in the plague cemeteries, as there were some open-air pulpits.[31] In some cases, the newly established plague cemeteries featured unique architectural features. In Weida in Thuringia there was a plague chancel (*Pestkanzel*) in the cemetery. In Dresden, such a chancel was attached to the outside of St. Bartholomew's church.[32] In other instances there are indications of open-air pulpits, likely to limit the spread of disease, while still allowing the delivery of sermons in an appropriate manner. Owing to the understanding of many diseases being spread through the air, victims of plague had to be buried quickly, and rituals were performed in abbreviated form or not at all. These changes to rituals also resulted in complaints by families and friends of the deceased. In order to counteract these concerns, town ordinances stressed the importance of the common good (*Gemeinwohl*) and orderliness.[33] Many preachers also adapted the contents of their sermons, like giving them a focus on divine punishment, sin, and redemption, or preaching on particular biblical passages that focused on resurrection, like that of Lazarus.[34] In Catholic sermons, priests advocated for saintly intercession, a feature that was lacking in Protestant ones.[35]

Considering these responses to the plague, it should be noted that there were some urban locations struck by plague or similar diseases that were able to accommodate the dead in regular cemeteries. Other towns opened plague cemeteries on the outskirts for only a short period of time. Once the outbreak of plague was over, the space was no longer used and the bodies were left to decompose, many of them lying in graves without markers.

The Nuremberg Plague Cemeteries

Nuremberg was one of the most important cities of the Holy Roman Empire in the later Middles Ages and early modern period. It was an economic hub, center of printing and the arts, and an important political player.[36] The town was also a center of medicine, as we know from the works of Hannah Murphy.[37] Due to the significant population size, plague epidemics could affect a particularly large number of people in towns like Nuremberg.[38] In such cases, the churchyards where the dead were normally buried could overflow. A lack of space and the resulting hygienic problems led to the establishment of burial spaces beyond the town walls. In Nuremberg this move away from churchyard burials influenced all major town churches, St. Sebald, St. Lorenz, St. Jakob, and the Heilig-Geist-Spital.[39]

In a mandate from 31 October 1518 Emperor Maximilian I ordered that burials during times of plague should be performed outside of the city walls. In 1517/18, the burial spaces that belonged to the churches of St. Lorenz and St. Sebald were moved to locations outside of the town, creating the cemeteries of St. Rochus and St. Johannis.[40] St. Rochus was named after one of the most important plague saints, illustrating the continued relevance of religion, even when cemeteries were no longer directly attached to churches. These cemeteries were deliberately moved outside of the city center to prevent the spread of the plague among the densely populated city. It was only possible to perform this move because there was significant support for it.

The city council enforced the movement of the cemeteries against the wishes of the clergy.[41] The cemetery of St. Rochus served the parish of St. Lorenz and the cemetery of St. Johannis was expanded so that it could accommodate more of the plague dead.[42] These new cemeteries also contained small chapels.[43] As early as 1520, the town council ordered that all regular burials should take place outside the city walls. This was extended in the 1540s to include a prohibition of burials inside the churches, the space traditionally reserved for the elites, who wanted to be buried inside the church, close to the altar. This meant that the two former plague cemeteries became the main burial sites until the nineteenth century.

Even the shift from urban burial sites to extramural plague cemeteries could not fully alleviate the scarcity of burial spaces. In order to accommodate the dead bodies of the inhabitants, numerous expansions were made to provide for an increasing urban population. The new pattern of occupancy meant that even during normal times there was little space in the extramural Nuremberg cemeteries, a problem that became even worse during the plague epidemics for which the cemeteries were originally designed. During the 1562 plague epidemic the cemetery was expanded to accommodate nine thousand dead, and in 1644 it was expanded once again.[44]

The case of Nuremberg is remarkable because in the space of only a few years the plague cemeteries outside of the city walls, initially intended to accommodate the increasing number of dead during outbreaks of disease, became the main urban burial sites. The town cemetery of Halle was used as a plague cemetery in the Middle Ages before it was used as the burial space for the whole town from 1557.[45] The space was used for mass graves for plague dead from 1350 onward, and when the town decided to establish this extramural space as the main burial site a wall was built and the space was beautified with arcades and sculptures. But, unlike in Nuremberg, it had been used as a plague cemetery for centuries before it was turned into the town's main burial space.

In Nuremberg, the new cemeteries were also enclosed and equipped with a small chapel, but not on the same scale as in Halle, making Nuremberg's quick move from plague cemetery to main cemetery of the town all the more remarkable. The town magistrates were able to enforce this change because they had the backing of the emperor and asserted the increasingly bad sanitary and spatial situation in inner-city churchyards. Moreover, the Nuremberg council was in a strong position and could enforce the change against the town clergy, who opposed it.[46] This would not have been possible in a city where the clergy were more powerful than the councilors.

In other towns, the space beyond the city walls continued to be associated with dishonorable burials. However, it seems that the Nuremberg city council's attempts to disassociate the burial spaces with plague and dishonor were successful. Later in the period, there was no longer a strong association between the cemeteries and plague, which is why in some accounts of Nuremberg cemeteries the fact that these spaces were established for plague victims was not always mentioned.[47] The transformation of a plague cemetery into the main urban burial space was not uncommon, but, as the example of Munich shows, this typically was a much longer process.

The Munich Plague Cemetery

As in Nuremberg, the city's ruler initiated the first discussions about extramural burials, especially during times of plague. As early as 1480 Duke Albrecht IV of Bavaria (1447–1508) requested that Munich should have extramural cemeteries.[48] This request was granted by the pope, who even banned burials inside the churches during plague epidemics. Between 1520 and 1560 there was rapid population growth in Munich, leading to problems with space and hygiene.[49] A new cemetery, called the southern cemetery (Südfriedhof), was established in 1563 as a plague cemetery. As it was outside of the city walls, it was also called Friedhof vor dem Sendlinger Tor.

Most plague cemeteries were located outside of the city walls, as was the case in Munich.[50] In some cases, those who died of other serious diseases were also included among those who had to be buried there. The gradual shift of graveyards in the early modern period meant that eventually everyone was buried outside of the compounds of towns and, to a lesser extent, villages. Burial sites in the center of towns not only provided an opportunity to display wealth and status, but they also excluded certain individuals from an honorable burial, symbolizing their ambiguous state within a congregation.

Munich's plague cemetery was not intended to be the town's main cemetery, but when a public campaign ensued in the late eighteenth century, in addition to pressure from the duke, to force urban dignitaries to move the cemetery from the town's center to the outskirts, there was discussion whether the plague cemetery should become the main urban resting place. Now, plague was no longer the main concern, but urban health in general. For medical considerations and a fear that diseases might spread, letters argued that "poisonous exhalations" would "damage the health of the town's inhabitants."[51] In another text, an anonymous author admonished that the burials underneath the church could harm people while they were worshipping: "The foul air locked in the crypts can even damage the people present in the church, the Temple of God."[52] In the margins the author wrote that the tombstones could be put into the church walls, as deemed fit, suggesting an awareness that many families would have wanted their family epitaphs and tombstones to survive any changes in the church space.

The campaign to relocate town cemeteries was successful and resulted in a shift in the necrogeography of Munich, where the southern cemetery, formerly a plague cemetery and reserved for diseased and dishonorable burials, became the only possible burial site in the whole city.[53] From 1788 to 1868, all corpses were buried in this space, including those of important dignitaries, like mayors or important scientists. The relocation of a cemetery from the churches to the outside of the town changed the layout and structure of the whole town. Similar moves of graveyards can be seen in other German and European cities. Formerly dishonorable burial sites turned into the sole cemeteries. The change in necrogeography in Munich came alongside other changes in the treatment of dead bodies. In the late eighteenth century Emperor Joseph II (1741–90) argued, for instance, that Bavaria as a whole would benefit from thorough postmortem examinations (*Leichenbeschau*) in order to ascertain why someone had died and to protect towns from further endemics.[54] Although plague was no longer a threat at this time, magistrates and rulers hoped to gain knowledge about the spread of diseases by examining corpses.

Munich follows a broader pattern of cemetery movements in the late eighteenth and nineteenth centuries.[55] For instance, in the course of the so-called Josephine reforms in the later eighteenth century, Emperor Joseph II ordered, among other things, that cemeteries should be moved to the outside of the towns because of the dangers to the health of the town. In August and September 1784, Joseph II had these decrees proclaimed for Austria. The attempts led to significant resistance, both from the citizens and from the clerics, who feared that they might lose a significant source of income. The case of Vienna is all the more interesting because cemeteries had already been moved to the outskirts of the town in the early sixteenth century. Clearly, it was not the general idea of moving a cemetery from the center of town that enraged the citizens. Rather, it was the closing of specific and long-established cemeteries which concerned the urban citizenry. In the case of Vienna, the opposition was ultimately futile, but the significant resistance to none other than the emperor shows how much was at stake when it came to the reordering of the dead in urban communities. In both Munich and Vienna, the connotations of extramural burial as dishonorable survived, but ultimately the burials took place there, regardless.

Within the complex interactions between clergy and councilors, other actors also played their part. Doctors increasingly advocated for extra-urban burials and cited outbreaks of disease as one of the most pressing concerns for towns. In Frankfurt in 1573 Joachim Strupp (1530–1606) argued that it would be beneficial for the town to have such extramural burial sites.[56] Concerns about outbreaks of plague and other epidemics resulted in public campaigns and medical experts' calls to move cemeteries. Many of the extramural cemeteries were first established as cemeteries for the poor or the plague dead. This was probably the case in Bamberg, Düsseldorf, Heidelberg, Lübeck, and Wiesbaden. *Camposanto* cemeteries, burial spaces surrounded by a wall with arcades, had niches in the walls to enable the elites to have a separate burial space, making these spaces more attractive.[57] In many cases, town councilors took the relocation of cemeteries as an opportunity to assert their authority over the urban space.

Munich as a center of Catholicism enables us to make comparisons with Lutheran and Reformed towns. Martin Luther himself promoted burials outside city centers, arguing that the place of burial no longer mattered and that the benefits of burials beyond the city center outweighed any drawbacks. Through the absence of altars, chapels, and other features of medieval sacred landscapes, it was possible to move cemeteries more easily than before.[58] Craig Koslofsky has argued that this was an expression and result of a "separation of the living and the dead."[59] By this he means that both theologically and spatially the living and the dead were separated by important evangelical reformers. As prayers for the souls of the deceased no longer functioned to decrease the time of souls spent in purgatory, cemeteries could now be moved outside the city walls. Instead of indulgences and saintly intercession, men and women were supposed to focus on the promise of eternal life and divine mercy. In the course of the sixteenth century, most towns established a burial space outside of the city walls for reasons of hygiene or space, but sometimes also motivated by religious change.[60]

With the increasing discussions around new extramural burial spaces, some Catholics were afraid of being forgotten too quickly. Georg Witzel wrote, "What should they [the corpses] do out in the field, if one hardly passes there two or three times a year? If one no longer sees the grave diggers daily and fewer people dying, the rough people will think one no longer dies."[61] Witzel accused the Lutherans of "Zartheit" (delicacy) because they could not bear to see the dead inside the walls.[62] But even among Protestants, a fear of change and desire for continuity meant that in many places burials inside the churches remained important until at least 1800.[63] Likewise, as we have seen in Munich, in later periods these concerns no longer played a role when it came to the changing meaning of plague cemeteries in Catholic towns.

While Witzel and other Catholic theologians opposed the establishment of cemeteries outside the city walls, there was much less resistance to extramural plague cemeteries. The establishment of plague cemeteries cut across confessional boundaries, and there is no clear indication that the confessional set-up of a town played a decisive role when it came to the establishment of such cemeteries.[64] Catholic magistrates and rulers also proposed to have plague cemeteries outside the city walls, to protect the congregation from the spread of diseases.

When magistrates forced townspeople to bury their dead in plague cemeteries, resistance could increase. As many of the extramural burial spaces had to be established quickly, they did not contain walls or hedges separating them from the surrounding area and not all of them were consecrated, making them less attractive burial spaces. The town council of Constance even punished families who refused to bury their dead in a plague cemetery with a hefty fine of 100 gulden. To further incentivize the burial, they officially allowed burials in unconsecrated ground.[65] Both these instructions and what we know of the regular extramural burial grounds point to a significant reluctance on the part of the urban population to bury their dead away from the center. In many cases, arguments around tradition and continuity were used to justify the refusal to bury the dead in different space than their ancestors.

Plague Cemeteries in Small Towns and Villages

It is especially hard to trace plague cemeteries in small towns and villages, where fewer sources survive. Yet they can provide a fascinating comparison to major urban centers.[66] There is some evidence that similar patterns to the large urban centers discussed above can be detected. The plague cemetery of Zitzschewig, Saxony, was established in 1637 on the eastern border of the town. In 1637, around forty plague dead were buried there. The last burial was that of a French soldier in 1813. In Hachenburg, a small town in the West of the Holy Roman Empire, the outbreak of plague in 1636 was recorded in the town book, where the burial of six people was marked specifically as related to the outbreak of the plague.[67] In the village of Reute, Breisgau, parishioners refused point blank to be buried in the new plague cemetery outside of the city gates and continued to bury their dead in the churchyard.[68] In these cases, similar processes to those in major urban centers are visible: the movement of cemeteries to the outskirts and some resistance to the burial of the plague dead in these newly established spaces.

One particularly striking example is that of Kötzschenbroda, a small town near Meißen in Saxony. The main churchyard was used for burials from around 1273, with a significant extension completed in 1602. This extension also included a program of beautifying the space. In the same year, a plague cemetery is mentioned for the first time, though it was likely already used in the middle of the sixteenth century. This plague cemetery functioned as a second burial space in the village. In this case, the execution site, where the gallows (*Galgenberg*) may also have been located, was in close proximity to the cemetery, reinforcing the impression of a dishonorable burial space outside the city gates. As is often the case for villages and small towns, sources are scarce, but comparing the case from Kötzschenbroda with other examples, it is likely that the burials around the church were considered to be more honorable, and particularly the elites were generally buried there. This changed at the end of the seventeenth century, when the former plague cemetery became the town's main burial space. Thus the cemetery continued to be used after the plague epidemics.[69] As the space in the cemetery was no longer sufficient in the nineteenth century, a new one was opened in 1874.

We might expect that, due to the higher density and generally higher number of deaths, dedicated plague cemeteries were more common in major urban centers. However, the examples from villages and small towns illustrate that magistrates there also established plague cemeteries. While the overall number of dead was much higher in towns than in the countryside, in terms of death rates, villages and small towns could be affected just as badly as larger settlements. Here, too, ways of dealing with the dead might no longer be sufficient to deal with the increased pressure on the town population, leading to an adaptation and change in the use of space and associated rituals. The outbreak of plague could have devastating consequences for small towns and villages. During the plague epidemic in Bad Wörishofen (Allgäu), nearly the whole population died, making it necessary to quickly open a new burial ground.[70] In a list of likely plague and leprosy cemeteries compiled by Reiner Sörries for early modern Germany, we find big cities as well as small towns.[71] The examples of small towns and villages illustrate that the main motivation behind the movement of the cemeteries was fear of the spread of disease as well as a lack of space, although this was more common in urban centers.

The opening of plague cemeteries in smaller towns runs counter to the opening of general extramural burial spaces in small towns and villages. Many of these relocations took longer to implement in the countryside, and churchyards continued to be the main burial space, in some cases until the present.[72] But the evidence suggests that when it came to the opening of plague cemeteries, small towns and villages were not significantly slower or worse equipped than larger urban settlements. Just as the plague itself, the challenges faced by large urban centers and small towns were similar.

There seems to have been one significant difference between urban and rural plague cemeteries. While urban density and population growth meant that plague cemeteries eventually became the main town cemeteries, some of the rural ones were used for only short periods of time and then closed again, as was the case in Ochtrup near Münster. Or, to name another example, the plague cemetery of Naundorf, Saxony, was opened in 1637, with the last known burial, in 1689, indicating that the cemetery operated only during a short time period. It was extremely rare for urban cemeteries to be closed without a larger replacement. In rural settings, there was not such a great need for space, meaning that cemeteries could be closed again and the space left to be grown over.

The temporary establishment of rural plague cemeteries raises the issue of the use of plague cemeteries after an epidemic. As we have seen, one possibility was to turn the cemetery into the main urban burial space, but it was also possible to continue using the space for slightly different purposes. The plague cemetery of Constance was turned into a cemetery for strangers and unbaptized children.[73] It is likely no coincidence that the space was now used for unbaptized children, a group who were also liminal and did not always receive honorable burials, much like the plague dead.[74] Many of the urban plague cemeteries were completely restructured in the course of these initiatives, including a neater order of graves or the building of small chapels.[75] The meaning of these burial sites was therefore never fixed and what may have been an honorable and desirable burial space in one century could be turned into an undesirable spot in the next.

Conclusion

One of the biggest challenges of a serious outbreak of plague was the increased number of dead bodies. The higher mortality resulted in a range of problems for urban magistrates and clerics, which led to different responses, depending on the precise circumstances and the severity of the outbreak. During epidemics, graves had to be dug quickly so as to accommodate the rising number of corpses.[76] In many instances, they were dug outside of the city walls, to prevent the spread of fumes or vapors that might infect other people, regardless of previous discussions about the problems of extramural burials. These examples illustrate that in extreme circumstances magistrates acted quickly to solve specific problems. It was after such events that more long-lasting changes were implemented and cemeteries moved to the outskirts of the towns permanently, as was the case with Munich's former plague cemetery. It was constructed in the mid-sixteenth century, but later became the main burial space for the whole city.[77]

When plague burials occurred, concerns about quick burials, the correct disinfection of spaces, or the assessment of bodies became more important than during quieter times, when seemingly mundane things, such as clothes, were discussed in decrees and orders.[78] Similar concerns were voiced during the outbreak of the COVID-19 pandemic, when quick burials were also a defining feature of the management of the disease. The examples from Nuremberg, Munich, and smaller towns show particularly well how variable responses to plague were in early modern towns and villages. In Nuremberg, a plague cemetery became the main urban burial space in a matter of years, while in Munich this occurred only after centuries and a large campaign, while many smaller places opened plague cemeteries that were closed again later. Constructing plague cemeteries helped urban magistrates and territorial princes to create a narrative of good rulership in difficult times.

The establishment of plague cemeteries was only one of many ways in which urban magistrates and clergy responded to the outbreak of plague. Quarantine, medicine, or fleeing the plague were all contained in the toolkit available to early modern polities. For example, England's King George II, elector of Hanover, ordered in 1738 that all travelers to Hanover had to pass through specific towns, where they would be checked for symptoms of the plague.[79] The assessment of the dead and measures to stop the spread of vapors also influenced the behavior of magistrates and rulers during serious outbreaks of plague or other diseases.

It should also be noted that the establishment of plague cemeteries was not a universal feature of early modern polities. There were large cities and small towns, which, as far as we know, never established plague cemeteries, whether for short-term use or in the long run. This was normally the case when the available normal burial spaces were still sufficient for burials. One striking example of the responses to plague comes from Lauban in Upper Lusatia. During a plague epidemic in 1613, a later account informs us, around 650 people died. But the gravediggers simply put the dead bodies onto the pews inside the church when the rapidly increasing number of deaths overwhelmed the town's infrastructure, since there was no specific plague cemetery in Lauban. This contaminated the pews, which had to be removed once the outbreak had abated.[80] The example suggests that even if there was no cemetery for the plague dead, adaptations had to be made.

But, when plague cemeteries were established, temporary solutions could become permanent fixtures of urban life. In many cases there was significant resistance to permanent changes in the burial culture and placement of the dead, as it meant that families had to bury their dead in new spaces, far removed from their ancestors. It was only later, in the eighteenth and nineteenth centuries, that most of these plague cemeteries lost some of their dishonorable reputation and were turned into main town cemeteries. Much like notions about honor, the meaning of plague cemeteries could change over the years. But, whether they became the main cemeteries of a city, town, or village, or were only temporary features, they deeply influenced early modern settlements and illustrate how important understanding responses to outbreaks of disease is to understanding early modern society at large.

Martin Christ is Junior Fellow and Post-Doctoral Researcher at the Max Weber Centre of the University of Erfurt in the Centre for Advanced Studies in Humanities and Social Sciences, "Religion and Urbanity: Reciprocal

Formations," funded by the German Research Foundation (DFG, FOR 2779). His monograph *Biographies of a Reformation. Religious Change and Confessional Coexistence in Upper Lusatia, c. 1520–1635* was published by Oxford University Press in 2021. He has published on religious coexistence in Central Europe, the Reformation of the Sorbs, and Catholic responses to Lutheranism. His current project focuses on the urban dead in Munich and London, ca. 1550–1850.

Notes

1. On the literature on plague, see, for example Zapnik, *Pest und Krieg*; Bulst, "Krankheit und Gesellschaft in der Vormoderne," 17–47.
2. See, for example, Henderson, "The Invisible Enemy," 263–74; Pouget, "Quarantine," 302–10; Schmauder "Leben in der Isolation," 120–42; Cohn, "The Black Death," 703–38; Cohn, *The Black Death Transformed*; Naphy and Spicer, *The Black Death*; Herlihy, *The Black Death*.
3. For the links between religion and outbreaks of disease, see Mormando and Worcester, *Piety and Plague*.
4. Haugland, "Guilds, Death and Funeral Arrangements," 152–83; Cremers, "Totenweiber und Totengräber," 181–88.
5. Slack, "Responses to Plague in Early Modern Europe," 409.
6. Muchembled, *Smells*, 93–97. On the related issue of bodily fluids, see Rublack, "Fluxes," 1–16.
7. Sörries, "Leprosen- und Pestfriedhöfe," 53.
8. Brademann, *Mit den Toten und für die Toten*.
9. Sörries, *Raum für Tote*; Fischer and Herzog, *Nekropolis*.
10. Illi, *Wohin die Toten gingen*.
11. On the concept of necrogeographies, see Laqueur, *The Work of the Dead*.
12. See Illi, *Wohin die Toten gingen*.
13. Happe, "Trennung von Kirche und Grab," 64. Further examples include Heilbronn (1502), Zwickau (1521), Isny (1522), Altdorf (1527).
14. Sörries, "Leprosen- und Pestfriedhöfe," 55.
15. Cole, "Of Mice and Moisture," 65–84.
16. Seiler, "Pest."
17. Wagner, *Von der Pestilentz*. All translations are mine.
18. On the deathbed, see von Thiessen, "Das Sterbebett als normative Schwelle," 625–59; Karant-Nunn, *The Reformation of Feeling*. For an English comparison of these last moments, see Wunderli and Broce, "The Final Moment before Death," 259–75.
19. Wagner, *Von der Pestilentz*.
20. For a contemporary depiction of such burials in a regular churchyard, see Seiler, "Pest."
21. Sörries, "Leprosen- und Pestfriedhöfe," 54–55.
22. Harding, "Burial of the Plague Dead," 53–64.
23. Sörries, "Leprosen- und Pestfriedhöfe." 57.
24. See Dirmeier, *Organisierte Barmherzigkeit*.
25. Happe, "Trennung von Kirche und Grab," 74.
26. Happe, "Trennung von Kirche und Grab," 66.
27. Happe, "Trennung von Kirche und Grab," 66.

28. Sieber, *Der konfessionelle Gottesacker*, especially 29–39 and 412–17; Brademann, *Mit den Toten und für die Toten*, 293–466.
29. See, for example, Illi, *Wohin die Toten gingen*.
30. Seifert, "Mikroevolution und Geschichte der Pest," 46.
31. Heinzmann, *Die Ringackerkapelle*; Burkhardt, *Domat/Ems*.
32. Weck, "Die dritte Kirche so gleicher Gestalt," 272.
33. See, for example, Rat der Stadt Elbing, *Kurtze Verordnung*.
34. Hallauer, *Pest-Predig*; Górska, "Das frühneuzeitliche Pestpredigeramt," 127–47; Górska, *Theatrum atrocissimorum fatorum*.
35. For a medieval comparison, see Sudhoff, "Pestschriften," 129–68.
36. On medieval Nuremberg, see Pope, "Nuremberg's Noble Servant," 159–80.
37. Murphy, *A New Order of Medicine*.
38. Rittgers, "Protestants and Plague," 132–55.
39. Pilz, *St. Johannis und St. Rochus in Nürnberg*.
40. On the Reformation in Nuremberg, see Seebaß, "Stadt und Kirche in Nürnberg"; Sehling, *Die evangelischen Kirchenordnungen des XVI. Jahrhunderts*, 16–20.
41. Diefenbacher and Landois, "*Hingeht die Zeit, herkommt der Todt.*"
42. Liedel and Dollhopf, *Der Johannisfriedhof zu Nürnberg*; Glossner, *Der St.-Johannisfriedhof zu Nürnberg*.
43. See Zahn, "Die Epitaphien der alten Nürnberger Friedhöfe," 203–11.
44. Trechsel, *Verneuertes Gedächtnis des Nürnbergischen Johannis-Kirch-Hofs*.
45. Happe, "Trennung von Kirche und Grab." 80.
46. See, for example, Meyer, *Die Stadt als Thema*.
47. Gugel, *Norischer Christen Freydhöfe Gedächtnis*.
48. Sörries, "Kirchhof oder Coemeterium?" 33; Dunst, *Der Friedhof im Mittelalter*, 27–28.
49. Happe, "Trennung von Kirche und Grab," 66.
50. See also Thewes and Uhrmacher, *Extra muros: Vorstädtische Räume in Spätmittelalter und Früher Neuzeit*.
51. Hauptstaatsarchiv München, GL Fasz. 2706/549; see also Hauptstaatsarchiv München, GR 1190/69; Hauptstaatsarchiv München, GL Fasz. 2707.
52. Hauptstaatsarchiv München, GL Fasz. 2706/540, Polizeirat I.
53. Archiv der Erzdiözese München-Freising, Realia. VN 3752 Erhebung des Mortuariums & Beerdingungsrecht 1760–1819; Realia VN 3209 Erhebung des Mortuariums & Beerdingungsrecht 1729–1877.
54. Hauptstaatsarchiv, München, GR Fasz. 1191, Nr. 26.
55. See Sörries, *Ruhe sanft*; Fischer and Herzog, *Nekropolis*.
56. Happe, "Trennung von Kirche und Grab," 69.
57. Happe, "Trennung von Kirche und Grab," 76.
58. Happe, "Trennung von Kirche und Grab," 71.
59. Koslofsky, *Reformation of the Dead*.
60. Happe, "Trennung von Kirche und Grab"; Koslofsky, *Reformation of the Dead*.
61. Koslofsky, *Reformation of the Dead*; Happe, "Trennung von Kirche und Grab," 73.
62. Happe, "Trennung von Kirche und Grab," 73.
63. Happe, "Trennung von Kirche und Grab," 81.
64. For a discussion of this topic in cemeteries more generally, see Sieber, *Konfessionelle Gottesacker*.
65. Sörries, "Leprosen- und Pestfriedhöfe," 60.

66. On the urban/rural dynamics regarding plague, see Curtis, "Was Plague an Exclusively Urban Phenomenon?" 139–70.
67. Fuchs, "Hachenburg," 108.
68. Sörries, "Leprosen- und Pestfriedhöfe," 59.
69. Deaconesses were buried there in the twentieth century, hence the alternative name *Diakonissenfriedhof*.
70. Sörries, "Leprosen- und Pestfriedhöfe," 58.
71. Sörries, "Leprosen- und Pestfriedhöfe," 62.
72. Brademann, *Mit den Toten und für die Toten*.
73. Sörries, "Leprosen- und Pestfriedhöfe," 60. See Coster, "Tokens of Innocence," 266–87.
74. Pfeifer, "Auswertung von Taufmatrikeln in München und Passau," 57–58.
75. Sörries, "Leprosen- und Pestfriedhöfe," 61.
76. Harding, "Burial of the Plague Dead," 53–64.
77. Denk and Ziesemer, *Kunst und Memoria*.
78. Harding, "Burial of the Plague Dead," 53–64.
79. Georg II, *Wir Georg der Andere*.
80. Dietmann, *Gesamte der ungeänderten Augsb. Confession zugethane Priesterschaft*, 471.

Bibliography

Archival Sources

Hauptstaatsarchiv München

GL Fasz. 2706/549.
GR 1190/69.
GL Fasz. 2707.
GL Fasz. 2706/540.
GR Fasz. 1191, Nr. 26.

Archiv der Erzdiözese München-Freising

Realia. VN 3752 Erhebung des Mortuariums & Beerdingungsrecht 1760–1819.
Realia VN 3209 Erhebung des Mortuariums & Beerdingungsrecht 1729–1877.

Primary Sources

Dietmann, Karl Gottlob. *Die gesamte der ungeänderten Augsb. Confeßion zugethane Priesterschaft in dem Marggrafthum Oberlausitz*. Lauban and Leipzig: Wirthgen, 1777.

Georg II. *Wir Georg der Andere, von Gottes Gnaden König von Groß-Britannien ... Nachdem Wir wegen der in Ungarn, Siebenbürgen, Bannat Temeswar ... grassirenden Pest bewogen worden, auf diejenige, so in Unsere Teutsche Lande kommen, genaue Obacht nehmen zu lassen*. Hannover: no publisher, 1738.

Gugel, Christoph Friedrich. *Norischer Christen Freydhöfe Gedächtnis. Das ist: Richtige Vorstellung und Verzeichnis aller derjenigen Monumenten, Epitaphien und Grabschrifften*. Nuremberg: Christian Sigmund Froberg, 1682.

Hallauer, Franz Xaver. *Pest-Predig Bey der, von einer Löblichen S. Michaels Bruderschafft zu Berg … Von München nach Ebersperg, zu dem Heiligen Martyrer Sebastiano, Umb Abwendung der laydigen Sucht, auf den ersten Sonntag in dem Advent angestellten heiligen Wahlfahrt*. Munich: Heinrich Thedor von Cölln, 1720.

Rat der Stadt Elbing. *Kurtze Verordnung/ Wie ein Jedweder bey dieser Zeit/ wegen besorglicher Pest-Gefahr/ Negst Göttlicher Hülffe sich præserviren/ und in der Cur verhalten solle: Mit Zulaß E. Wol Edl. und Hochw. Rahts der Königl. Stadt Elbing*. Elbing: Preuss, 1708.

Sehling, Emil, ed. *Die evangelischen Kirchenordnungen des XVI. Jahrhunderts. Bd. 11 Bayern. 1. Teil. Franken. Markgrafschaft Brandenburg-Ansbach-Kulmbach. Reichsstädte Nürnberg. Rothenburg. Schweinfurt. Weißenburg. Windsheim. Grafschaften Castell. Rieneck und Wertheim. Herrschaft Thüngen*, Tübingen: J. C. B. Mohr (Paul Siebeck), 1961.

Trechsel, Johann Martin, genannt Großkopf. *Verneuertes Gedächtnis des Nürnbergischen Johannis-Kirch-Hofs mit Anhang Ordentliche Verzeichnüß und Beschreibung aller und jeder Monumenten und Epitaphien, so der Zeit auf dem Nürnbergischen Gottes-Acker bey S. Johannis, und in dasiger Kirche … zu finden und anzutreffen sind*. Frankfurt am Main: Felsecker, 1736.

Wagner, Bartholomeus. *Von der Pestilentz/ Nützliche vnd gründliche vnterrichtunge wie man sich mit Gottes hülffe vor der vergifftung bewaren*. Danzig: Jakob Rhode, 1564.

Weck, Anton. "Die dritte Kirche so gleicher Gestalt ietztgedachtem Thore ist die Capell zu S. Bartholomaei." In *Der Chur-Fürstlichen Sächsischen weitberuffenen Residentz- und Haupt-Vestung Dresden Beschreib- und Vorstellung*, 271–72. Nuremberg: Froberger, 1680.

Secondary Sources

Brademann, Jan. *Mit den Toten und für die Toten. Zur Konfessionalisierung der Sepulkralkultur im Münsterland (16. bis 18. Jahrhundert)*. Münster: Rhema Verlag, 2013.

Bulst, Neithard. "Krankheit und Gesellschaft in der Vormoderne. Das Beispiel der Pest." In *Maladies et Société (XIIe–XVIIIe siècles). Actes du colloque de Bielefeld*, edited by Neithard Bulst and Robert Delort, 17–47. Paris: Ed. du Centre National de la Recherche Scientifique, 1989.

Burkhardt, Lorena, ed. *Domat/Ems, Sogn Pieder: Vom frühmittelalterlichen Herrenhof zum neuzeitlichen Pestfriedhof*. Chur: Somedia-Buchverlag, 2020.

Cohn, Samuel. "The Black Death: End of a Paradigm." *American Historical Review* 107, no. 3 (2002): 703–38.

Cohn, Samuel. *The Black Death Transformed: Disease and Culture in Early Renaissance Europe*. London, New York: Arnold and Oxford University Press, 2002.

Cole, Lucinda. "Of Mice and Moisture: Rats, Witches, Miasma, and Early Modern Theories of Contagion." *Journal for Early Modern Cultural Studies* 10, no. 2 (2010): 65–84.

Coster, Will. "Tokens of Innocence: Infant Baptism, Death and Burial in Early Modern England." In *The Place of the Dead: Death and Remembrance in Late Medieval and Early Modern Europe: Death and Remembrance in Late Medieval and Early Modern Europe*, edited by Peter Marshall and Bruce Gordon, 266–87. Cambridge: Cambridge University Press, 2000.

Cremers, Dietmar. "Totenweiber und Totengräber in einer mittelhessischen Kleinstadt. Zwei Beispiele zum Umgang mit dem Leichnam im 19. Jahrhundert." In *Körper ohne Leben. Begegnung und Umgang mit Toten*, edited by Norbert Stefenelli, 181–88, Vienna: Böhlau, 1997.

Curtis, Daniel R. "Was Plague an Exclusively Urban Phenomenon? Plague Mortality in the Seventeenth-Century Low Countries." *The Journal of Interdisciplinary History* 47, no. 2 (2016): 139–70.

Denk, Claudia and John Ziesemer. *Kunst und Memoria—Der Alte Südliche Friedhof in München*. Berlin, Munich: Deutscher Kunstverlag, 2014.

Diefenbacher, Michael and Antonia Landois, eds. *"Hingeht die Zeit, herkommt der Todt"—500 Jahre Johannis- und Rochusfriedhof 1518–2018*. Neustadt, Aisch: Schmidt, 2018.

Dirmeier, Artur, ed. *Organisierte Barmherzigkeit. Armenpflege und Hospitalwesen in Mittelalter und Früher Neuzeit*. Regensburg: Pustet, 2010.

Dunst, Jenny. *Der Friedhof im Mittelalter—mit Beispielen aus dem Alpen-Adria-Raum*. Klagenfurt: Diplomarbeit, 2012.

Fischer, Norbert, and Markwart Herzog, eds. *Nekropolis: der Friedhof als Ort der Toten und der Lebenden*. Stuttgart: Kohlhammer, 2005.

Fuchs, Konrad. "Hachenburg—ehemalige Residenzstadt im Oberwesterwald." *Lebendiges Rheinland-Pfalz* 8, no. 4 (1971): 106–11.

Glossner, Otto. *Der St.-Johannisfriedhof zu Nürnberg*. Munich and Berlin: Deutscher Kunstverlag, 1991.

Górska, Liliana. "Das frühneuzeitliche Pestpredigeramt." *Barok: Historia—Literatura—Sztuka* 16, no. 1 (2009): 127–47.

Górska, Liliana. *Theatrum atrocissimorum fatorum: Religiöse Pestbewältigung in Danzig 1709*. Tönning: Der Andere Verlag, 2010.

Happe, Barbara. "Die Trennung von Kirche und Grab: Außerstädtische Begräbnisplätze im 16. und 17. Jahrhundert." In *Raum für Tote: Die Geschichte der Friedhöfe von den Gräberstraßen der Römerzeit bis zur anonymen Bestattung*, edited by Reiner Sörries, 62–83. Braunschweig: Thalacker Medien, 2003.

Harding, Vanessa. "Burial of the Plague Dead in Early Modern London." In *Epidemic Disease in London*, edited by J. A. I. Champion, 53–64. London: Centre for Metropolitan History, 1993.

Haugland, Håkon. "'To Help the Deceased Guild Brother to His Grave.' Guilds, Death and Funeral Arrangements in Late Medieval and Early Modern Norway, ca. 1300–1900." In *Cultures of Death and Dying in Medieval and Early Modern Europe*, edited by Mia Korpiola and Anu Lahtinen, 152–83. Helsinki, 2015.

Heinzmann, Josef. *Die Ringackerkapelle. Das barocke Marienheiligtum auf dem ehemaligen Pestfriedhof bei Leuk-Stadt / VS (Schweiz). Ihre Geschichte, ihre Sehenswürdigkeiten*. Visp: Neue Buchdruckerei, 1968.

Henderson, John. "The Invisible Enemy: Fighting the Plague in Early Modern Italy." *Centaurus* 62, no. 2 (2020): 263–74.

Herlihy, David. *The Black Death and the Transformation of the West*, edited by Samuel K. Cohn, Jr. Cambridge: Harvard University Press, 1997.

Illi, Martin. *Wohin die Toten gingen. Begräbnis und Kirchhof im alten Zürich*. Zürich: Chronos Verlag, 2000.

Karant-Nunn, Susan C. *The Reformation of Feeling: Shaping the Religious Emotions*. Oxford: Oxford University Press, 2010.

Koslofsky, Craig. *The Reformation of the Dead. Death and Ritual in Early Modern Germany, 1450–1700*. New York: Saint Martin's Press, 2000.

Laqueur, Thomas W. *The Work of the Dead: A Cultural History of Mortal Remains*. Princeton: Princeton University Press, 2015.

Liedel, Herbert and Helmut Dollhopf. *Der Johannisfriedhof zu Nürnberg*. Würzburg: Stürtz, 1984.

Meyer, Carla. *Die Stadt als Thema. Nürnbergs Entdeckung in Texten um 1500*. Ostfildern: Jan Thorbecke Verlag, 2009.

Mormando, Franco, and Thomas Worcester, eds. *Piety and Plague from Byzantium to the Baroque*. University Park: Pennsylvania State University Press, 2007.

Muchembled, Robert. *Smells: A Cultural History of Odours in Early Modern Times*. Translated by Susan Pickford. Cambridge: Cambridge University Press, 2020.

Murphy, Hannah. *A New Order of Medicine: The Rise of Physicians in Reformation Nuremberg*. Pittsburgh: University of Pittsburgh Press, 2019.

Naphy, William G., and Andrew Spicer. *The Black Death and the History of Plagues 1345–1730*. Stroud: Tempus Publishing, 2000.

Pfeifer, Gabriele. "Auswertung von Taufmatrikeln in München und Passau in der Zeit von 1600 bis 1820—unter besonderer Berücksichtigung der Münchner Findelkinder." PhD thesis. Munich, 2015.

Pilz, Kurt. *St. Johannis und St. Rochus in Nürnberg. Die Kirchhöfe mit den Vorstädten St. Johannis und Gostenhof*. Nuremberg: H. Carl, 1984.

Pope, Ben. "Nuremberg's Noble Servant: Werner von Parsberg (d. 1455) between Town and Nobility in Late Medieval Germany." *German History* 36, no. 2 (2018): 159–80.

Pouget, Benoit. "Quarantine, Cholera, and International Healthspaces: Reflections on 19th-Century European Sanitary Regulations in the Time of SARS-CoV-2." In *Centaurus* 62, no. 2 (2020): 302–10.

Rittgers, Ronald K. "Protestants and Plague: The Case of the 1562/63 Pest in Nürnberg." In *Piety and Plague from Byzantium to the Baroque*, edited by Franco Mormando and Thomas Worcester, 132–55. University Park: Pennsylvania State University Press, 2007.

Rublack, Ulinka. "Fluxes: The Early Modern Body and the Emotions." Translated by Pamela Selwyn. *History Workshop Journal* 53 (2002): 1–16.

Schmauder, Andreas. "Leben in der Isolation: Lepra, Pest und Syphilis." In *Die Macht der Barmherzigkeit. Lebenswelt Spital*, edited by Andreas Schmauder, 120–42. Constance: Universitätsverlag Konstanz, 2000.

Seebaß, Gottfried. "Stadt und Kirche in Nürnberg im Zeitalter der Reformation." In *Stadt und Kirche im 16. Jahrhundert*, edited by Bernd Moeller, 66–86. Gütersloh: Gütersloher Verlagshaus, 1978.

Seifert, Lisa. "Mikroevolution und Geschichte der Pest: Paläogenetische Detektion und Charakterisierung von Yersinia pestis, gewonnen aus historischem Skelettmaterial." PhD thesis. Munich, 2014.

Seiler, Roger. "Pest." In *Historisches Lexikon der Schweiz (HLS)*, version from 27 September 2010. Retrieved 27 June 2021 from https://hls-dhs-dss.ch/de/articles/007980/2010-09-27/.

Sieber, Dominik Gerd. *Der konfessionelle Gottesacker. Katholische und protestantische Sepulkralkultur in den oberschwäbischen Reichsstädten in der Frühen Neuzeit*. Stuttgart: Kohlhammer, 2018.

Slack, Paul. "Responses to Plague in Early Modern Europe: The Implications of Public Health." *Social Research: An International Quarterly* 87, no. 2 (2002): 409–28.

Sörries, Reiner. "Kirchhof oder Coemeterium? Anmerkungen zum mittelalterlichen Friedhof, zu den Sonderfriedhöfen und zur Auslagerung vor die Stadt." In

Nekropolis: der Friedhof als Ort der Toten und der Lebenden, edited by Norbert Fischer and Markwart Herzog, 23–35. Stuttgart: Kohlhammer, 2005.

Sörries, Reiner. "Leprosen- und Pestfriedhöfe und ihre Bedeutung für die nachmittelalterlichen Friedhöfe." In *Raum für Tote: Die Geschichte der Friedhöfe von den Gräberstraßen der Römerzeit bis zur anonymen Bestattung*, edited by Reiner Sörries, 53–62. Braunschweig: Thalacker Medien, 2003.

Sörries, Reiner, ed. *Raum für Tote: Die Geschichte der Friedhöfe von den Gräberstraßen der Römerzeit bis zur anonymen Bestattung*. Braunschweig: Thalacker Medien, 2003.

Sörries, Reiner. *Ruhe sanft: Kulturgeschichte des Friedhofs*. Darmstadt: Wissenschaftliche Buchgesellschaft, 2011.

Sudhoff, Karl. "Pestschriften aus den ersten 150 Jahren nach der Epidemie des 'Schwarzen Todes' 1348. XV. Pesttraktate aus dem östlichen Süddeutschland, Böhmen und Österreich in der 2. Hälfte des 15. Jahrhunderts." *Archiv Für Geschichte Der Medizin* 14, no. 5–6 (1923): 129–68.

Thewes, Guy and Martin Uhrmacher, eds. *Extra muros: Vorstädtische Räume in Spätmittelalter und Früher Neuzeit. Espaces suburbains au bas Moyen Âge et à l'époque moderne*. Cologne: Böhlau, 2019.

Thiessen, Hillard von. "Das Sterbebett als normative Schwelle. Der Mensch in der Frühen Neuzeit zwischen irdischer Normenkonkurrenz und göttlichem Gericht." *Historische Zeitschrift* 295, no. 3 (2012): 625–59.

Wunderli, Richard, and Gerald Broce. "The Final Moment before Death in Early Modern England." *The Sixteenth Century Journal* 20, no. 2 (1989): 259–75.

Zahn, Peter. "Die Epitaphien der alten Nürnberger Friedhöfe: Quellen zur Sozialgeschichte." In *Mitteilungen des Vereins für Geschichte der Stadt Nürnberg* 88 (2001): 203–11.

Zapnik, Jörg. *Pest und Krieg im Ostseeraum. Der Schwarze Tod in Stralsund während des Großen Nordischen Krieges (1700–1721)*. Hamburg: Kovac, 2007.

Pandemics—Theirs and Ours

An Afterword

PETER HESS

Living with plague was a common reality in Germany from 1348 until the early eighteenth century. Yet, historians, theologians, and literary scholars have not contemplated the impact of plague on early modern physical and emotional lives, as well as on related intellectual and epistemological concerns. The historian Lyndal Roper conceded: "I've written a biography of Luther, but until the COVID-19 pandemic I had never thought deeply about the impact of plague on him. I had assumed plague was something early modern people took in their stride, and its history the territory of specialist medical historians." Early modern people appreciated, she continued, "as we have had to learn, that economic exchange, friendships, social life, can suddenly be undone by disease."[1]

Plague was a recurring issue in Central Europe for almost four centuries. The 1490 founding charter of the St. Sebastian plague hospital in Nuremberg noted that plague "commonly occurs approximately every ten to twelve years in this honorable city of Nuremberg."[2] Some outbreaks were massive, others mild; some affected large regions, others spread only locally. The Nuremberg writer Hans Sachs (1494–1576) witnessed nine significant outbreaks of plague in his native city during his lifetime.[3] Being exposed to plague periodically was part of early modern life. Furthermore, older diseases, like cholera, smallpox (devastating the Indigenous populations in the Americas), typhoid, and leprosy, were circulating in early modern Europe as well. In addition, two new diseases appeared and spread through Europe: English sweat beginning in 1485 and the French pox, or syphilis, beginning in 1495.

Giovanni Boccaccio's *The Decameron*, probably written between 1349 and 1352, is the first literary text to describe the traumatic impact of this disease and its effect on human society:

> What made this pestilence all the more virulent was that it was spread by the slightest context between the sick and the healthy just as a fire will catch dry or oily materials when they are placed right beside it. In fact, this evil went further, for not only did it infect those who merely talked or spent any time with the sick, but it also appeared to transfer the disease to anyone who merely touched the clothes of other objects that had been handled or used by those who were its victims.[4]

From the outset, managing and surviving plague became a primary concern, as Boccaccio confirmed: "These things and many others like them, or even worse, caused all sorts of fears and fantasies in those who remained alive, almost all of whom took one utterly cruel precaution, namely, to avoid the sick and their belongings, fleeing far away from them, for in doing so they all thought they could preserve their own health."[5]

From the very beginning, plague was disruptive to human lives and forced people to respond and make choices: how to protect themselves and their families, whether to stay or to leave for a safer place, whether to engage with others or to isolate themselves, and how to deal with family members or neighbors who were infected. It is the plague's impact on the emotional and social lives that we as historians had missed. In Boccaccio's tale, ten young, privileged people decided to flee the city of Florence to sit out the plague in an isolated, posh country estate where they told stories to each other. Martin Luther faced the same dilemma when Elector John of Saxony on 10 August 1527 ordered the evacuation of Wittenberg University to Jena because of plague. While Justus Jonas and Philipp Melanchthon left with their families, Martin Luther and Johannes Bugenhagen refused to comply so that they could minister to the sick and dying.[6] These two examples suffice to illustrate just how invasive plague was in early modern daily life.

This volume was conceived in the darkest moments of the COVID-19 pandemic when most of the world was on lockdown and when we spent most of our time in isolation. While the privileged left cities for their country estates, we engaged in disorienting discussions on whether to lock down, whether to wear masks, how to track the disease, whether to quarantine the infected, and how to bury the dead. While internet technology allowed many to work remotely, some workers were declared "essential," meaning that they could be asked to risk exposure while performing their duties. We were struck by how this inexplicable pandemic completely ruled our lives and by how helpless we felt in the face of this mysterious disease that claimed so many lives. Only in this moment, did the traumatic experience of previous generations with plague and other pandemics become relatable. Our experience with COVID-19 revealed a blind spot, as we had neglected to raise relevant research questions and to integrate the early modern plague experience into our scholarly work.

It was in this moment that the question arose how previous generations experienced pandemics, how they sought to prevent outbreaks, and how they attempted to manage pandemics once they flared up in their communities. We were not primarily interested in medical theories surrounding pandemics, nor in religious explanations for the spread of disease, although the idea of diseases as divine punishments or threats from outside would have been interesting to investigate, as so many of these ideas infused political arguments surrounding COVID-19. However, pointing to similarities between COVID-19 and past pandemics was not a primary objective of this volume. Rather, the aim was to understand pandemics in their specific historicity, that is, in terms of evolving early modern health literacy and within their political, cultural, and religious contexts.

Some of the basic questions were: how did communities react and what forces were set in motion when plague arrived? How did authorities seek to control the spread of epidemic disease and to mitigate its effects? How could individuals protect themselves? What discussions did outbreaks of plague set off? How was information about plague shared within and between communities? What were the policies and measures that were discussed and implemented? What institutions, like health boards or plague hospitals, were created to address plague? What resistance was offered against certain policies? What did non-compliance with public health rules look like, and how could authorities respond?

The rapid rise in printed plague advice literature, peaking in the 1560s, shaped the public discourse surrounding plague. Erik Heinrichs identified a total of 943 vernacular German plague books and pamphlets that were printed between 1473 and 1682.[7] By publishing plague pamphlets, health professionals enhanced their profiles, generated extra income for authors and printers, and often promoted their own cures for plague. In Chapter 1 Christopher Hutchinson examined two 1482 plague treatises by Hans Folz, one in prose and one in verse. Folz, a pioneer of the genre, understood the value of print to promote the circulation of valuable information, while conceding that the uncontrolled spread of printed texts could boost errors or misinformation—just as falsehoods have been an integral part of the current COVID-19 discussion.

Peter Hess added in Chapter 2 that early writers, like Hans Folz, wrote as citizens who expressed their own opinions and focused on actions individuals could take, while in later texts the focus shifted to how authorities could formulate public policy to protect the common good. Generally, the demand for an increased government role in the sixteenth century coincided with the rise of territorial and urban administrations around 1500. It is in this context that governments were establishing regulatory frameworks to manage periodic outbreaks of plague. Inversely, the rise of plague also gave governments cause to advance the role of government in general.

The early responses to the French pox by municipal authorities in Nuremberg and Frankfurt, the focus of Monica O'Brien in Chapter 4, revealed a similar pattern of expanding government authority. The assumed possibility of non-sexual transmission, like by contagious vapors, prompted cities to develop protection mechanisms that were similar to those against plague, including the establishment of pox hospitals. Like measures against plague, those against French pox showed how municipal authorities became increasingly involved in health care and poor relief, but also how they used health crises to assert control over their cities.

Mandates to limit attendance at church services and in funeral processions so as to curb infections, for example, were seen as government overreach by some clerics. During the COVID-19 crisis, church services were widely seen as "superspreader" events, yet many clerics resisted the suspension of in-person services. Plague, just as COVID-19 much later, was also instrumentalized for religious purposes. Erik Heinrichs explored in Chapter 3 how Bavarian physicians and political leaders used plague pamphlets to promote Catholic piety between the Reformation and the middle of the seventeenth century by linking the struggle against sin and heresy with the fight against plague. The chapters by Hutchinson, Hess, and Heinrichs also demonstrated how plague texts, the discussion of public policy, and the pursuit of other political objectives were intertwined.

In Chapter 5 Thomas Wozniak compiled detailed and precise demographic data to track the course of plague in the two separate jurisdictions of Quedlinburg, both governed by the abbess of Quedlinburg Abbey, and compared these records with the political measures taken by the abbess. Due to a high mortality rate, against the pleas of the city council in September 1598, Abbess Anna III ordered a lockdown that turned out to be effective. However, her lockdown faced resistance, particularly because of the ban on markets and because she allegedly did not open up the territory fast enough. Balancing the preservation of life and the maintenance of economic activity was one of the most difficult and controversial issues during plague years, as it was during the COVID-19 pandemic.

Finding this balance was also a concern in Franconia and in Bavaria during the devastating plague outbreak of 1634, as Sigrun Haude argued in Chapter 6. Quarantine measures may have saved lives, but they also created anxieties about the disruption of commerce. Furthermore, enforcement of established rules was difficult, and consequences against violations of restrictions were often difficult to implement, particularly in times of war. Haude points to an increasing attention to recordkeeping and scientific data to help authorities curb the spread of the disease. The ability to collect data and track the disease turned out to be critical during COVID-19 as well; the inability to do so was a key factor why the United States experienced such a high mortality rate, while their experience with tracking other infectious diseases helped many African countries fare much better. As Haude asserted, the ongoing Thirty Years' War gravely complicated efforts to contain plague, as established mechanisms failed in war-torn areas, particularly in Franconia.

Epizootics—epidemic disease among animals—and human epidemics often spread parallel to each other, due to trade and military activities, as Ansgar Schanbacher, Philip Knäble, and Malte de Vries argued in Chapter 9. Their chapter found an interdependence of contagion discourses and measures regarding animals and humans throughout epidemics in the sixteenth and seventeenth centuries. Not surprisingly, there was a high convergence between fighting animal and human diseases. Recipes and prevention measures against such diseases were similar, such as fumigation, separation of individual animals, quarantine for sick animals, and the prohibition on trading contaminated animal products.

With the rise of absolutism, territorial states were able to develop firm but flexible responses to plague and thus to further expand government authority. In Chapter 7 Ulf Wendler traced the dynamic response by the Electorate of Hanover to restrain sporadic outbreaks of plague during the plague campaign of 1709–16. In periods of peak infection, authorities gradually implemented quarantine, cordoning off, and isolation measures, resembling how many jurisdictions responded to COVID-19. They protected external borders and established internal checkpoints to repress the circulation of contagion and of undesirable people. In Wendler's analysis, an absolutistic central government had the option to act decisively and consistently to contain disease. Furthermore, the central government could rely on local authorities to comply with their directives in times of serious outbreaks.

Plague became the subject of academic debates as well. In Chapter 8 Benjamin Wallura traced the debates at the University of Helmstedt during the plague years of 1681–83. Based on the analysis of a large number of academic writings, Wallura argued that late seventeenth-century academic discourse and knowledge of plague were much more complex than the discussion in the public domain that drove policy. Threats of plague catalyzed the discussions among scholars and professors from the faculties of philosophy, medicine, law, and theology who discussed what was considered "right" or "wrong" within the frameworks of their disciplines and intellectual traditions, arriving at different and sometimes conflicting conclusions.

During the peak of the COVID-19 pandemic, authorities struggled with a large number of human remains which had to be buried quickly to prevent a further spread of the disease. Martin Christ makes the point in Chapter 10 that early modern authorities faced the same problem during pandemic emergencies. Burial practices had to be modified and elaborate ceremonies curtailed. Standard communications surrounding death between families, magistrates, clergy, and the general public frequently could not take place. In many jurisdictions, plague cemeteries were established outside the city walls to contain contagion, raising objections to extramural burials, particularly from the elites with prestigious burial plots within the city. Christ argues that responses to the management of corpses in early modern towns and villages varied greatly, depending on available burial space in the settlement and on political constellations. In many cities and towns, burial grounds outside the city became permanent cemeteries, like in Nuremberg.

The ten chapters of this volume enhance our scholarly insights into pandemic response mechanisms in early modern Germany and thus add to our understanding of the premodern world. We no longer assume that the experience of plague was "something early modern people took in their stride," in Roper's words. While the value of this volume for early modern scholarship is indisputable, we cannot assume that its results apply directly to our own concerns with pandemics. To be sure, authorities and citizens in early modern Europe dealt with some of the same issues that we dealt with during COVID-19, and sometimes arrived at similar conclusions. Studying and investigating premodern pandemics thus can give us valuable insight, although we cannot count on a linearity of history that would allow us to deduce direct conclusions.

Scientific advances give us tools today that did not exist in the early modern period. The bacterium that causes plague, *Yersinia pestis*, was discovered only in 1894, long after pragmatic measures had all but eradicated the disease. The coronavirus SARS-CoV-2, on the other hand, was identified quickly, and an effective vaccine was developed and administered within a year. Yet, we were utterly unprepared when COVID-19 started to spread at the end of 2019. It was sobering to realize that little of the insight generated during the plague centuries had a lasting effect, exactly because we did not trust the pragmatic insights generated in a pre-scientific age. Even scientific evidence was discarded, and the validity and efficacy of the vaccine were questioned quickly by a vast disinformation campaign.

The early modern experience tells us how much of the response to pandemics was politicized. That was even truer for COVID-19. Five years on, the sobering insight is that we have not even learned the lessons from COVID-19. The world still is litigating the COVID-19 pandemic, its causes, its consequences, and the lockdowns that undoubtedly saved lives but also hindered economic progress and curtailed individual liberties. Pandemic responses have been weakened, particularly in the United States, as have global organizations like the World Health Organization. Sadly, we will be less prepared for the next pandemic as a consequence. Some potential pandemics are looming already, like bird flu, Ebola virus, Marburg virus, and Mpox.[8] The French writer Michel Houellebecq said in May 2020 that after the coronavirus "everything will remain exactly the same, only a bit worse."[9] He may be right.

Peter Hess is Professor Emeritus of German and European Studies at the University of Texas at Austin. From 2009 to 2018 he served as department chair. Recent publications are *Resisting Pluralization and Globalization in German Culture, 1490–1540: Visions of Nation in Decline* (De Gruyter, 2020) and *Violent First Contact in Venezuela: Nikolaus Federmann's Indian History* (Penn State University Press, 2021). He is currently working on a book on Ulrich Schmidel's service as a mercenary in the Río de la Plata region, 1534–54.

Notes

1. Roper, "When Plague Came to Wittenberg."
2. Quoted in Bühl, "Die Pestepidemien," 123.
3. Dross, "'es flohen die reichen leud,'" 306–7.
4. Boccaccio, *The Decameron*, 6.
5. Boccaccio, *The Decameron*, 7.
6. Roper, *Martin Luther*, 307.
7. Heinrichs, *Plague, Print, and the Reformation*, 5–11.
8. Mpox was a name the World Health Organization chose in 2022, replacing the term monkeypox. This was done primarily for political reasons, to de-emphasize the African origin of the virus.
9. France Info, "Coronavirus."

Bibliography

Boccaccio, Giovanni. *The Decameron*, translated and with an introduction by Wayne A. Rebhorn. New York, London: W. W. Norton, 2013.

Bühl, Charlotte. "Die Pestepidemien des ausgehenden Mittelalters und der Frühen Neuzeit in Nürnberg (1483/84 bis 1533/34)." In *Nürnberg und Bern: Zwei Reichsstädte und ihre Landgebiete*, edited by Rudolf Endres, 121–68. Erlangen: Universitätsbund Erlangen-Nürnberg, 1990.

Dross, Fritz. "'es flohen die reichen leud alle auß der stat/ darinnen sturben 10345 Menschen.' Seuchen in der frühneuzeitlichen Stadt." In *Ingolstadt in Bewegung: Grenzgänge am Beginn der Reformation*, edited by Susanne Greiter and Christine Zengerle, 303–24. Göttingen: Optimus Verlag, 2015.

France Info. "Coronavirus: pour Michel Houellebecq, le monde d'après 'sera le même, en un peu pire'." *France Info, Radio France*, 4 May 2020. Retrieved 24 June 2025 from https://www.franceinfo.fr/sante/maladie/coronavirus/coronavirus-pour-michel-houellebecq-le-monde-d-apres-sera-le-meme-en-un-peu-pire_3948117.html.

Heinrichs, Erik A. *Plague, Print, and the Reformation: The German Reform of Healing, 1473–1573*. London, New York: Routledge, 2018.

Roper, Lyndal. *Martin Luther: Renegade and Prophet*. New York: Random House, 2016.

Roper, Lyndal. "When Plague Came to Wittenberg." *London Review of Books, LRB Blog*, 6 July 2020. Retrieved 4 March 2021 from https://www.lrb.co.uk/blog/2020/july/when-plague-came-to-wittenberg.

INDEX

www.ingramcontent.com/pod-product-compliance
Ingram Content Group UK Ltd.
Pitfield, Milton Keynes, MK11 3LW, UK
UKHW021836100926
8556IPUK00004B/375

9 781836 95425